First Aid, CPR, and AED Advanced

Sixth Edition

Alton L. Thygerson, EdD, FAWM
Medical Writer

Steven M. Thygerson, PhD, MSPH, CIH
Medical Writer

Benjamin Gulli, MD, FAAOS
Medical Editor

Gina Piazza, DO, FACEP
Medical Editor

American College of
Emergency Physicians®
ADVANCING EMERGENCY CARE

JONES & BARTLETT
LEARNING

AMERICAN ACADEMY OF ORTHOPAEDIC SURGEONS

World Headquarters
Jones & Bartlett Learning
40 Tall Pine Drive
Sudbury, MA 01776
978-443-5000
info@jblearning.com
www.jblearning.com

Jones & Bartlett Learning Canada
6339 Ormindale Way
Mississauga, Ontario L5V 1J2
Canada

Jones & Bartlett Learning International
Barb House, Barb Mews
London W6 7PA
United Kingdom

Substantial discounts on bulk quantities of Jones & Bartlett Learning publications are available to corporations, professional associations, and other qualified organizations. For details and specific discount information, contact the special sales department at Jones & Bartlett Learning via the above contact information or send an email to specialsales@jblearning.com.

Jones & Bartlett Learning books and products are available through most bookstores and online booksellers. To contact Jones & Bartlett Learning directly, call 800-832-0034, fax 978-443-8000, or visit our website, www.jblearning.com.

Production Credits
Chairman, Board of Directors: Clayton Jones
Chief Executive Officer: Ty Field
President: James Homer
Sr. V.P., Chief Operating Officer: Don W. Jones, Jr.
V.P., Design and Production: Anne Spencer
V.P., Manufacturing and Inventory Control: Therese Connell
V.P., Sales, Public Safety Group: Matthew Maniscalco
Executive Publisher: Kimberly Brophy
Executive Vice President: Lawrence D. Newell
Executive Acquisitions Editor—EMS: Christine Emerton
Director of Sales, Public Safety Group: Patricia Einstein

Associate Managing Editor: Amanda Brandt
Associate Production Editor: Lisa Cerrone
Marketing Manager: Brian Rooney
Composition: Shepherd, Inc.
Cover Design: Kristin E. Parker
Photo Research and Permissions Supervisor: Christine Myaskovsky
Associate Photo Researcher: Jessica Elias
Cover Image: © Tony West/Alamy Images
Printing and Binding: Courier Kendallville
Cover Printing: Courier Kendallville

Copyright © 2012 by Jones & Bartlett Learning, LLC

The first aid, CPR, and AED procedures and protocols in this book are based on the most current recommendations of responsible medical sources. The American Academy of Orthopaedic Surgeons and the publisher, however, make no guarantee as to, and assume no responsibility for, the correctness, sufficiency, or completeness of such information or recommendations. Other or additional safety measures may be required under particular circumstances.

Reviewed by the American College of Emergency Physicians. The American College of Emergency Physicians (ACEP) makes every effort to ensure that its reviewers are knowledgeable content experts. Readers are nevertheless advised that the statements and opinions expressed in this publication are provided as recommendations at the time of publication and should not be construed as official College policy. ACEP is not responsible for, and expressly disclaims all liability for, damages of any kind arising out of use, reference to, reliance on, or performance of such information. The materials contained herein are not intended to establish policy, procedure, or a standard of care. To contact ACEP, write to: PO Box 619911, Dallas, TX 75261-9911; call toll-free 800-798-1822, or 972-550-0911.

Additional illustrations and photographic credits appear on page 470, which constitutes a continuation of the copyright page.

To order this product, use ISBN: 978-1-4496-3505-3

Library of Congress Cataloging-in-Publication Data Not Available at Time of Printing
ISBN: 978-1-4496-0946-7

6048
Printed in the United States of America
15 14 13 12 11   10 9 8 7 6 5 4 3 2

brief contents

contents

EMERGENCY CARE & SAFETY INSTITUTE

Welcome to the Emergency Care & Safety Institute

Welcome to the Emergency Care & Safety Institute (ECSI), brought to you by the American Academy of Orthopaedic Surgeons (AAOS) and the American College of Emergency Physicians (ACEP).

ECSI is an internationally renowned organization that provides training and certifications that meet job-related requirements as defined by regulatory authorities such as OSHA, The Joint Commission, and state offices of EMS, Education, Transportation, and Health. Our courses are delivered throughout a range of industries and markets worldwide, including colleges and universities, business and industry, government, public safety agencies, hospitals, private training companies, and secondary school systems.

ECSI programs are offered in association with the AAOS and ACEP. AAOS, the world's largest medical organization of musculoskeletal specialists, is known as the original name in EMS publishing with the first EMS textbook ever in 1971, and ACEP is widely recognized as the leading name in all of emergency medicine.

About the AAOS

The AAOS provides education and practice management services for orthopaedic surgeons and allied health professionals. The AAOS also serves as an advocate for improved patient care and informs the public about the science of orthopaedics. Founded in 1933, the not-for-profit AAOS has grown from a small organization serving less than 500 members to the world's largest medical organization of musculoskeletal specialists. The AAOS now serves about 36,000 members internationally.

About ACEP

ACEP was founded in 1968 and is the world's oldest and largest emergency medicine specialty organization. Today it represents more than 28,000 members and is the emergency medicine specialty society recognized as the acknowledged leader in emergency medicine.

ECSI Course Catalog

Individuals seeking training from ECSI can choose from among various traditional classroom-based courses or alternative online courses such as:

- Advanced Cardiac Life Support
- Automated External Defibrillation (AED)
- Bloodborne and Airborne Pathogens
- Babysitter Safety
- Driver Safety
- CPR (Layperson and Health Care Provider Levels)
- Emergency Medical Responder
- First Aid (Multiple Courses Available)
- Oxygen Administration, and more!

ECSI offers a wide range of student manuals, instructor support materials, and interactive technology, including online courses. ECSI student manuals are the center of an integrated teaching and learning system that offers resources to better support instructors and train students. The instructor supplements provide practical hands-on, time-saving tools like PowerPoint presentations, DVDs, and web-based administrative tools. Technology resources provide interactive exercises and simulations to help students become prepared for any emergency.

Documents attesting to ECSI's recognitions of satisfactory course completion will be issued to those who successfully meet the course requirements. Written acknowledgement of a participant's successful course completion is provided in the form of a Course Completion Card, issued by the Emergency Care & Safety Institute.

Visit www.ECSInstitute.org today!

This concise student manual is designed to give laypersons the education and confidence they need to effectively provide emergency care. Features that reinforce and expand on essential information include:

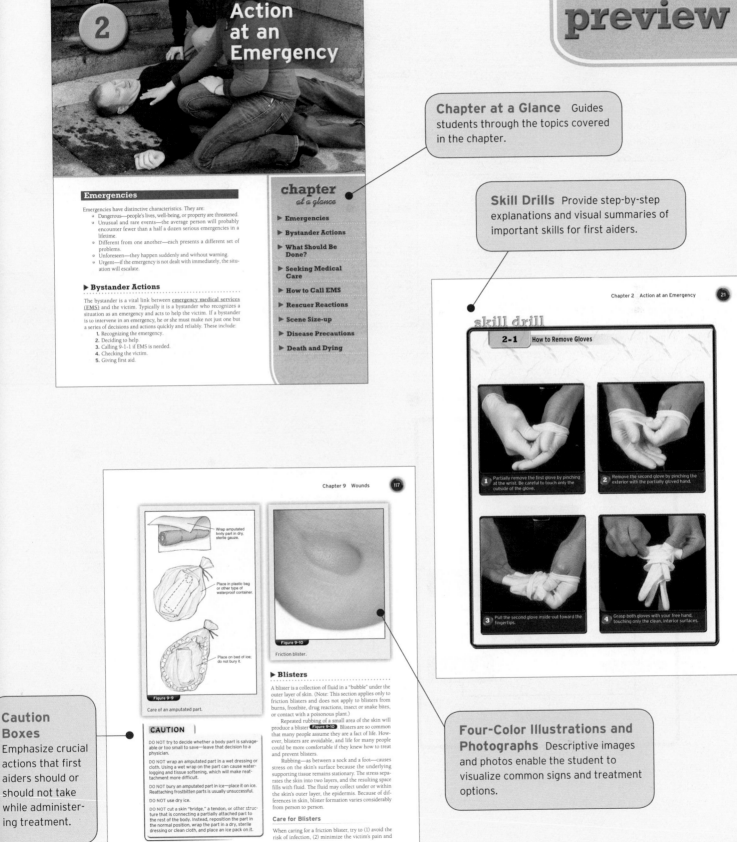

Chapter at a Glance Guides students through the topics covered in the chapter.

Skill Drills Provide step-by-step explanations and visual summaries of important skills for first aiders.

Caution Boxes Emphasize crucial actions that first aiders should or should not take while administering treatment.

Four-Color Illustrations and Photographs Descriptive images and photos enable the student to visualize common signs and treatment options.

From the chapter opener image (Chapter 2)

Action at an Emergency

Emergencies

Emergencies have distinctive characteristics. They are:
- Dangerous—people's lives, well-being, or property are threatened.
- Unusual and rare events—the average person will probably encounter fewer than a half dozen serious emergencies in a lifetime.
- Different from one another—each presents a different set of problems.
- Unforeseen—they happen suddenly and without warning.
- Urgent—if the emergency is not dealt with immediately, the situation will escalate.

▶ Bystander Actions

The bystander is a vital link between emergency medical services (EMS) and the victim. Typically it is a bystander who recognizes a situation as an emergency and acts to help the victim. If a bystander is to intervene in an emergency, he or she must make not just one but a series of decisions and actions quickly and reliably. These include:
1. Recognizing the emergency.
2. Deciding to help.
3. Calling 9-1-1 if EMS is needed.
4. Checking the victim.
5. Giving first aid.

chapter *at a glance*

- ▶ Emergencies
- ▶ Bystander Actions
- ▶ What Should Be Done?
- ▶ Seeking Medical Care
- ▶ How to Call EMS
- ▶ Rescuer Reactions
- ▶ Scene Size-up
- ▶ Disease Precautions
- ▶ Death and Dying

From the Skill Drill (Chapter 2, page 21)

Chapter 2 Action at an Emergency 21

skill drill

2-1 How to Remove Gloves

1. Partially remove the first glove by pinching at the wrist. Be careful to touch only the outside of the glove.

2. Remove the second glove by pinching the exterior with the partially gloved hand.

3. Pull the second glove inside-out toward the fingertips.

4. Grasp both gloves with your free hand, touching only the clean, interior surfaces.

From the Wounds chapter (Chapter 9, page 117)

Chapter 9 Wounds 117

Wrap amputated body part in dry, sterile gauze.

Place in plastic bag or other type of waterproof container.

Place on bed of ice; do not bury it.

Figure 9-9
Care of an amputated part.

CAUTION

DO NOT try to decide whether a body part is salvageable or too small to save—leave that decision to a physician.

DO NOT wrap an amputated part in a wet dressing or cloth. Using a wet wrap on the part can cause waterlogging and tissue softening, which will make reattachment more difficult.

DO NOT bury an amputated part in ice—place it on ice. Reattaching frostbitten parts is usually unsuccessful.

DO NOT use dry ice.

DO NOT cut a skin "bridge," a tendon, or other structure that is connecting a partially attached part to the rest of the body. Instead, reposition the part in the normal position, wrap the part in a dry, sterile dressing or clean cloth, and place an ice pack on it.

Figure 9-10
Friction blister.

▶ Blisters

A blister is a collection of fluid in a "bubble" under the outer layer of skin. (Note: This section applies only to friction blisters and does not apply to blisters from burns, frostbite, drug reactions, insect or snake bites, or contact with a poisonous plant.)

Repeated rubbing of a small area of the skin will produce a blister **Figure 9-10**. Blisters are so common that many people assume they are a fact of life. However, blisters are avoidable, and life for many people could be more comfortable if they knew how to treat and prevent blisters.

Rubbing—as between a sock and a foot—causes stress on the skin's surface because the underlying supporting tissue remains stationary. The stress separates the skin into two layers, and the resulting space fills with fluid. The fluid may collect under or within the skin's outer layer, the epidermis. Because of differences in skin, blister formation varies considerably from person to person.

Care for Blisters

When caring for a friction blister, try to (1) avoid the risk of infection, (2) minimize the victim's pain and

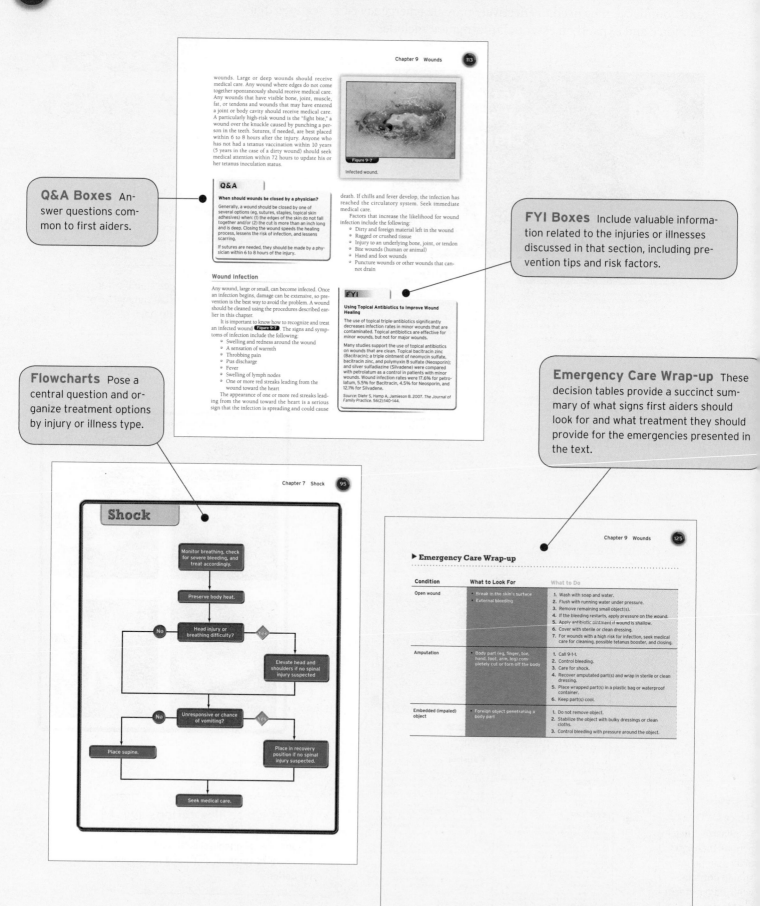

Q&A Boxes Answer questions common to first aiders.

FYI Boxes Include valuable information related to the injuries or illnesses discussed in that section, including prevention tips and risk factors.

Flowcharts Pose a central question and organize treatment options by injury or illness type.

Emergency Care Wrap-up These decision tables provide a succinct summary of what signs first aiders should look for and what treatment they should provide for the emergencies presented in the text.

Prep Kit End-of-chapter activities reinforce important concepts and improve students' comprehension.

Assessment in Action Brief case study followed by critical thinking questions that allow students to apply what they've learned.

Check Your Knowledge Questions quiz students on the chapter's core concepts.

Key Terms List of the key terms and definitions from the chapter.

142

prep kit

▶ Ready for Review

- A dressing covers an open wound; it touches the wound.
- Dressings used in most first aid situations are commercially prepared, but dressings may need to be improvised.
- A bandage should be clean but need not be sterile.
- The basic types of bandages are roller bandages; self-adhering, conforming bandages; gauze rollers; elastic roller bandages; triangular bandages; adhesive tape; and adhesive strips.
- With a little ingenuity, you can apply a roller bandage to almost any body part.

▶ Vital Vocabulary

adhesive strips A combination of both a sterile dressing and a bandage.

adhesive tape Come in rolls and in a variety of widths.

elastic roller bandages Used for compression on sprains, strains, and contusions and come in various widths.

gauze pads Used for small wounds, sterile, and available in separately wrapped packages of various sizes. Some have a special coating to keep them from sticking to the wound.

gauze rollers Cotton and nonelastic that come in various widths.

roller bandages Come in various widths, lengths, and types of material.

self-adhering, conforming bandages Come as rolls of slightly elastic, gauzelike material in various widths.

trauma dressings Made of large, thick, absorbent, sterile materials.

triangular bandages Available commercially or can be made from a 36" to 40" square of preshrunk cotton muslin material.

▶ Assessment in Action

You are enjoying a fly-fishing trip along a popular trout fishing river. It is a Saturday and there are several others fishing the same area. You and your friend decide to descend a steep riverbank to access a less crowded spot. Your friend slips down the river bank. You hurry down the bank and find her clutching her arm, which is bleeding. Another bystander arrives with a first aid kit.

Directions: Circle Yes if you agree with the statement; circle No if you disagree.

Yes No 1. You should wash your hands with sanitizer and apply exam gloves from the first aid kit.

Yes No 2. A dressing goes directly on the wound.

Yes No 3. You can apply a roller bandage on the arm using spiral turns.

Yes No 4. You should start bandaging from the upper part of the arm and progress down to the wrist.

Yes No 5. After applying the bandage, you see that your friend's fingers are blue. This is a sign that the bandage is too tight.

▶ Check Your Knowledge

Directions: Circle Yes if you agree with the statement; circle No if you disagree.

Yes No 1. A dressing does not touch an open wound.

Yes No 2. Adhesive strips are used for small cuts and abrasions.

Yes No 3. A bandage should be clean but need not be sterile.

Yes No 4. Roller bandages come in only one size.

Yes No 5. Roller bandages can be used only on the arm.

Yes No 6. A square knot is the preferred knot for bandages.

Yes No 7. Check the victim's lips for signs of a too-tight bandage.

Yes No 8. If the victim can wiggle his or her fingers, the bandage is not on correctly.

Yes No 9. Elastic roller bandages are used for compression on sprains, strains, and contusions.

Yes No 10. The figure-eight method is used to apply a roller bandage to hold dressings or to provide compression at or near a joint.

Acknowledgments

Jones & Bartlett Learning would like to thank the following individuals for their review of the manuscript and topics presented.

Les Chatelain
Center for Emergency Programs
Health Promotion & Education Department
University of Utah
Salt Lake City, Utah

Francine M. Oran, MA, BS, RMA, LRT, PBT (ASCP)
Southeast Community College
Lincoln, Nebraska

Stuart Rosenhaus
City University of New York—Brooklyn College
Brooklyn, New York

Leland Yarger, MS ED
Ball State University
Muncie, Indiana

Background Information

1

▶ Why Is First Aid Important?

A large truck swings around a corner, crashes into an automobile, and pushes it over an embankment. Bystanders rush to the rescue. They remove the driver of the car from the vehicle, lift the injured man to his feet, stop a passing car, and send the injured driver to a nearby hospital in a sitting position. Because of the lack of knowledge and unskilled handling, the man's spinal cord is injured by the sharp edge of a broken vertebra, and he will remain paralyzed for the rest of his life. This tragic outcome could have been avoided if someone had known what to do in an emergency.

A backcountry hiker is bitten by a rattlesnake. Her frantic companion "cuts and sucks" the bitten area, not realizing that this is an obsolete and harmful procedure. A trained first aider would have known the proper procedures for taking care of the victim.

An unresponsive swimmer is pulled from the water. No one helps because no one knows cardiopulmonary resuscitation (CPR). The emergency medical service (EMS) ambulance arrives too late to revive the swimmer. CPR would have served as an interim action and preserved life for the few minutes needed until the ambulance arrived.

Late at night, a man who had earlier smashed a finger in a car door can no longer stand the excruciating pain caused by the pressure of blood accumulating underneath the fingernail. He drives himself to a hospital emergency department where a blood clot is relieved. He later receives a bill for more than $100. If he had known the proper first aid procedure, he could have relieved the pain sooner and saved money.

These cases clearly point out the need for first aid training. *It is better to know it and not need it than to need it and not know it.* Everyone should be able to perform first aid, because most people will eventually find themselves in a situation requiring it for another person or for themselves. First aiders do not diagnose (this is what medical doctors do), but they can suspect what the problem is and then give first aid.

▶ Who Needs First Aid?

Although heart disease and cancer continue to be critical health problems in the United States, injuries—both unintentional and intentional—constitute a major threat to public health. This threat has been called the neglected epidemic. shows the role of injury as a cause of death by age group and ranking compared with other causes of death.

Death statistics do not always reflect the extent or severity of the injury problem. Most people who are injured do not die of their injuries. The scope of injuries can best be appreciated if thought of as a pyramid. Deaths from injuries and hospital discharges, traditionally where the most available data have been, are only

Table 1-1 Leading Causes of Death

					Age Groups						
Rank	<1	1-4	5-9	10-14	15-24	25-34	35-44	45-54	55-64	65+	Total
1	Congenital Anomalies 5,785	Unintentional Injury 1,588	Unintentional Injury 965	Unintentional Injury 1,229	Unintentional Injury 15,897	Unintentional Injury 14,977	Unintentional Injury 16,931	Malignant Neoplasms 50,167	Malignant Neoplasms 103,171	Heart Disease 496,095	Heart Disease 616,067
2	Short Gestation 4,857	Congenital Anomalies 546	Malignant Neoplasms 480	Malignant Neoplasms 479	Homicide 5,551	Suicide 5,278	Malignant Neoplasms 13,288	Heart Disease 37,434	Heart Disease 65,527	Malignant Neoplasms 389,730	Malignant Neoplasms 562,875
3	SIDS 2,453	Homicide 398	Congenital Anomalies 196	Homicide 213	Suicide 4,140	Homicide 4,758	Heart Disease 11,839	Unintentional Injury 20,315	Chronic Low. Respiratory Disease 12,777	Cerebro-vascular 115,961	Cerebro-vascular 135,952
4	Maternal Pregnancy Comp. 1,769	Malignant Neoplasms 364	Homicide 133	Suicide 180	Malignant Neoplasms 1,653	Malignant Neoplasms 3,463	Suicide 6,722	Liver Disease 8,212	Unintentional Injury 12,193	Chronic Low. Respiratory Disease 109,562	Chronic Low. Respiratory Disease 127,924
5	Unintentional Injury 1,285	Heart Disease 173	Heart Disease 110	Congenital Anomalies 178	Heart Disease 1,084	Heart Disease 3,223	HIV 3,572	Suicide 7,778	Diabetes Mellitus 11,304	Alzheimer's Disease 73,797	Unintentional Injury 123,706
6	Placenta Cord Membranes 1,135	Influenza & Pneumonia 109	Chronic Low. Respiratory Disease 54	Heart Disease 131	Congenital Anomalies 402	HIV 1,091	Homicide 3,052	Cerebro-vascular 6,385	Cerebro-vascular 10,500	Diabetes Mellitus 51,528	Alzheimer's Disease 74,632
7	Bacterial Sepsis 820	Septicemia 78	Influenza & Pneumonia 48	Chronic Low. Respiratory Disease 64	Cerebro-vascular 195	Diabetes Mellitus 610	Liver Disease 2,570	Diabetes Mellitus 5,753	Liver Disease 8,004	Influenza & Pneumonia 45,941	Diabetes Mellitus 71,382
8	Respiratory Distress 789	Perinatal Period 70	Benign Neoplasms 41	Influenza & Pneumonia 55	Diabetes Mellitus 168	Cerebro-vascular 505	Cerebro-vascular 2,133	HIV 4,156	Suicide 5,069	Nephritis 38,484	Influenza & Pneumonia 52,717
9	Circulatory System Disease 624	Benign Neoplasms 59	Cerebro-vascular 38	Cerebro-vascular 45	Influenza & Pneumonia 163	Congenital Anomalies 417	Diabetes Mellitus 1,984	Chronic Low. Respiratory Disease 4,153	Nephritis 4,440	Unintentional Injury 38,292	Nephritis 46,448
10	Neonatal Hemorrhage 597	Chronic Low. Respiratory Disease 57	Septicemia 36	Benign Neoplasms 43	Three Tied* 160	Liver Disease 384	Septicemia 910	Viral Hepatitis 2,815	Septicemia 4,231	Septicemia 26,362	Septicemia 34,828

*The three causes are: Complicated Pregnancy, HIV, Septicema

Source: National Vital Statistics System, National Center for Health Statistics, CDC.

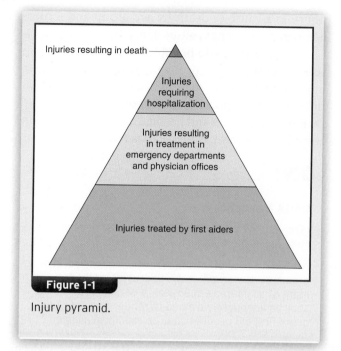

Figure 1-1

Injury pyramid.

Pyramid labels (top to bottom):
- Injuries resulting in death
- Injuries requiring hospitalization
- Injuries resulting in treatment in emergency departments and physician offices
- Injuries treated by first aiders

the tip of the problem. There are a far greater number of injuries seen in emergency departments, clinics, and physician offices. An even greater number of injuries are treated by first aiders. This supports the need for first aid training **Figure 1-1**.

Table 1-2 shows the leading causes of nonfatal, unintentional injury by age group in the United States. Each year, one in four people experiences a nonfatal injury serious enough to need medical care or to restrict activity for at least 1 day. More sports-related nonfatal injuries are treated in hospital emergency departments than any other type of unintentional injury.

A delay of as little as 4 minutes when a person's heart stops can mean death. Therefore, what a bystander does can mean the difference between life and death. Fortunately, most injuries do not require lifesaving efforts. During their entire lifetimes, most people will see only one or two situations involving life-threatening conditions. Most injuries do not

Table 1-2 Ten Leading Causes of Nonfatal Injuries

Rank	<1	1-4	5-9	10-14	15-24	25-34	35-44	45-54	55-64	65+	All Ages
1	Unintentional Fall 125,097	Unintentional Fall 8778,612	Unintentional Fall 639,091	Unintentional Fall 607,365	Unintentional Struck by/ Against 1,031,192	Unintentional Fall 813,125	Unintentional Fall 584,738	Unintentional Fall 913,341	Unintentional Fall 742,735	Unintentional Fall 2,114,113	Unintentional Fall 8,551,037
2	Unintentional Struck by/ Against 37,010	Unintentional Struck by/ Against 371,404	Unintentional Struck by/ Against 399,995	Unintentional Struck by/ Against 583,948	Unintentional Fall 918,574	Unintentional Overexertion 675,349	Unintentional Overexertion 584,738	Unintentional Overexertion 448,656	Unintentional Struck by/ Against 230,874	Unintentional Struck by/ Against 229,304	Unintentional Struck by/ Against 3,278,300
3	Unintentional Other Bite/ Sting 13,092	Unintentional Other Bite/ Sting 134,920	Unintentional Cut/ Pierce 106,907	Unintentional Overexertion 283,813	Unintentional MV-Occupant 743,738	Unintentional Struck by/ Against 654,918	Unintentional Struck by/ Against 529,223	Unintentional Struck by/ Against 424,305	Unintentional Overexertion 213,174	Unintentional Overexertion 178,344	Unintentional Overexertion 3,278,300
4	Unintentional Foreign Body 11,035	Unintentional Foreign Body 123,360	Unintentional Other Bite/ Sting 83,107	Unintentional Cut/ Pierce 135,610	Unintentional Overexertion 735,400	Unintentional MV-Occupant 528,751	Unintentional MV-Occupant 412,047	Unintentional MV-Occupant 350,291	Unintentional MV-Occupant 197,380	Unintentional MV-Occupant 176,571	Unintentional MV-Occupant 2,581,605
5	Unintentional Fire/Burn 9,101	Unintentional Cut/ Pierce 81,571	Unintentional Pedal Cyclist 80,743	Unintentional Pedal Cyclist 108,016	Other Assault Struck By/Against 475,386	Unintentional Cut/Pierce 411,514	Unintentional Cut/ Pierce 320,785	Unintentional Cut/Pierce 289,857	Unintentional Cut/ Pierce 156,046	Inintentional Cut/ Pierce 112,015	Unintentional Cut/ Pierce 2,072,604
6	Unintentional Other Specified 8,271	Unintentional Overexertion 78,018	Unintentional Overexertion 75,796	Unintentional Unknown/ Unspecified 100,842	Unintentional Cut/ Pierce 452,297	Other Assault Struck by/Against 308,662	Unintentional Other Specified 228,808	Unintentional Other Specified 225,469	Unintentional Other Specified 95,934	Unintentional Poisoning 74,623	Other Assault Struck by/Against 1,297,555
7	Unintentional Unknown/ Unspecified 6,722	Unintentional Other Specified 69,043	Unintentional MV-Occupant 57,236	Unintentional MV-Occupant 75,969	Unintentional Other Specified 203,484	Unintentional Other Specified 196,247	Other Assault Struck by/Against 198,019	Unintentional Poisoning 169,088	Unintentional Poisoning 84,040	Unintentional Other Bite/ Sting 73,062	Unintentional Other Specified 1,109,782
8	Unintentional Cut/ Pierce 5,916	Unintentional Fire/Burn 50,708	Unintentional Foreign Body 56,624	Other Assault Struck By/Against 73,372	Unintentional Unknown/ Unspecified 191,276	Unintentional Other Bite/Sting 146,982	Unintentional Poisoning 132,444	Other Assault Struck by/Against 152,308	Unintentional Other Bite/Sing 72,088	Unintentional Unknown/ Unspecified 65,524	Unintentional Other Bite/Sting 993,923
9	Unintentional Inhalation/ Suffocation 4,975	Unintentional Unknown/ Unspecified 45,017	Unintentional Other Transport 45,158	Unintentional Other Transport 57,597	Unintentional Other Bite/Sting 167,310	Unintentional Unknown/ Unspecified 126,719	Unintentional Other Bite/ Sting 128,813	Unintentional Other Bite/Sting 122,059	Other Assault Struck by/Against 46,004	Unintentional Other Transport 60,997	Unintentional Unknown/ Unspecified 806,819
10	Unintentional MV Occupant 4,818	Unintentional Dog Bite 38,214	Unintentional Unknown/ Unspecified 41,967	Unintentional Other Bite/Sting 52,489	Unintentional Other Transport 125,828	Unintentional Poisoning 103,881	Unintentional Unknown/ Unspecified 101,767	Unintentional Unknown/ Unspecified 81,359	Unintentional Unknown/ Unspecified 45,563	Unintentional Other Specified 44,520	Unintentional Poisoning 732,316

Source: Office of Statistics and Programming, National Center for Injury Prevention and Control, CDC.

require lifesaving efforts. Knowing what to do for less severe injuries demands greater attention during first aid instruction.

Each year, the injuries of millions of Americans go unreported. For many of them, the injury causes temporary pain and inconvenience; for others, however, the injury leads to disability, chronic pain, and a profound change in lifestyle. Given the size of the injury and sudden illness problem, everyone should be prepared to deal with an emergency.

Value to Self

Although many people learn first aid to help others, the training primarily helps oneself. It enables a person to give proper immediate care to one's own injuries and sudden illnesses. If victims are too seriously injured to help themselves, they could be able to direct others in proper care. First aid training also helps develop safety awareness. Discussing injuries teaches people how injuries occur and thus promotes injury prevention.

Value to Others

People with first aid training are more likely to give proper assistance to injured family members. Although the main beneficiaries are the trained person and his or her family, the benefits of knowing appropriate first aid techniques extend further, usually to coworkers, acquaintances, and strangers.

Value in Remote Areas

Should an injury or sudden illness require medical care, time, distance, and availability are major considerations. EMS can reach most victims who are severely injured or suddenly ill within 10 to 20 minutes. However, some victims are long distances from medical care. Although most people associate long distances and lack of medical care with wilderness settings involving outdoor recreational activities (for example, hiking, camping, hunting, and snowmobiling), other settings also demand that people be prepared to give first aid for an extended time. The following are some examples:

- Urban areas after a disaster that destroys or overwhelms the EMS
- Remote occupations (for example, farming, ranching, commercial fishing, and forestry)
- Remote communities
- Developing countries

First aid needed in remote locations is similar to that needed in urban settings, but extra skills are sometimes required. See Chapter 24, *Wilderness First Aid*, for information on delivering first aid in remote locations.

▶ What Is First Aid?

First aid is the immediate care given to an injured or suddenly ill person. First aid does not take the place of proper medical care. It consists only of giving temporary help until proper medical care, if needed, is obtained or until the chance for recovery without medical care is ensured. Most injuries and illnesses do not require medical care.

Properly applied, first aid might mean the difference between life and death, between rapid recovery and a long hospitalization, or between a temporary and a permanent disability. First aid involves more than doing things for others; it also includes treatments that people can give themselves.

Recognizing a serious medical emergency and knowing how to get help could be crucial in saving a life. Recognition of an emergency can be delayed because neither the victim nor bystanders know basic symptoms (for example, a heart attack victim might wait hours after the onset of symptoms before seeking help). Moreover, too many people do not know first aid; even if they do, they might panic in an emergency.

▶ First Aid Supplies

The supplies in a first aid kit should be customized to include those items likely to be used on a regular basis **Figure 1-2**. A kit for the home is often different than one for the workplace. A home kit may contain personal medications and a smaller number of items. A workplace kit will need more items (such as bandages) and will not include personal medications. **Table 1-3** lists the basic items that should be stocked in a workplace first aid kit.

Although a first aid kit may have some medications, such as antihistamines and topical ointments, there might be local requirements that restrict the use of these items by first aiders without prior written approval. For example, teachers, activity leaders, and bus drivers in certain areas might not be able to administer these items to children without specific written permission signed by a child's parent or guardian.

Figure 1-2

Sample first aid kit contents.

▶ First Aid and the Law

Legal and ethical issues concern all first aiders. For example, is a first aider required to stop and give care at an automobile crash? Can a child with a broken arm be treated even when the parents cannot be contacted for their consent? These and many other legal and ethical questions confront first aiders.

A first aider can be sued. Do not become overly concerned about being sued—it rarely happens. Ways to minimize the risk of a suit include:

- Obtaining the victim's consent before touching him or her.
- Following this book's guidelines and not exceeding your training level.
- Explaining any first aid you are about to give.
- Once starting to care for a victim, stay with that person. You are legally bound to remain with the victim until care is turned over to an equally or better trained person.

Table 1-3 Sample First Aid Kit

Items	Minimum Quantity
Adhesive strip bandages (1″ × 3″)*	20
Triangular bandages* (muslin, 36″–40″ × 36″–40″ × 52″–56″)	4
Sterile eye pads (2″ × 2″)	2
Sterile gauze pads (4″ × 4″)	6
Sterile gauze pads (3″ × 3″)*	6
Sterile gauze pads (2″ × 2″)*	6
Sterile nonstick pads (3″ × 4″)*	6
Sterile trauma pads (5″ × 9″)*	2
Sterile trauma pads (8″ × 10″)	1
Sterile conforming roller gauze (2″ width)	3 rolls
Sterile conforming roller gauze (4.5″ width)	3 rolls
Waterproof tape (1″ × 5 yards)	1 roll
Porous adhesive tape (2″ × 5 yd)*	1 roll
Elastic roller bandages (4″ and 6″)	1 of each
Antiseptic skin wipes, individually wrapped*	10 packets
Antibiotic ointment, individual packets*	6 packets
Disposable (medical exam) gloves (various sizes)*	2 pairs per size
Mouth-to-barrier device (either a face mask with a one-way valve or a disposable face shield)	1
Disposable instant cold packs	2
Sealable plastic bags (quart size)	2
Padded malleable splint (SAM Splint, 4″ × 36″)	1
Emergency blanket	1
Scissors	1
Tweezers	1
Hand sanitizer (61% ethyl alcohol)	1 bottle
Biohazard waste bag (3.5 gallon capacity)	2
Mini flashlight and batteries	1
List of local emergency telephone numbers	1
First aid guide*	1

*Item meets the ANSI/ISEA Z308.1-2009 minimum standard for the workplace first aid kit. Optional items and sizes may be added based on the potential hazards.

Consent

A first aider must have the victim's **consent** (permission) before giving first aid. Touching another person without his or her consent is unlawful (known as **battery**) and could be grounds for a lawsuit. Likewise, giving first aid without the victim's consent is unlawful.

Expressed Consent

Consent must be obtained from every alert, mentally competent (able to make a rational decision) person of legal age. Tell the victim that you have first aid training and explain what you will be doing. The victim may give permission verbally or with a nod of the head, which would indicate **expressed consent**.

Implied Consent

Implied consent involves an unresponsive victim with a life-threatening condition. It is assumed or implied that an unresponsive victim would consent to lifesaving interventions. An alert victim who does not resist the administrations of a first aider is also assumed to have given implied consent.

Children and Mentally Incompetent Adults

Consent must be obtained from the parent or guardian of a child victim, as legally defined by the state. The same is true for an adult who is mentally incompetent. When life-threatening situations exist and a parent or legal guardian is not available for consent, first aid should be given based on implied consent. Do not withhold first aid from a minor just to obtain consent from a parent or guardian.

Psychiatric emergencies present difficult problems of consent. Under most conditions, a police officer is the only person with the authority to restrain and transport a person against that person's will. A first aider should not intervene unless directed to do so by a police officer or unless it is obvious that the victim is about to do life-threatening harm to himself or herself or to others.

Q&A

How can I avoid a lawsuit resulting from giving first aid?

Before giving first aid, get the victim's consent or permission. Then provide good care, keep within your training level, be nice to the victim, have witnesses, and afterward, write down what you did, names of witnesses, and who took over the victim's care from you.

Refusing Help

Although it seldom happens, a person might refuse assistance for countless reasons, such as religious grounds, avoidance of possible pain, or the desire to be examined by a physician rather than by a first aider. Whatever the reason for refusing medical care, or even if no reason is given, the alert and mentally competent adult can reject help.

Generally, the wisest approach is for you to inform the victim of his or her medical condition, what you propose to do, and why the help is necessary. If the victim understands the consequences and still refuses treatment, there is little else you can do. Call 9-1-1 and, while awaiting arrival:

- Try again to persuade the victim to accept care and encourage others at the scene to persuade the victim. A victim could change his or her mind after a short time.
- Make certain you have witnesses. A victim could refuse consent and then deny having done so.
- Consider calling for law enforcement assistance. In most locations, the police can place a person in protective custody and require him or her to go to a hospital.

Abandonment

Abandonment means leaving a victim after starting to give help without first ensuring that the victim will receive continued care at the same level or higher. Once you have responded to an emergency, you must not leave a victim who needs continuing first aid until another competent and trained person takes responsibility for the victim. This might seem obvious, but there have been cases in which critically ill or injured victims were left unattended and then died. Thus, a first aider must stay with the victim until another equally or better trained person takes over.

Negligence

Negligence means not following the accepted standards of care, resulting in further injury to the victim. Negligence involves:

1. Having a duty to act (required to give first aid)
2. Breaching that duty (either by giving no care or by giving substandard care)
3. Causing injury and damages
4. Exceeding your level of training

Duty to Act

No one is required to give first aid unless a legal **duty to act** exists. For example, you do not have to help a stranger unless you have a legal obligation to that person, or you were involved in the events that led to the victim's injuries, regardless of who was at fault. The decision to help in an emergency is usually an ethical (moral) one. Duty to act could apply in the following situations:

- *When employment requires it.* If your employer designates you as the person responsible for providing first aid to meet Occupational Safety and Health Administration (also known as OSHA) requirements and you are called to an injury scene, you have a duty to act. Examples of occupations that involve a legal obligation to give first aid include law enforcement officers, park rangers, athletic trainers, lifeguards, flight attendants, and fire fighters.
- *When on duty (and sometimes when off duty).* Some states require certain people who are licensed by the state to give emergency care regardless of their on- or off-duty status. In other words, these people are considered to be always on duty. Other states require them to act when on duty but not generally when they are off duty, unless they are in uniform or have other visible insignia and appear to be on duty—in which case these people must respond.
- *When a preexisting responsibility exists.* You might have a preexisting relationship with other persons that makes you responsible for them, which means that you must give first aid should they need it. For example, a parent has a preexisting responsibility for a child, and a driver for a passenger.

Duty to act means following guidelines for standards of care. Standards of care ensure quality care and protection for injured or suddenly ill victims. The elements that make up standards of care include the following:

- *The type of rescuer.* A first aider should provide the level and type of care expected of a reasonable person with the same amount of training and in similar circumstances. Different standards of care apply to physicians, nurses, emergency medical technicians (EMTs), and first aiders.
- *Published guidelines.* Emergency care-related organizations and societies publish rec-

ommended first aid procedures. For example, the American Heart Association publishes guidelines for giving CPR, and the Wilderness Medical Society publishes guidelines for assisting victims who are in remote locations.

Breach of Duty

A **breach of duty** happens when a first aider fails to provide the type of care that would be given by a person having the same or similar training. There are two ways to breach one's duty: acts of omission and acts of commission. An **act of omission** is the failure to do what a reasonably prudent person with the same or similar training would do in the same or similar circumstances. An **act of commission** is doing something that a reasonably prudent person would not do under the same or similar circumstances. Forgetting to put on a dressing is an act of omission; cutting a snake-bite site is an act of commission.

Injury and Damages Inflicted

In addition to physical damage, injury and damage can include physical pain and suffering, mental anguish, medical expenses, and sometimes loss of earnings and earning capacity.

Confidentiality

First aiders might learn confidential information. It is important that you be extremely cautious about revealing information you learn while caring for someone. The law recognizes that people have the right to privacy. Do not discuss what you know with anyone other than those who have a medical need to know. The exception to this is when state laws require the reporting of certain incidents, such as rape, abuse, and gunshot wounds.

Good Samaritan Laws

Starting in the late 1950s, a number of states (beginning with California in 1959) enacted laws designed to protect physicians and other medical personnel from legal actions that might arise from emergency treatment they provided while not in the line of duty. These laws, known as **Good Samaritan laws**, encourage people to assist others in distress by granting them immunity against lawsuits. Although the laws vary from state to state, Good Samaritan immunity generally applies only when the rescuer is (1) acting during an emergency; (2) acting in good faith, which means he or she has

Q&A

What is the rescue doctrine?

The rescue doctrine is an unfamiliar concept to most rescuers and emergency personnel. The rescue doctrine says that a person who is injured while performing a rescue may, unless he or she has acted rashly or recklessly, recover from the person whose negligence created the peril that necessitated the rescue in the first place. In other words, in some cases an injured rescuer has the right to recover for injuries sustained while attempting to assist others who caused the dangerous rescue.

good intentions; (3) acting without compensation; and (4) not guilty of malicious misconduct or gross negligence toward the victim (deviating from rational first aid guidelines).

Although Good Samaritan laws primarily cover health care providers, many states have expanded them to include laypersons serving as first aiders. In fact, some states have several Good Samaritan laws that cover different types of people in various situations. Many legal experts believe Good Samaritan laws have given first aiders a false sense of security. These laws will not protect first aiders who have caused further injury to a victim. Good Samaritan laws are not a protection for poorly given first aid or for exceeding the scope of your training. Fear of lawsuits has made some people hesitant of becoming involved in emergency situations. First aiders, however, are rarely sued.

▶ Injury Prevention

"An ounce of prevention is worth a pound of cure" refers to the fact that it is easier to prevent an injury or illness than it is to treat one. Effective prevention requires a combination of interventions that can be shown as the 3Es: education, enforcement, and engineering.

Educational interventions are the most well known because they are the easiest to implement. Education attempts to change behavior by informing a target group about potential hazards, explaining risks, and persuading people to adopt safer behavior.

Enforcement tries to reduce dangerous behaviors through enforcing laws and regulations. For most laws to be effective, they should have the following elements:

- A perceived high likelihood of apprehension
- Swift penalty delivery
- Penalties that do not always have to be extreme or severe

Engineering makes changes to the environment or product design to protect everyone automatically. This is called a passive or automatic intervention because it requires no work on the part of the individual.

Examples of interventions are listed in Table 1-4.

Haddon Matrix

The Haddon Matrix is a strategy for identifying interventions that can be applied to any type of illness or injury. The three major phases go horizontally left to right and can be viewed as time phases:

- Pre-event phase interventions attempt to stop or hinder an event (eg, drowning) from happening—this involves prevention efforts.
- Event phase attempts to modify the consequences of such events either to prevent or to reduce the severity of an injury (eg, air bag inflating on impact).

Table 1-4 Examples of Interventions

Education/Persuasion	Enforcement/Laws	Engineering/Technology
Swimming lessons	Laws requiring seat belt and helmet use	Air bags in cars
Gun safety course	Prohibition of fireworks	Helmets
DVD showing a safety procedure or message	Laws requiring personal flotation devices (PFDs) be worn when boating	Child-resistant packaging on medications and chemicals
Weather and road condition alerts for drivers	Building codes and inspections	Smoke and carbon monoxide detectors

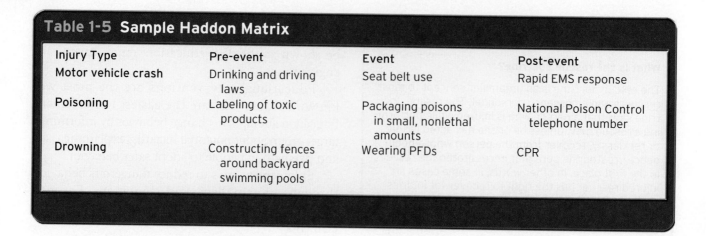

Table 1-5 Sample Haddon Matrix

Injury Type	Pre-event	Event	Post-event
Motor vehicle crash	Drinking and driving laws	Seat belt use	Rapid EMS response
Poisoning	Labeling of toxic products	Packaging poisons in small, nonlethal amounts	National Poison Control telephone number
Drowning	Constructing fences around backyard swimming pools	Wearing PFDs	CPR

- Post-event phase focuses on returning the victim to the fullest of functioning in society after an injury or illness. This phase involves rescue, first aid, medical treatment, and rehabilitation.

Table 1-5 shows examples of interventions related to crashes, poisoning, and drowning.

▶ Ready for Review

- Everyone should be able to perform first aid because most people will eventually find themselves in a situation requiring it for another person or for themselves.
- First aid is the immediate care given to an injured or suddenly ill person. First aid does not take the place of proper medical care.
- The supplies in a first aid kit should be customized to include those items likely to be used on a regular basis.
- Legal and ethical issues concern all first aiders.
- A first aider must have the victim's consent (permission) before giving first aid.
- First aiders might learn confidential information. It is important that you be extremely cautious about revealing information you learn while caring for someone.
- Varying from state to state, Good Samaritan laws encourage people to assist others in distress by granting them immunity against lawsuits.

▶ Vital Vocabulary

abandonment Failure to continue first aid until relieved by someone with the same or a higher level of training.

act of commission Doing something that a reasonably prudent person would not do under the same or similar circumstances.

act of omission Failure to do what a reasonably prudent person with the same or similar training would do in the same or similar circumstances.

battery Touching a person or providing first aid without consent.

breach of duty When a first aider fails to provide the type of care that would be given by a person having the same or similar training.

consent An agreement by a patient or victim to accept treatment offered as explained by medical personnel or first aiders.

duty to act A person's responsibility to provide victim care.

expressed consent Permission for care that a victim gives verbally or with a head nod.

first aid Immediate care given to an injured or suddenly ill person.

Good Samaritan laws Laws that encourage people to voluntarily help an injured or suddenly ill person by minimizing the liability for errors made while rendering emergency care in good faith.

implied consent An assumed consent given by an unconscious adult when emergency lifesaving treatment is required.

negligence Deviation from the accepted standard of care that results in further injury to the victim.

▶ Assessment in Action

Toward the end of the ski season you hear that a ski resort in a neighboring state is almost vacant of skiers, and the resort is offering reduced fees during weekdays. You decide to take advantage of reduced ski fees and take a few days off to go skiing. As you ski down the mountain on a run with trees bordering on both sides, you come across a man lying motionless in the snow near a tree he may have crashed into. No other skiers are in sight and you are alone. As you approach the victim, you see no obvious injuries. You have no first aid supplies. Your first aid certification is still current.

Directions: Circle Yes if you agree with the statement; circle No if you disagree.

Yes   No   **1.** You have to stop to help the man.

Yes   No   **2.** You have implied consent to help this man.

Yes   No   **3.** After tapping on the man's shoulder to see if he is OK, he remains unresponsive but breathing. You can leave and assume that the ski patrol will be coming shortly.

Yes   No   **4.** You decide to help. Before assessing the victim, you roll him over, causing him to slide down the hill and hit a tree. Good Samaritan laws protect you even if you cause further harm to the victim.

prep kit

▶ Check Your Knowledge

Directions: Circle Yes if you agree with the statement; circle No if you disagree.

Yes   No   **1.** Because an ambulance can arrive within minutes in most locations, most people do not need to learn first aid.

Yes   No   **2.** Correct first aid can mean the difference between life and death.

Yes   No   **3.** During your lifetime, you are likely to encounter many life-threatening emergencies.

Yes   No   **4.** All injured victims need medical care.

Yes   No   **5.** Before giving first aid to an alert, competent adult, you must get consent (permission) from the victim.

Yes   No   **6.** If you ask an injured adult if you can help, and she says "No," you can ignore her and proceed to provide care.

Yes   No   **7.** People who are designated as first aiders by their employers must give first aid to injured employees while on the job.

Yes   No   **8.** First aiders who help injured victims are rarely sued.

Yes   No   **9.** Good Samaritan laws provide a degree of protection for first aiders who act in good faith and without compensation.

Yes   No   **10.** You are required to provide first aid to any injured or suddenly ill person you encounter.

2 Action at an Emergency

Emergencies

Emergencies have distinctive characteristics. They are:

- Dangerous—people's lives, well-being, or property are threatened.
- Unusual and rare events—the average person will probably encounter fewer than a half a dozen serious emergencies in a lifetime.
- Different from one another—each presents a different set of problems.
- Unforeseen—they happen suddenly and without warning.
- Urgent—if the emergency is not dealt with immediately, the situation will escalate.

▶ Bystander Actions

The bystander is a vital link between <u>emergency medical services (EMS)</u> and the victim. Typically it is a bystander who recognizes a situation as an emergency and acts to help the victim. If a bystander is to intervene in an emergency, he or she must make not just one but a series of decisions and actions quickly and reliably. These include:

1. Recognizing the emergency.
2. Deciding to help.
3. Calling 9-1-1 if EMS is needed.
4. Checking the victim.
5. Giving first aid.

Compared with health care providers, ordinary bystanders are significantly less likely to offer help in emergencies that occur in public places. Some reasons for this include:

- Lack of knowledge
- Confusion about what is an emergency
- Characteristics of the emergency (for example, unpleasant physical appearance of the victim, the presence of other bystanders)

Lack of Knowledge and Helping Behavior

The average layperson is unaware of many aspects of emergency care and has difficulty recognizing common medical emergencies and deciding to call 9-1-1 for help. Also, a person who does not feel competent to deal with an emergency is not likely to offer even minimal help. The person who does not feel competent can escape this uncomfortable feeling by failing to acknowledge the situation as an emergency. The implication is that bystanders who are uncertain of their ability to deal with a seriously injured victim are more likely to assume that the victim is not seriously injured.

Confusion About What Is an Emergency

Sometimes, laypersons have a great deal of difficulty deciding when an emergency exists **Figure 2-1**. For example, motor vehicle crashes can be easier to recognize as emergencies than heart attacks. This can lead to delays in calling 9-1-1 and to inappropriate decisions, such as transporting victims with life-threatening problems by private vehicles rather than calling 9-1-1.

Figure 2-1

It is not always clear at first glance whether an emergency exists.

Other Factors That Influence Whether a Bystander Helps

In addition to lack of knowledge and confusion, bystanders encounter other barriers that can slow or prevent action in an emergency. Many people are put off by unpleasant physical characteristics such as blood, vomitus, or alcohol on the breath. Reluctance to help might reflect an unwillingness to approach or touch a bloody victim. Public attention on human immunodeficiency virus (HIV) and acquired immunodeficiency syndrome (AIDS) can make this problem more difficult. Another factor involved in helping behavior is the bystander's time of arrival. A bystander who sees the emergency happen is more likely to help than a bystander who arrives after the event.

Quality of Help Provided by Bystanders

First aid and other assistance given by bystanders can be inadequate or potentially dangerous. Failure to keep an open airway and the decision to transport the victim in a private vehicle rather than by EMS are two examples. Many people, trained decades ago or remembering a home remedy, might use outdated and unproven first aid procedures for various injuries or sudden illnesses. A few examples include:

- Putting butter on a burn
- Treating a nosebleed by tilting the head back
- Using hydrogen peroxide to clean a wound
- Sticking an object between the teeth of a seizure victim to prevent the victim from biting his or her tongue
- Giving syrup of ipecac for a swallowed poison

▶ What Should Be Done?

As stated at the beginning of this chapter, victims would benefit if bystanders could quickly and reliably do the following:

1. Recognize the emergency.
2. Decide to help.
3. Call 9-1-1 if EMS is needed.
4. Check the victim.
5. Give first aid.

Recognize the Emergency

To help in an emergency, the bystander first has to notice that something is wrong. Noticing that something is wrong is related to four factors:

- *Severity*. Severe, catastrophic emergencies such as a motor vehicle crash involving an overturned car or several vehicles attract attention.
- *Physical distance*. The closer a bystander is to an emergency situation, the more likely he or she will notice it.
- *Relationship*. Knowing the victim increases the likelihood of noticing an emergency. For example, you would notice your child's injuries before you might notice the same injuries on a stranger.
- *Time exposed*. Evidence indicates that the longer a bystander is aware of the situation, the more likely he or she will notice it as an emergency.

Decide to Help

At some time, everyone will have to decide whether to help another person. Unless the decision to act in an emergency is considered well in advance of an actual emergency, the many obstacles that make it difficult or unpleasant for a bystander to help a stranger are almost certain to impede action. One important strategy that people use to avoid action is to refuse (consciously or unconsciously) to acknowledge the emergency. Many emergencies do not look like the ones portrayed on television, and the uncertainty of the real event can make it easier for the bystander to avoid acknowledging the emergency.

Making a quick decision to get involved at the time of an emergency is more likely to occur if the bystander has previously considered the possibility of helping others. Thus, the most important time to make the decision to help is before you ever encounter an emergency. Deciding to help is an attitude about emergencies and about one's ability to deal with emergencies. It is an attitude that takes time to develop and is affected by a number of factors. Developing such a helping attitude means that you must:

- Appreciate the importance of bystander help to an injured or suddenly ill person.
- Feel confident enough about helping someone who is seriously injured or suddenly ill even if someone else is present.
- Be willing to take the time to help.
- Be able to put the potential risks of helping in perspective.
- Feel comfortable about taking charge at an emergency scene.
- Feel comfortable about seeing or touching a victim who is bleeding or vomiting or who appears dead.

Deciding Not to Help

A bystander could always find excuses for not helping in emergency situations. The following are reasons that people do not aid others:

- *It could be harmful*. Bystanders have lost their lives or been severely injured while attempting to rescue others. The fear of being sued or contracting a disease such as HIV or tuberculosis (TB) can also act as a deterrent. And some would-be rescuers have been attacked by dogs protecting their disabled owners.
- *Helping doesn't matter*. Some bystanders might feel that the victim is getting what he or she deserves. Rewards, if any, are not significant for rescuers, possibly consisting of a newspaper write-up or a small cash prize. Often the rescuer gets nothing more than a hurried, "Thanks," and in some cases, rescuers are never known.
- *Obstacles can prevent helping*. Many bystanders do not know how to help. They cannot swim, do not know how to control bleeding or perform cardiopulmonary resuscitation (CPR), or do not have other necessary rescue and first aid skills. Some would-be rescuers are adversely affected by the sight of blood, vomit, and other unpleasant conditions sometimes found at emergency scenes.
- *No other bystanders are helping*. The likelihood that an individual will help in an emergency decreases as the number of bystanders increases. When bystanders see that others are not taking action, they may conclude that the situation is not serious. The presence of other bystanders may also cause a person to believe that others can help just as well.

Call 9-1-1 if EMS Is Needed

Wrong decisions about calling 9-1-1 can be made. Examples include a delay in calling 9-1-1 until callers are absolutely sure that an emergency exists, or deciding to bypass EMS and to transport the victim to medical care in a private vehicle. Such actions can endanger a victim. Fortunately, most injuries and sudden illnesses do not require medical care—only first aid.

Check the Victim

You must decide whether life-threatening conditions exist and what kind of help a victim needs. See Chapter 4, *Finding Out What's Wrong*, for details.

FYI

Actual Versus Perceived EMS Response Time
Patients' perceptions of ambulance response times are inaccurate. They tend to overestimate response time while underestimating scene time and time to medical care.
Source: Harvey AH, Gerard WC, Rice GF, Finch H. 1999. Actual vs. perceived EMS response time. *Prehosp Emerg Care* 3(1):11-14.

Give First Aid

Often the most critical life support measures are effective only if started immediately by the nearest available person. That person usually will be a layperson—a bystander.

Q&A

Should the family be present during resuscitation?

Controversy exists regarding this question. Studies indicate that most family members want to be present. However, first aiders, emergency medical responders, and emergency medical technicians appear to be more uncomfortable with family present.

▶ Seeking Medical Care

Knowing when to call 9-1-1 for help from EMS is important. To know when to call, you must be able to tell the difference between a minor injury or illness and a life-threatening one. For example, upper abdominal pain can be indigestion, ulcers, or an early sign of a heart attack. Wheezing could be related to a person's asthma, for which the person can use his or her prescribed inhaler for quick relief, or it can be as serious as a severe allergic reaction from a bee sting.

Not every cut needs stitches, nor does every burn require medical care. It is, however, always best to err on the side of caution. According to the American College of Emergency Physicians (ACEP), if the answer to any of the following questions is "yes," or if you are unsure, call 9-1-1 for help.

- Is the victim's condition life threatening?
- Could the condition get worse and become life threatening on the way to the hospital?
- Does the victim need the skills or equipment of EMS?

- Could the distance or traffic conditions cause a delay in getting the victim to the hospital?
- Is a spinal injury suspected?

ACEP also recommends immediate transport to the hospital emergency department, by EMS or by private vehicle, for the following conditions that are warning signs of more serious conditions:

- Chest pain lasting 2 minutes or more
- Uncontrolled bleeding (see the following list of wounds needing immediate medical care)
- Any sudden or severe pain
- Coughing or vomiting blood
- Difficulty breathing, shortness of breath
- Sudden dizziness, weakness, fainting
- Changes in vision
- Difficulty speaking
- Severe or persistent vomiting or diarrhea
- Change in mental status (for example, confusion, difficulty arousing)
- Suicidal or homicidal feelings
- Wounds needing immediate medical care include (see Chapter 9, *Wounds*, for additional wounds needing medical care) those in which:
  - Bleeding from a cut does not slow during the first 15 minutes of steady direct pressure.
  - Signs of shock occur.
  - Breathing is difficult because of a cut to the neck or chest.
  - A deep cut to the abdomen causes moderate to severe pain.
  - There is a cut to the eyeball.
  - A cut amputates or partially amputates an extremity.

When a serious situation occurs, call 9-1-1 *first*. Do *not* call your doctor, the hospital, a friend, relatives, or neighbors for help before you call 9-1-1. Calling anyone else first only wastes time. Calling 9-1-1 has several advantages over driving to the hospital emergency department by private vehicle:

- Many victims should not be moved except by trained personnel.
- The EMS personnel who arrive with the ambulance know what to do. In addition, they are in radio contact with hospital physicians.
- Care provided by EMS personnel at the scene and on the way to the hospital can increase a victim's chances of survival and rate of recovery. The condition could get worse and become life threatening on the way to the hospital.
- An EMS ambulance usually can get a victim to the hospital quicker.

If the situation is not an emergency, call your doctor. However, if you have *any* doubt about whether the situation is an emergency, call 9-1-1. Later chapters identify when to call 9-1-1 for specific problems.

▶ How to Call EMS

In most communities, to receive emergency assistance of any kind, call 9-1-1 **Figure 2-2**. Check to see if this is true in your community. Emergency telephone numbers are usually listed on the inside front cover of telephone directories. Keep these numbers near or on every telephone. Dial 0 (the operator) if you do not know the emergency number. A community 9-1-1 number has some benefits:

- There is only one number to remember.
- Calls are received by specially trained personnel.
- Response time is reduced.

When you call 9-1-1, speak slowly and clearly. Be ready to give the dispatcher the following information:

1. *The victim's location.* Give the address, names of intersecting roads, and other landmarks, if possible. This information is the most important thing you can give. Also, tell the specific location of the victim. (For example, "in the basement" or "in the backyard.")
2. *The phone number you are calling from and your name.* This allows dispatchers to detect false reports, thus minimizing their frequency, and it allows a dispatch center without the enhanced 9-1-1 system to call back if disconnected or for additional information if needed.

3. *What happened.* State the nature of the emergency. (For example, "My husband fell off a ladder and is not moving.")
4. *Number of persons needing help and any special conditions.* (For example, "There was a car crash involving two cars. Three people are trapped.")
5. *Victim's condition.* (For example, "My husband's head is bleeding.") List any first aid you have tried (such as pressing on the site of the bleeding).

Do *not* hang up the phone unless the dispatcher instructs you to do so. Enhanced 9-1-1 systems can track a call, but some communities lack this technology. Also, the EMS dispatcher could tell you how best to care for the victim. If you send someone else to call, have the person report back to you so you can be sure the call was made. Other tips include:

- Teach children what 9-1-1 is for and how and when to call. Refer to "nine-one-one," not "nine-eleven," because children might expect to find an eleven on the dial or on the push buttons.
- Do not hang up without explanation if you call 9-1-1 by mistake, or the dispatcher will have to call back to see if you need help.
- If your area does not have a 9-1-1 system, add EMS, fire, and police numbers to a list by your phones. During an emergency, you might not have the time or presence of mind to find a directory listing.

▶ Rescuer Reactions

The sight of blood and the cries of victims can be upsetting to people attempting to rescue and help an injured person. Seeing a grotesque amputation, being splattered with vomit or blood, or smelling disagreeable odors from urine and feces can be unnerving. More than one rescuer has felt nauseated and weak, vomited, or fainted when helping injured victims. Even the toughest of physicians and emergency medical technicians (EMTs) have difficult moments when exposed to certain situations.

It is essential that first aiders stay alert and working at an injury scene. A first aider who collapses while aiding an injured person detracts attention from the original victim, whose condition is usually more serious. All the knowledge and skills a rescuer has are useless if he or she collapses or has to leave the scene because of weakness or fainting.

Some emergency care providers seem to have ice in their veins. They always appear calm and unaffected by even the worst injuries. These people might seem

Figure 2-2

For help, call 9-1-1 or the local emergency number.

callous, but the proper psychological term is *desensitized*. A specialty within psychology deals with desensitization and suggests ways of overcoming anxieties caused by unpleasant sights and sounds. Desensitization is a deconditioning or a counterconditioning process that can be effective in eliminating fears and anxieties. The idea is to weaken an undesirable response such as fainting by strengthening an incompatible response. When responses are incompatible (calmness versus anxiety), the occurrence of either one prevents the occurrence of the other. By desensitizing, you learn to associate relaxation with situations that elicit anxiety so that eventually you do not experience anxiety. But you first need to learn how to invoke relaxation before gradually exposing yourself to anxiety-producing situations such as the sight of blood.

A simple way to desensitize (calm) yourself while helping another person is to change your thought patterns from the unpleasant to the pleasant by singing a favorite song to yourself (not out loud, of course, for the obvious reason of how you might appear to the victim or observers). You can begin a process of gradual exposure to unpleasant scenes by viewing television programs, DVDs, or pictures of injuries in medical journals. You might eventually consider volunteering at a hospital emergency department where you can see injuries.

In a number of cases, a first aider who fainted had failed to eat breakfast. It is strongly recommended that everyone maintain an adequate blood glucose level through proper eating habits, especially eating breakfast.

Postcare Reactions

After giving first aid for severe injuries, a person might feel an emotional letdown, which is frequently overlooked. A stressful event can be psychologically overwhelming and can result in a condition known as **posttraumatic stress disorder (PTSD)**. Its symptoms include depression and flashbacks of the event.

Discussing your feelings, fears, and reactions within 24 to 72 hours of helping at an emergency helps prevent later emotional problems. You could discuss your feelings with a trusted friend, a mental health professional, or a member of the clergy. Bringing out your feelings quickly can relieve personal anxieties and stress.

▶ Scene Size-up

If you are at the scene of an emergency situation, do a 10-second **scene size-up** **Figure 2-3**, looking for three

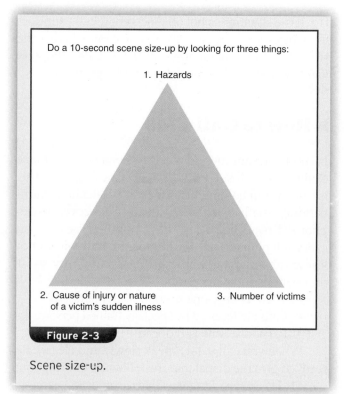

Do a 10-second scene size-up by looking for three things:

1. Hazards

2. Cause of injury or nature of a victim's sudden illness

3. Number of victims

Figure 2-3

Scene size-up.

Figure 2-4

The scene size-up includes evaluating the scene for hazardous conditions.

things: (1) hazards that could be dangerous to you, the victim(s), or bystanders; (2) the cause of the injury or illness; and (3) the number of victims. As you approach an emergency scene, scan the area for immediate dangers to yourself or to the victim **Figure 2-4**. For example, if a car crash is obstructing traffic, you have to consider whether you can safely go to that vehicle to help the victim. Or you might notice that gasoline is dripping from the gas tank and that the battery has shorted out and is sparking. Other conditions include hazardous conditions such as chemical spills, toxic fumes, explosives, gas leaks, or live electric wires. Some locations might have a danger of an avalanche, landslides, fires, flash floods, or attack dogs. If the scene is dangerous, stay away and call 9-1-1. You are not being cowardly, merely realistic. Never attempt a rescue that you have not been specifically trained to do. You cannot help another person if you also become a victim. For details about hazards at an emergency scene, refer to Chapter 26, *Disaster Preparedness*.

The second step is to try to determine the cause of the injury. For example, if the emergency department physician knows that a victim was thrown against a steering wheel, he or she will check for liver, spleen, and cardiac injuries. Be sure to tell EMS personnel about your findings so they can identify the extent of any injuries. Finally, determine how many people are involved. There could be more than one victim, so look around and ask about others involved.

Figure 2-5

Use a waterless handwashing solution if there is no running water available.

Q&A

Should a first aider's headlights be left on at a scene?

Unless your headlights are needed to light up the scene, turn off your headlights when parked at the scene. Your headlights can blind approaching vehicles, making it difficult for the drivers to see rescue personnel walking around the scene.

▶ Disease Precautions

First aiders must understand the risks from infectious diseases, which can range in severity from mild to life threatening. First aiders should know how to reduce the risk of contamination to themselves and to others.

An **infectious disease** is a medical condition caused by the growth and spread of small, harmful organisms within the body. A **communicable disease** is a disease that can spread from one person to another. Immunizations, protective techniques, and handwashing can minimize the risk of infection. Because there are so many different infectious diseases to be concerned about, the Centers for Disease Control and Prevention (CDC) developed a set of **standard precautions**, which advise you to assume that all victims are infected and can spread an organism that poses a risk for transmission of infectious diseases. These protective measures are designed to prevent first aiders from coming into direct contact with infectious agents.

Handwashing

Handwashing is one of the simplest, yet most effective ways to control disease transmission. Even if you are wearing gloves, you should wash your hands before, if possible, and definitely after every victim contact. The longer the germs remain with you, the greater their chance of infecting you.

The proper procedure for washing your hands is as follows:

1. Use soap and warm water, if possible. All types of soap are acceptable when washing with water.
2. Rub your hands together for 15 to 20 seconds to work up a lather. Wash all surfaces well, including wrists, palms, backs of hands, and fingers. Clean the dirt from under your fingernails.
3. Rinse the soap from your hands.
4. Dry your hands completely with a clean towel if possible (this helps remove the germs). If towels are not available, however, it is okay to allow your hands to air dry.

If soap and water are not available, use an alcohol-based hand sanitizer to clean your hands . Apply the gel to one hand and rub hands together, covering all surfaces of hands and fingers, until the hands are dry. If your mucous membranes (for example, your eyes, nose, or mouth) are splashed by a bloody fluid, immediately flush the area with clean water.

Personal Protective Equipment

Personal protective equipment (PPE) includes exam gloves, mouth-to-barrier devices, eye protection, and gowns. PPE provides a barrier between the first aider and infectious diseases.

Q&A

Why is the use of latex gloves a concern?

Natural latex, which is used in latex gloves, contains natural proteins that have been shown to sensitize and cause allergic reactions in some persons over a period of time with repeated use. During the processing and manufacturing of latex gloves, many impurities are left in the gloves and eventually attach to the cornstarch that is placed in the gloves for ease of donning. When the gloves are removed, the natural proteins, which are attached to the cornstarch, are aerosolized into the air and inhaled by everyone nearby. The person who just took off the gloves may further sensitize himself or herself by touching the nose, eyes, or mucous membranes while the powder is still on the hands.

Persons who are sensitive or allergic to latex may experience a wide variety of symptoms, including rash, asthma, severe food allergies, anaphylaxis, and death. There is a large amount of literature available regarding concerns over the use of latex gloves. Alternatives to latex gloves are nitrile, neoprene, and vinyl.

FYI

Do Gloves Really Protect?

A study tested the effectiveness of vinyl and latex gloves as barriers to hand contamination. Gloves were checked according to the American Society for Testing and Materials, and leaks occurred with 43% of vinyl gloves and 9% of latex gloves. The researchers concluded that latex gloves and, to a lesser extent, vinyl gloves provide substantial protection during hand contact with moist body substances, functioning as a barrier even when leaks are present. Because leaks are not always detected by the wearer, handwashing should routinely follow the use of disposable gloves.

Source: Olsen RJ, et al. 1993. Examination gloves as barriers to hand contamination in clinical practice. *JAMA* 270:350-353.

Exam Gloves

Exam gloves are the most common type of PPE and should always be worn when there is any possibility of exposure to blood or body fluids. The Food and Drug Administration (FDA), the CDC, and the Occupational Safety and Health Administration (OSHA) have stated that both vinyl and latex gloves provide adequate protection. Research indicates that latex has fewer micropores (very small holes) and, thus, offers the most protection. However, latex tends to break down faster (within several years) while the gloves are in a first aid kit waiting to be used. Another option is nitrile gloves. All first aid kits should contain several pairs of gloves. Because some rescuers have allergic reactions to latex, latex-free gloves should also be available.

It is important to use the proper technique when removing used gloves so you do not contaminate yourself. When removing used gloves, do not touch their outside surface ▶Skill Drill 2-1◀. The proper method of removing gloves is as follows:

1. Begin by partially removing one glove. With the other gloved hand, pinch the first glove at the wrist—being certain to touch only the outside of the first glove—and start to roll it back off the hand, inside out. Leave the exterior of the fingers on that first gloved hand exposed (**Step** ❶).

2. Use the still-gloved fingers of the first hand to pinch the wrist of the second glove and begin to pull it off, rolling it inside-out toward the fingertips as you did with the first glove (**Step** ❷).

3. Continue pulling the second glove off until you can pull the second hand free (**Step** ❸).

4. With your now-ungloved second hand, grasp the exposed inside of the first glove and pull it free of your first hand and over the now-loose second glove. Be sure that you touch only clean, interior surfaces with your ungloved hand (**Step** ❹).

You might consider putting on a second pair of gloves over the first if there is major, significant external bleeding or body fluid. If the gloves are cut or torn, replace them.

skill drill

2-1   **How to Remove Gloves**

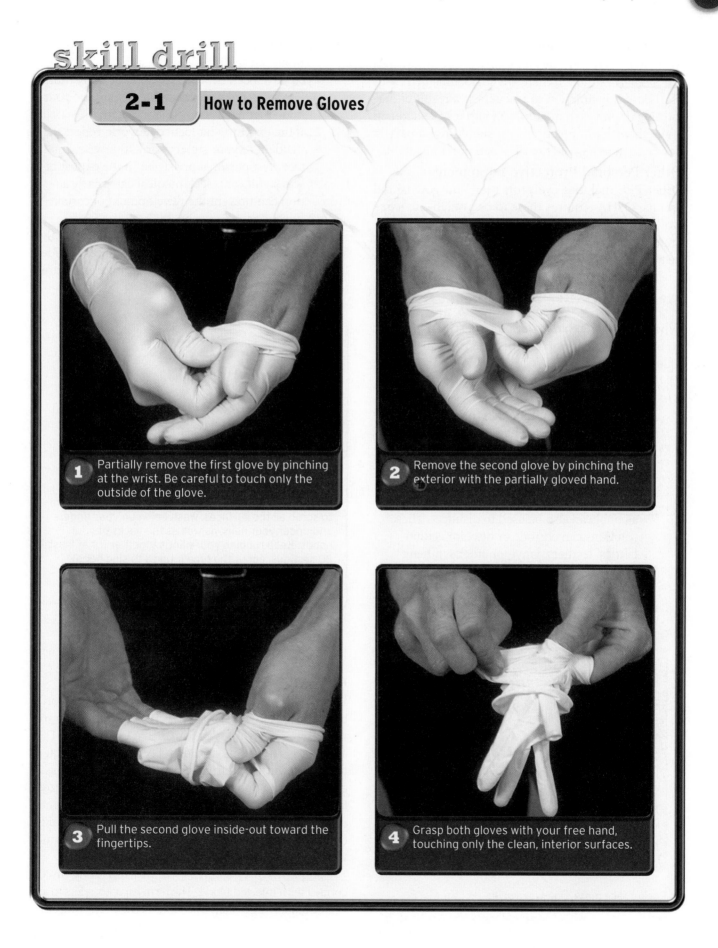

1 Partially remove the first glove by pinching at the wrist. Be careful to touch only the outside of the glove.

2 Remove the second glove by pinching the exterior with the partially gloved hand.

3 Pull the second glove inside-out toward the fingertips.

4 Grasp both gloves with your free hand, touching only the clean, interior surfaces.

Mouth-to-Barrier Devices

Mouth-to-barrier devices are recommended **Figure 2-6**. Although there are no documented cases of disease transmission to rescuers as a result of performing unprotected mouth-to-mouth resuscitation on a victim with an infection, you should use a barrier device such as a pocket mask when providing CPR.

Other Personal Protective Equipment

Other PPE includes eye protection and gowns and aprons. OSHA requires these to be available in some workplaces, especially for health care workers. These are not required for first aiders and usually will not be available.

Cleaning Up After an Emergency

When cleaning up blood or other body fluids, protect yourself and others against disease transmission by following these steps:

1. Wear heavier gloves than lightweight latex or vinyl.
2. If you have been trained in the correct procedures, use absorbent barriers to soak up blood or other infectious materials.
3. Clean the spill area using soap and water. After cleaning, disinfect with a bleach and water solution at a 1:10 dilution. Isopropyl alcohol can also be used to disinfect. These solutions can corrode or discolor certain fabrics, leathers, vinyl, or other synthetic materials.

Figure 2-6

Pocket face mask, one-way valve.

4. Discard contaminated materials in an appropriate waste disposal container.

If you have been exposed to blood or body fluids:

1. Use soap and water to wash the parts of your body that have been contaminated.
2. If the exposure happened at work, report the incident to your supervisor. Otherwise, contact your personal physician. If the exposure was significant, seek medical care. Early action can prevent the development of certain infections.

The best protection against disease is using the safeguards described here. By following these guidelines, first aiders can decrease their chances of contracting bloodborne illnesses.

FYI

Handwashing

After you touch something that might be contaminated, you need to wash your hands as soon as possible. Wearing gloves does not excuse you from the need to wash your hands.

Wash your hands with clean, warm, running water. Apply soap and rub your hands together to make a substantial lather. The soap you use does not have to be antibacterial; regular soap is sufficient. Be sure to scrub all the surfaces; wash between your fingers and under your nails, as well as the backs of your hands. Keep rubbing your hands together for at least 20 seconds, about the time it takes to sing happy birthday to yourself. Thoroughly rinse your hands and dry them with a paper towel.

Some Diseases of Special Concern

Bloodborne Diseases

Some diseases are carried by an infected person's blood (**bloodborne diseases**). **HIV (human immunodeficiency virus)** is the virus that can cause AIDS. The virus is transmitted by direct contact with infected blood, semen, or vaginal secretions; there is no scientific documentation that the virus is transmitted by contact with sweat, saliva, tears, sputum, urine, feces, vomitus, or nasal secretions, unless these fluids contain visible signs of blood. There is currently no vaccine available to prevent HIV infection.

Hepatitis B virus (HBV) is also spread by direct contact with infected blood. The term *hepatitis* refers to an inflammation (and often infection) of the liver. A vaccine

On-the-Job Protection

People infected with HBV or HIV might not show symptoms and might not even know they are infected. For that reason, all human blood and body fluids should be considered potentially infectious, and precautions should be taken to avoid contact. Standard precautions recommend you assume that *all* body fluids are a possible risk. EMS personnel routinely follow standard precautions, even if blood or body fluids are not visible.

OSHA requires any company with employees who are expected to give first aid in an emergency to follow standard precautions. OSHA applies the "Good Samaritan" definition to an employee who assists another with a nosebleed or a cut. Such acts, however, are not considered occupational exposure unless the employee who provides the assistance is a member of a first aid team or is designated or expected to provide first aid as part of his or her job. In essence, OSHA's requirement excludes unassigned employees who perform unanticipated first aid.

Whenever there is a chance that you could be exposed to bloodborne pathogens, your employer must provide appropriate PPE, which might include eye protection, gloves, gowns, and masks. The PPE must be accessible, and your employer must provide training to help you choose the right PPE for your work.

EMS personnel follow standard precautions, and OSHA requires designated work-site first aiders to follow standard precautions—but what procedures should a typical first aider follow? It makes sense for first aiders to follow standard precautions and assume that *all* blood and body fluids are infectious and follow appropriate protective measures.

Emergency Medical Service

If you or someone you know is ever sick or injured and needs emergency help, remember, there are lots of people who are specially trained to help you!

Emergency medical technicians: Emergency medical technicians, sometimes called EMTs, have different amounts of training, depending on their jobs. Sometimes EMTs are dispatchers who answer calls for help and send ambulances and rescue vehicles to the scene of the emergency. Other EMTs drive the ambulance, assist with rescues, and perform basic emergency medical care. An EMT course requires about 150 hours of training.

Paramedics: Paramedics are EMTs with the highest level of training. They are able to perform many medical procedures at the scene of the emergency or in the ambulance on the way to the hospital. Using a radio to communicate, paramedics often get instructions from a doctor at the emergency room or at the base station (the paramedic's headquarters).

Emergency nurses: If you were a patient in the emergency department, an emergency nurse would probably be the first person you'd see. One of the nurse's jobs is to ask you questions about your problem and help decide when you can see the doctor. Emergency nurses are specially trained to help treat emergency patients.

Emergency physicians: Emergency physicians are doctors who are specially trained to take care of a certain type of patient: emergency patients. Doctors who are specially trained are often called specialists. Emergency physicians specialize in helping people who are injured or who become sick very suddenly, such as someone who is having a heart attack or has a very high fever.

Emergency medical responders: Police officers and fire fighters are some of the other people who might help you, especially if you have to be rescued.

Source: American College of Emergency Physicians.

is available for HBV and is recommended for all infants and for adults who might have contact with carriers of the disease or with blood. <u>Hepatitis C virus (HCV)</u> can cause liver disease or cancer. It cannot be cured, and there is no vaccine.

Airborne Diseases

<u>Airborne diseases</u> are transmitted through the air by coughing or sneezing. <u>Tuberculosis</u>, a chronic bacterial disease that usually affects the lungs, is becoming a common problem and is hard to distinguish from other diseases. Victims who present the highest risk often have a cough. Tuberculosis is more common in people who have lived in a homeless shelter, or in a developing country. <u>SARS (severe acute respiratory syndrome)</u> is a potentially life-threatening viral infection. It is thought to be transmitted by close person-to-person contact. If a surgical mask is available, wear it or wrap a handkerchief over your nose and mouth.

▶ Death and Dying

There are few incidents that involve more emotional stress than the life-and-death situations that you might face. Seeing death and dying are the unfortunate parts of providing emergency care.

The Dying Victim

A dying person presents a difficult situation. To assist such a victim:

- Avoid negative statements about the victim's condition. Even an unresponsive person can hear what is being said.
- Assure the victim that you will locate and inform his or her family of what has happened. Attempt to have family members present—they can provide great comfort to the victim.
- Allow some hope. Don't tell the victim that he or she is dying. Instead, say something like, "I won't give up on you, so don't give up on yourself."

- Do not volunteer information about the victim or others who might also be injured. However, if the victim asks a question about a family member, tell the truth. Provide simple, honest, clear information if it is requested and repeat it as often as necessary.
- Use a gentle tone of voice.
- Use a reassuring touch, if appropriate.
- Let the person know that everything that can be done to help will be done.

The Stages of Grieving

People who lose a loved one go through a <u>grieving process</u>. This process generally involves five stages, but not all people move through the process in the same way or at the same pace.

1. *Denial* ("Not me."). The person cannot believe what is happening. This stage serves as a buffer for the person experiencing the situation. This reaction is normal.
2. *Anger* ("Why me?"). First aiders and bystanders could be the target of the anger. Do not take the anger or insults personally. Be tolerant, use good listening skills, and be empathetic.
3. *Bargaining* ("OK, but first let me . . ."). In the victim's mind, an agreement will postpone an unpleasant event (such as death).
4. *Depression* ("OK, but I haven't . . ."). This stage is characterized by sadness and despair. The person is usually silent and retreats into his or her own world.
5. *Acceptance* ("OK, I am not afraid."). This does not mean a person is happy about the situation. The family often requires more support during this stage than the victim does.

With an understanding of these five stages, you can better understand the reactions of those who are grieving and also your reactions to stressful situations.

Dealing With Survivors

Deal with the family members of a dead or dying victim as follows:

- Do not pronounce death; leave the confirmation of death to a physician.
- Allow survivors to grieve in whatever way seems right to them (anger, rage, crying).
- Provide simple, honest, clear information as it is requested, and repeat it as often as necessary.
- Offer as much support and comfort as possible by your presence and by your words. Do not leave an individual survivor alone, but respect that person's right to privacy.
- Use a gentle tone of voice.
- Use a reassuring touch, if appropriate.

prep kit

▶ Ready for Review

- Emergencies are dangerous, unusual, rare, unforeseen, and must be dealt with before the situation becomes worse.
- A bystander is a vital link between EMS and the victim.
- Victims would benefit if bystanders could quickly and reliably do the following:
  - Recognize the emergency.
  - Decide to help.
  - Call 9-1-1 if EMS is needed.
  - Check the victim.
  - Give first aid.
- Knowing when to call 9-1-1 is important. To do so, you must be able to tell the difference between a minor injury or illness and a life-threatening one.
- In most communities, call 9-1-1 to receive emergency assistance.
- The sight of blood and the cries of victims can be upsetting, but it is essential that first aiders remain alert and working at an injury scene.
- If you are at the scene of an emergency situation, do a 10-second scene size-up looking for hazards, the cause of the injury or illness, and the number of victims.
- First aiders should take precautions to protect against infectious diseases.
- There are few incidents that involve emotional stress like the life-and-death situations that you might face.

▶ Vital Vocabulary

airborne diseases Infections transmitted through the air, such as tuberculosis.

bloodborne diseases Infections transmitted through the blood, such as HIV or HBV.

communicable disease A disease that can spread from person to person, or from animal to person.

emergency medical services (EMS) A system that represents the combined efforts of several professionals and agencies to provide emergency medical care.

grieving process Feelings and emotions after a stressful situation that cause personal pain. People go through several stages of grieving.

hepatitis B virus (HBV) A viral infection of the liver for which a vaccine is available.

hepatitis C virus (HCV) A viral infection of the liver for which no vaccine is available.

human immunodeficiency virus (HIV) The virus that can cause acquired immunodeficiency syndrome (AIDS).

infectious disease A medical condition caused by the growth of small, harmful organisms within the body.

personal protective equipment (PPE) Equipment, such as exam gloves, used to block the entry of an organism into the body.

posttraumatic stress disorder (PTSD) A delayed stress reaction to a prior emergency event.

SARS (severe acute respiratory syndrome) A potentially life-threatening viral infection that usually starts with flu-like symptoms.

scene size-up Steps taken when approaching an emergency scene. Steps include checking for hazards, noting the cause of the injury or illness, and determining the number of victims.

standard precautions Protective measures that have traditionally been developed by the Centers for Disease Control and Prevention (CDC) for use in dealing with objects, blood, body fluids, or other potential exposure risks of communicable disease.

tuberculosis A bacterial disease usually affecting the lungs.

▶ Assessment in Action

You are walking from house to house in an unfamiliar neighborhood collecting donated clothing for a local charitable organization. You find no one home at a particular house but hear a loud explosion in the garage. You decide to see what happened. Upon entering the garage you find a teenage boy lying on the ground.

There is a strong gasoline odor. You have a cellular telephone with you.

Directions: Circle Yes if you agree with the statement; circle No if you disagree.

Yes   No   **1.** This scene could be dangerous.

Yes   No   **2.** You should not be concerned about other possible victims.

Yes   No   **3.** In most communities, 9-1-1 can be used to contact EMS.

Yes   No   **4.** If you do not know the exact address of the emergency, be prepared to give a description of the location as best as you can.

▶ Check Your Knowledge

Directions: Circle Yes if you agree with the statement; circle No if you disagree.

Yes   No   **1.** A scene survey should be done before giving first aid to an injured victim.

Yes   No   **2.** For a severely injured victim, call the victim's doctor before calling for an ambulance.

Yes   No   **3.** Dial 0 (for the telephone operator) if you do not know the emergency telephone number.

Yes   No   **4.** First aiders should assume that blood and all body fluids are infectious.

Yes   No   **5.** If you are exposed to blood while on the job, report it to your supervisor, and if off the job, to your personal physician.

Yes   No   **6.** First aid kits should contain exam gloves.

Yes   No   **7.** Wash your hands with soap and water after giving first aid.

Yes   No   **8.** Vaccinations are available for both HBV and HCV.

Yes   No   **9.** Exam gloves can be made of almost any material as long as they fit the hand well.

Yes   No   **10.** Tuberculosis is a bloodborne disease.

The Human Body

The Human Body

To assess a victim's condition adequately and to give effective first aid, a first aider must be familiar with the basic structure and functions of the human body. This knowledge provides a solid cornerstone for building the essentials of quality victim assessment and emergency first aid. By using the proper medical terms, you will be able to communicate more effectively with medical care providers.

In injuries and illnesses, most life-threatening conditions affect the respiratory, circulatory, and nervous systems. These three body systems include the most important and sensitive organs: the lungs, the heart, the brain, and the spinal cord. The other body systems are also important, and thorough assessment of the victim can locate injury and/or sudden illnesses affecting them as well. The major body systems described in this chapter are the respiratory, circulatory, nervous, skeletal, and muscular systems. The skin is also described. The other body systems—the endocrine, gastrointestinal, and genitourinary systems—are not discussed.

▶ The Respiratory System

The body can store food to last several weeks and water to last several days, but it can store enough oxygen for only a few minutes. Ordinarily, this does not matter because we only have to inhale air to get the

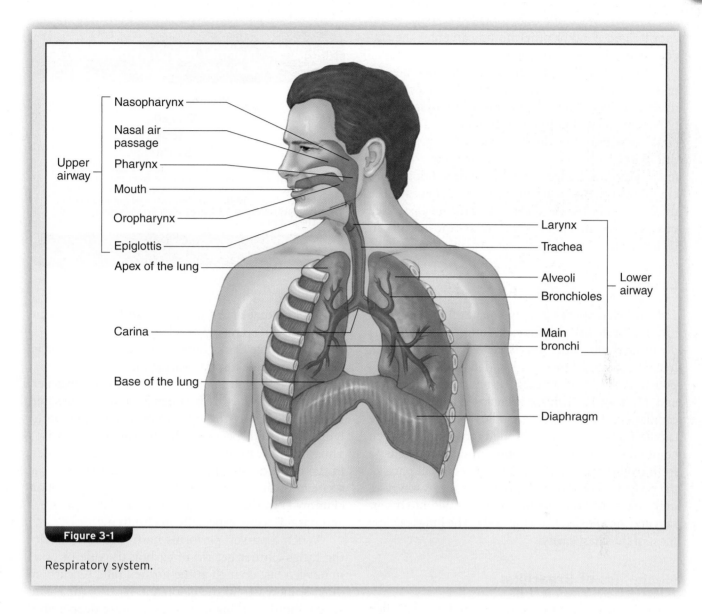

Figure 3-1

Respiratory system.

oxygen we need. If the body's oxygen supply is cut off, as in drowning, choking, or smothering, death will result in about 4 to 6 minutes unless the oxygen intake is restored. Oxygen from air is made available to the blood through the **respiratory system** and then to the body cells by the circulatory system.

Nose

Air normally enters the body during inhalation through the nostrils. It is warmed, moistened, and filtered as it flows over the damp, mucous membrane (sticky lining) of the nose. When a person breathes through the mouth instead of the nose, there is less filtration and warming. After passing through the nasal passages, air enters the nasal portion of the pharynx (throat).

Pharynx and Trachea

From the back of the nose or the mouth, the air enters the throat or pharynx **Figure 3-1**. The pharynx is a common passageway for food and air. At its lower end, the pharynx divides into two passageways: one for food and the other for air. Muscular control in the back of the throat routes food to the **esophagus** (food tube), which leads to the stomach; air is routed from the pharynx to the **trachea** (windpipe), which leads to the lungs. The trachea and the esophagus are separated by a small flap of tissue, the epiglottis, which diverts food away from the trachea. Usually this diversion works automatically to keep food out of the trachea and to prevent air from entering the esophagus. If the muscles of the pharynx and larynx are not coordinated, food or other liquid can enter the trachea instead of the esophagus.

Normal swallowing controls do not operate if a person is unresponsive. That is why a first aider should never pour liquid into the mouth of an unresponsive person in an attempt to revive him or her. The liquid could flow into the windpipe and suffocate the victim. Foreign objects, such as false teeth or a piece of food, might also lodge in the throat or windpipe and cut off the passage of air. In the upper 2 inches of the trachea, just below the epiglottis, is the <u>larynx</u> (voice box), which contains the vocal cords. The larynx can be felt in the front of the throat (<u>Adam's apple</u>).

Lungs

The trachea branches into two main tubes (bronchial tubes or bronchi), one for each lung. Each bronchus divides and subdivides somewhat like the branches of a tree. The smallest bronchioles end in thousands of tiny pouches (<u>alveoli</u>, or air sacs), just as the twigs of a tree end in leaves. Each air sac is enclosed in a network of capillaries. The walls that separate the air sacs and the capillaries are very thin. Through those walls, oxygen combines with the hemoglobin in red blood cells to form oxyhemoglobin, which is carried to all parts of the body. Carbon dioxide and certain other waste gases in the blood move across the capillary walls into the air sacs and are exhaled from the body. The lungs occupy most of the chest cavity.

Mechanics of Breathing

The passage of air into and out of the lungs is called respiration. Breathing in is called inhalation; breathing out is called exhalation. Ventilation is a mechanical process brought about by alternately increasing and decreasing the size of the chest cavity. When the <u>diaphragm</u> (the dome-shaped muscle dividing the chest from the <u>abdomen</u>) contracts, the chest expands, drawing air into the lungs (inhalation). An exchange of oxygen and carbon dioxide takes place in the lungs. When the diaphragm relaxes, it exerts pressure on the lungs, causing air to flow out (exhalation).

Infants and children differ from adults. Their respiratory structures are smaller and more easily obstructed than those of adults. Infants' and children's tongues take up proportionally more space in the mouth than do the tongues of adults. The trachea is more flexible in infants and children. The primary cause of cardiac arrest in infants and children is an uncorrected respiratory problem.

The average rate of breathing in an adult at rest is 12 to 20 complete respirations per minute (Table 3-1). Normal rates for children are from 15 to 30 times per minute; infant rates are between 25 and 50 times per minute. Normally the rate slows when a person is lying down and speeds up during vigorous exercise. The rate of breathing is controlled by a nerve center in the brain. Signs of inadequate breathing include a rate of breathing outside the normal range, cool or clammy skin that is pale or cyanotic (blue-purple), and nasal flaring, especially in children.

When a person performs hard muscular work, the lungs cannot get rid of carbon dioxide or take in oxygen fast enough at the normal rate. As carbon dioxide increases in the blood and tissues, the brain sends impulses along its nerves to cause deeper and more rapid respirations. At the same time, the heart rate increases. This faster heart rate increases the supply of oxygen available to the body as the heart pumps more blood through the lungs.

▶ The Circulatory System

The <u>circulatory system</u> (Figure 3-2) is made up of the blood, the heart, and the blood vessels. Blood is the great delivery system for cells throughout the body. It carries nutrients and other products from the digestive tract in its plasma, and it carries oxygen from the lungs in its hemoglobin. It also transports wastes produced by the cells to the lungs, kidneys, and other excretory organs for removal from the body.

Table 3-1 Normal Respiration Rate Ranges

	Breaths per Minute*
Adults	12 to 20
Children	15 to 30
Infants	25 to 50

*To obtain the breathing rate in a person, count the number of breaths in a 30-second period and multiply by 2. A person's awareness that respirations are being counted can influence the respiratory rate, so avoid letting the person know you are counting respirations.

Figure 3-2

Circulatory system.

Figure 3-3

The heart. **A.** Circulation (internal view). **B.** The two main coronary arteries supply the heart with blood.

Heart

The human circulatory system is a completely closed circuit of tubelike vessels through which blood flows. The <u>heart</u> **Figure 3-3**, by contracting and relaxing, pumps blood through the vessels. It is a powerful, hollow, muscular organ about as big as a man's clenched fist, shaped like a pear, and located in the left center of the chest, behind the sternum (breastbone). The heart is divided by a wall in the middle. Right and left compartments are divided into two chambers, the atrium above and the ventricle below. Check valves are located between each atrium and its corresponding ventricle and at the exit of the major arteries leading out of each ventricle. The opening and shutting of these valves at just the right time in the heartbeat keeps the blood from backing up.

FYI

Did You Know?

The carotid arteries along the neck convey the blood to the head, and if pressure is applied to them, the individual becomes unconscious, seeming to drop off into a stupor or slumbers. Hence, the Greeks called these arteries the "karotides" from the Greek word karoun, meaning "to stupefy."

Source: Skinner HA: *The Origin of Medical Terms,* ed 2. Baltimore, MD, Williams & Wilkins. 1961.

Table 3-2 Normal Heart Rates

	Beats per Minute*
Adults	60 to 100
Children	80 to 100
Toddlers	100 to 120
Newborns	120 to 140

*To obtain a heart rate in most people, count the number of beats in a 30-second period and multiply by 2.

At each beat, or contraction, the heart pumps blood rich in carbon dioxide and low in oxygen from the right ventricle to the lungs and returns oxygen-rich blood to the left atrium of the heart from the lungs. The left ventricle pushes blood rich in oxygen freshly obtained to the rest of the body and returns oxygen-poor blood to the right atrium. At each relaxation of the heart, blood flows into the left atrium from the lungs and into the right atrium from the rest of the body **Table 3-2**.

Blood Vessels

The **arteries** are elastic, muscular tubes that carry blood away from the heart **Figure 3-4**. They begin at the heart as two large tubes: the pulmonary artery, which carries blood to the lungs for the carbon dioxide and oxygen exchange, and the **aorta**, which carries blood to all the other parts of the body. The aorta divides and subdivides until it ends in networks of extremely fine vessels (**capillaries**) smaller than hairs. Through the thin walls of the capillaries, oxygen and nourishment pass out of the bloodstream into the

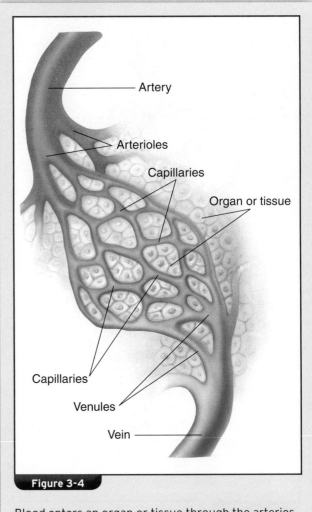

Figure 3-4

Blood enters an organ or tissue through the arteries and leaves through the veins. This process provides adequate blood flow to the tissue to meet the cells' needs.

FYI

Word Origins

Arteries received their name from the Greek term for windpipe because the Greek physician Praxagoras thought they carried air. In corpses, they are usually empty and that was probably where his observations were made.

Source: Skinner HA: *The Origin of Medical Terms,* ed 2. Baltimore, MD, Williams & Wilkins, 1961.

stationary cells of the body, while the body cells discharge their waste products into the bloodstream. In the capillaries of the lungs, carbon dioxide is released and oxygen is absorbed. Capillaries, having reached their limit of subdivision, begin to join together again into veins. The **veins** become larger and larger and finally form major trunks that empty blood returning from the body into the right atrium and blood from the lungs into the left atrium.

It is impossible to prick normal skin anywhere without puncturing capillaries. Because the flow of blood through the capillaries is relatively slow and under little pressure, blood merely oozes from a punctured capillary and usually has time to clot, promptly plugging the leak.

Each time the heart contracts, the surge of blood can be felt as a **pulse** at any point where an artery lies close to the surface of the body, near the skin surface and over a bone. When an artery is cut, blood spurts out. There is no pulse in a vein because the pulse is lost by the time the blood has passed through the capillaries. Hence, blood from a cut vein flows out in a steady stream. It has much less pressure behind it than blood from a cut artery.

Major locations for feeling pulses include the following **Figure 3-5**:

- **Carotid artery**: The major artery of the neck, which supplies the head with blood. Pulsations can be palpated (felt) on either side of the neck (do not try to feel both at the same time). Health care providers use the carotid artery to check an unresponsive person's pulse.
- **Femoral artery**: The major artery of the thigh, which supplies the lower extremities with blood. Pulsations can be palpated in the groin area (the crease between the abdomen and thigh).
- **Radial artery**: The major artery of the lower arm. Pulsations can be palpated at the palm side of the wrist on the thumb side. Use the radial location to check an alert person's pulse.
- **Brachial artery**: An artery of the upper arm. Pulsations can be palpated on the inside of the arm between the elbow and the armpit. Health care providers use the brachial location to determine a pulse in an infant.
- **Posterior tibial artery**: Located behind the inside ankle knob. Pulsations can be palpated behind the posterior surface of the medial malleolus.
- **Dorsalis pedis artery**: Pulsations can be palpated on the top surface of the foot (many people have no pulsations here).

Blood Pressure

Blood pressure is a measure of the pressure exerted by the blood on the walls of the flexible arteries. Blood pressure might be high or low according to the resistance offered by the walls to the passage of blood. This difference in resistance could have several causes. For example, if blood does not fill the system, as following hemorrhage, the pressure will be low (hypotension). High blood pressure (hypertension) might be present when the arterial walls have become hard and cannot expand readily.

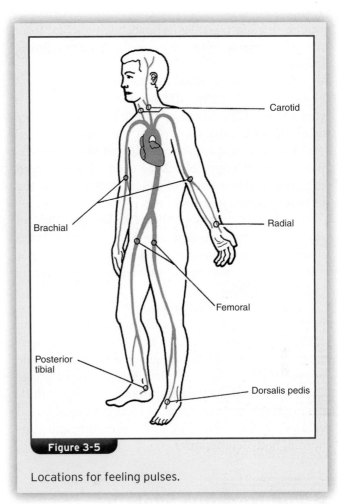

Figure 3-5

Locations for feeling pulses.

Blood

Blood has liquid and solid portions. The liquid portion is called plasma. The solid portion, which is transported by the plasma, includes disklike red blood cells; slightly larger, irregularly shaped white blood cells; and an immense number of smaller bodies called **platelets**.

Plasma, the liquid part of the blood, is about 90% water, in which minerals, sugar, and other materials are dissolved. Plasma carries food materials picked up from the digestive tract and transports them to the body cells. It also carries waste materials produced by cells to the kidneys, digestive tract, sweat glands, and lungs for elimination (excretion) in urine, feces, sweat, and expired breath.

The **red blood cells**, which give blood its color, carry oxygen to the organs. The **white blood cells** are part of the body's defense against infection. These cells can go wherever they are needed in the body to fight infection, for example, to a wound in the skin or other tissue that is diseased or injured. Pus, a sign of wound infection, gets its yellowish white color from the innumerable white blood cells that are fighting the invading bacteria.

Platelets are essential for the formation of blood clots. If blood plasma did not clot at the site of a wound, the slightest cut or abrasion would produce death from bleeding. Clots plug the openings through which blood escapes from punctured blood vessels. Bleeding from a large blood vessel could be too rapid to permit the formation of a clot. *Hemorrhage* is the term for profuse bleeding.

Perfusion refers to the circulation of blood through an organ or a structure. Hypoperfusion is the inadequate circulation of blood through an organ or a structure. The average-size man has about 6 quarts (12 pints) of blood.

Inadequate circulation is known as shock (hypoperfusion). Shock is a state of profound depression of the vital processes of the body and may be characterized by the following signs and symptoms: pale or cyanotic (bluish), cool, clammy skin; rapid pulse; rapid breathing; restlessness, anxiety, or mental dullness; nausea and vomiting; reduction in total blood volume; low or decreasing blood pressure; and subnormal body temperature.

▶ The Nervous System

The **nervous system** is a complex collection of nerve cells (neurons) that coordinate the work of all parts of the human body and keep the individual in touch with the outside world. Neurons receive stimuli from the environment and transmit impulses to nerve centers in the brain and spinal cord. Then, by a complicated process of thinking (reasoning) plus reflex and automatic reactions, they produce nerve impulses that regulate and coordinate all bodily movements and functions and govern behavior and consciousness.

Once neurons have been destroyed, the body cannot regenerate them. Some limited nerve repair is possible, however, as long as the vital cell body is intact. If a nerve fiber is cut or injured, the section attached to the cell body remains alive, but the part beyond the injury withers away.

The nervous system can be classified in different ways. From a structural standpoint, there are the **central nervous system (CNS)**, which includes the brain and the spinal cord, and the peripheral nervous system, a network of nerve cells that originates in the brain and spinal cord and extends to all parts of the body, including the muscles, the surface of the skin, and the special sense organs, such as the eyes and the ears. The peripheral nervous system is further subdivided into the voluntary and the autonomic (involuntary) nervous systems.

Central Nervous System

The CNS consists of the brain, which is enclosed within the skull, and the spinal cord, which is housed in a semiflexible bony column of vertebrae **Figure 3-6**. The CNS serves as the controlling organ of the body. The brain enables us to think, judge, and act. The spinal cord is a major communication pathway between the brain and the rest of the body.

Brain

The **brain**, which is the headquarters of the human nervous system, is probably the most highly specialized organ in the body. It weighs about 3 pounds in the average adult, is richly supplied with blood vessels, and requires considerable oxygen to perform effectively.

The brain has three main subdivisions: the **cerebrum** (large brain), which occupies nearly all (75%) of the cranial cavity; the **cerebellum** (small brain); and the **brain stem**. The cerebrum is divided into two hemispheres by a deep cleft. The outer surface of the cerebrum, the cerebral cortex, is about one eighth-inch thick, composed mainly of cell bodies of nerve cells, and often referred to as gray matter.

Certain sections of the cerebrum are localized to control specific body functions such as sensation, thought, and associative memory, which allows us to store, recall, and make use of past experiences. The sight center of the brain is located at the back of the cerebrum, which is called the occipital lobe. The temporal lobes, at the sides of the head, direct smell and hearing. The cerebellum is located at the back of the **cranium** (skull) and below the cerebrum. Its main function is to coordinate muscular activity and balance.

The third major area of the brain is the brain stem, which extends from the base of the cerebrum to the foramen magnum (a large opening at the base of the skull). The brain stem controls automatic functions such as breathing and heart rate.

Small cavities in the brain contain the **cerebrospinal fluid (CSF)**, a clear, watery solution similar to blood plasma. Circulating throughout the brain and

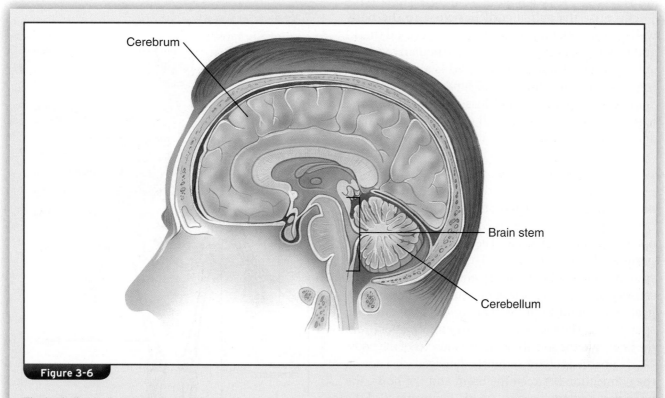

Figure 3-6

The brain lies well protected within the skull. Its principal subdivisions are the cerebrum, the cerebellum, and the brain stem.

the spinal cord, CSF serves as a protective cushion and exchanges food and waste materials. The total quantity of CSF in the brain–spinal cord system is 100 to 150 mL, although up to several liters can be produced daily. It is constantly being produced and reabsorbed.

Knowledge of nerve structure and function enables physicians to locate diseased brain sections. Because nerves from one side of the body eventually connect with the opposite side of the brain, a person whose left arm is paralyzed after a stroke will have suffered damage to the right side of the brain.

Spinal Cord

The **spinal cord** is a soft column of nerve tissue continuous with the lower part of the brain that is enclosed in the bony vertebral column **Figure 3-7**. The spinal cord exits the brain through the foramen magnum, which is a hole in the base of the skull. Thirty-one pairs of spinal nerves branch from the spinal cord. These nerves are large trunks that are similar to telephone cables because they house many nerve fibers. Some fibers carry impulses into the spinal cord; others carry impulses away from it. Spinal nerves at different levels of the cord regulate activities of various parts of the body.

Figure 3-7

The spinal cord is a continuation of the brain stem.

Because the spinal cord lies close to the bony walls of the vertebra, especially in the cervical (neck) and thoracic (chest) regions, it is particularly vulnerable to injury. Damage to the cord is almost always irreversible. An injury to the lumbar (lower back) spine causes paralysis and loss of sensation in the legs; an injury to the cervical cord causes paralysis and loss of sensation in the arms and the legs.

Peripheral Nervous System

At each vertebral level and on each side of the spinal cord, a spinal nerve exits the spinal cord through an opening in the bony canal. These nerves make up the peripheral nervous system. The peripheral nervous system consists of the sensory and motor nerves. The sensory nerves carry sensations such as smell, touch, heat, and sound from the body to the brain and the spinal cord. The motor nerves carry information from the brain and the spinal cord to the muscles of the body.

If a nerve is cut or seriously damaged, disrupting the connection between the brain and the body, the body part will not be able to work. For example, if the motor nerve going to the right leg is cut, the leg will be unable to move. This can be a permanent loss. Injuries to the nerves in the spinal cord can be very serious.

Fortunately, the CNS is well protected against injury. The brain is enclosed in the cranial cavity of the skull. The spinal cord is contained in the hollow space of the vertebrae. The brain and the spinal cord are also protected by three layers of tissue known as the meninges. The space between the layers of the meninges is filled with CSF, which also helps protect the brain and spinal cord from injury.

Autonomic Nervous System

The autonomic nervous system consists of a group of nerves that control heart rate, digestion, sweating, and other automatic body processes. These processes are not controlled by the conscious mind, but they can be influenced by the CNS to a limited extent.

▶ The Skeletal System

The human body is shaped by its bony framework. Without its bones, the body would collapse. The adult **skeleton** has 206 bones **Figure 3-8**. **Bones** are composed of living cells surrounded by hard deposits of calcium. The bone cells are well supplied by blood

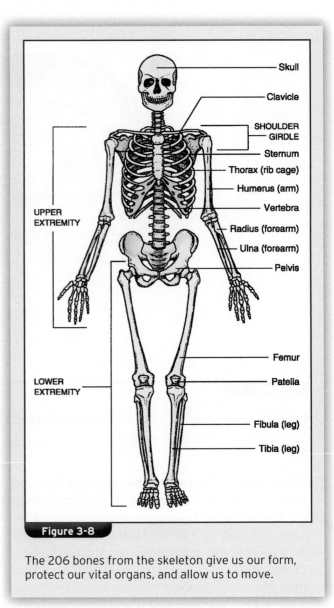

Figure 3-8

The 206 bones from the skeleton give us our form, protect our vital organs, and allow us to move.

vessels and nerves. The calcium deposits give bones their strength and rigidity. Broken bones are repaired by bone-building cells lying in the bone and its covering sheath, the periosteum. New bone is formed at the site of the break, much as two pieces of steel are welded together.

Skull

The skull rests at the top of the spinal column. It contains the brain, certain special-purpose glands (such as the pituitary and the pineal), and the centers of special senses—sight, hearing, taste, and smell. The skull has two parts, the brain case (cranium) and the face **Figure 3-9**. Blood vessels and nerve trunks pass to and from the brain through openings in the skull,

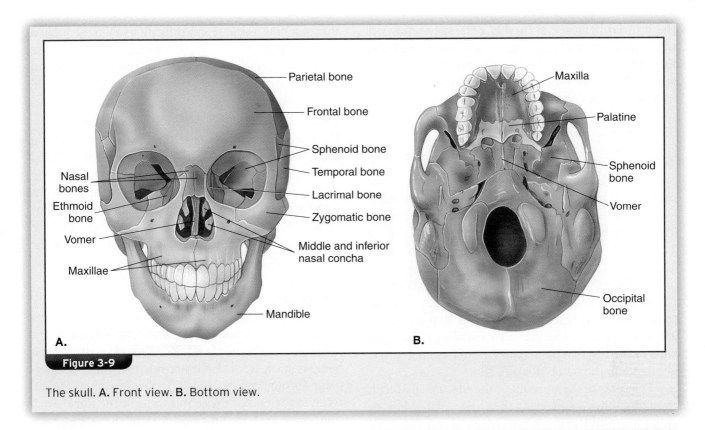

Figure 3-9

The skull. **A.** Front view. **B.** Bottom view.

mostly at the base. The largest opening is the foramen magnum, where the spinal cord exits the skull and joins the brain. The brain, which fits snugly in the cranium, is covered by the meninges. The very narrow spaces between the meninges are filled with CSF.

Although the skull is very tough, a blow can fracture it. Even if there is no fracture, a sudden impact can tear or bruise the brain and cause it to swell, just as any soft tissue swells following an injury or a bruise. Because the skull does not "give," injury to the brain is magnified by the contained pressure within the skull. Unresponsiveness or even death could result from swelling (edema), a tearing wound (laceration), bleeding, or other damage to the brain. The face extends from the eyebrows to the chin and contains the eyes, nose, cheeks, mouth, and lower jaw (mandible).

Spinal Column

The spinal column **Figure 3-10** is made up of irregularly shaped bones called vertebrae (singular is vertebra). Lying one on top of the other to form a strong, flexible column, the vertebrae are bound firmly together by strong **ligaments**. Between every two vertebrae is an intervertebral disk, a pad of tough elastic cartilage that acts as a shock absorber.

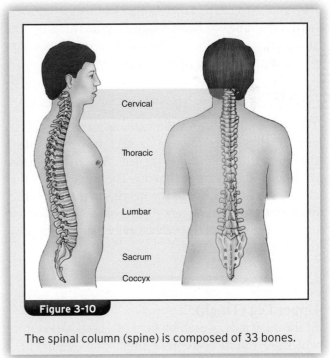

Figure 3-10

The spinal column (spine) is composed of 33 bones.

The spinal column can be damaged by disease or by injury. A crushed or displaced vertebra can squeeze, stretch, tear, or sever the spinal cord. Careless handling of an injured person by well-meaning but uninformed persons or movement of the disabled part by the injured person can further displace sections of the spinal column, resulting in additional injury to the cord and possibly permanent paralysis. For that reason, a person with a back or neck injury must be handled with extreme care.

Thorax

The thorax (rib cage) is made up of ribs and the sternum (breastbone). The sternum is a flat, narrow bone in the middle of the front wall of the chest. The collar bones and certain ribs are attached to the sternum. The 24 ribs are semiflexible arches of bone. There are 12 on each side of the chest. The back ends of the 12 pairs of ribs are attached to the 12 thoracic vertebrae. Strong ligaments bind the back ends of the ribs to the backbone but allow slight gliding or tilting movements. The front ends of the top 10 pairs of ribs are attached to the sternum by cartilage. The front ends of the last two pairs (pairs 11 and 12) hang free, giving them the name **floating ribs.**

Fractures of the sternum or the ribs usually result from crushing or squeezing the chest. A fall, blow, or penetration of the chest wall by an object can have the same effect. The chief danger from such injuries is that the lungs or heart might be punctured by the sharp ends of the broken bones. The lowest portion of the sternum is the **xiphoid process.**

Pelvis

The two hipbones and the sacrum form the pelvic girdle (pelvis). Muscles help connect the pelvic bones, the trunk, the thighs, and the legs. The pelvis forms the floor of the abdominal cavity. The lower part of the cavity, sometimes called the pelvic cavity, holds the bladder, rectum, and internal parts of the reproductive organs. The floor of the pelvic cavity helps to support the intestines.

Leg Bones

Upper Leg (Thigh)

At the outer side of each hipbone is a deep socket into which the round head of the thighbone (**femur**) fits, forming a ball-and-socket joint. The lower end of the femur is flat and has two knobs. These knobs articulate with the shinbone (tibia) at the knee joint. Although the femur is the longest and strongest bone in the skeleton, it is a common fracture site. A fractured femur is always serious because it is difficult to align the broken or splintered ends to create a strong union. Because of the force required to break the femur, laceration of the surrounding tissues, pain, and blood loss could be extensive.

Knee

The knee joint is the largest joint in the body and is a strong hinge joint **Figure 3-11**. The joint is protected and stabilized in the front by the kneecap (patella). The **patella** is a small, triangular-shaped bone in front of and between the femur and the tibia and within the tendon of the large muscle (the quadraceps) of the front of the thigh. Because the patella usually receives the force of falls or blows to the knee, it is frequently bruised or dislocated and sometimes fractured.

Lower Leg

The lower leg refers to the portion of the lower extremity between the knee and the ankle. Its two bones are the tibia and the fibula **Figure 3-12**. The **tibia** (shin bone) is at the front and inner side of the leg. It is palpable throughout its length. Its broad upper surface receives the end of the femur to form the knee joint. The lower end, much smaller than the upper end, forms the inner rounded knob of the ankle (medial malleolus). The fibula, which is not a part of the true knee joint, is attached at the top to the tibia. Its lower end forms the outside ankle knob (lateral malleolus). The fibula is more often fractured alone than is the tibia.

Ankles, Feet, and Toes

The ends of the tibia and fibula form the socket of the ankle joint. Both ankle knobs are easily palpated. The seven ankle bones (tarsals) are bound firmly together by tough ligaments. The heel bone (calcaneus) transmits the weight of the body to the ground and forms a base for the muscles of the calf of the leg when walking **Figure 3-13**. The sole and the instep of the foot are formed by the five long metatarsals. These articulate with the tarsals and with the front row of toe bones (phalanges).

Shoulder

The collar bone (clavicle) and the shoulder blade (scapula) form the shoulder girdle. Each **clavicle**—a long, slightly double-curved bone—is attached to the sternum at its inner end and to the scapula at its outer end. Each clavicle can be palpated throughout its length.

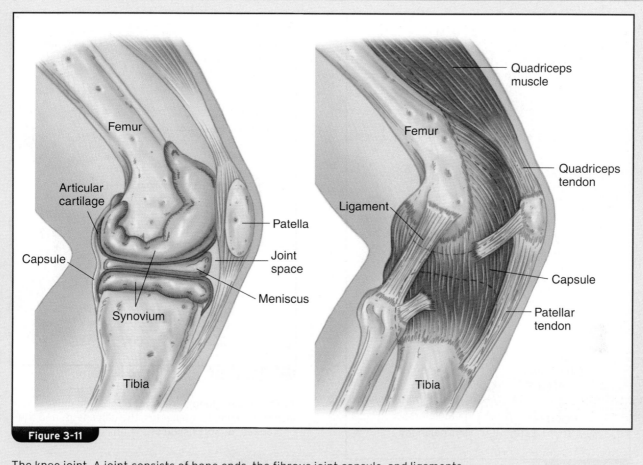

Figure 3-11

The knee joint. A joint consists of bone ends, the fibrous joint capsule, and ligaments.

Fractures are common because the clavicle lies close to the surface and must absorb blows. Each scapula—a large, flat, triangular bone—is located over the upper ribs at the back of the thorax.

Arm Bones

Upper Arm

The bone of the upper arm, the **humerus,** is the arm's largest bone. Its upper end (the head) is round; its lower end is flat. The round head fits into a shallow cup in the shoulder blade, forming a ball-and-socket joint. This is the most freely movable joint in the body and is easily dislocated. Dislocations can tear the capsule of the joint (synovial membrane) and cause damage. Improper manipulation during attempts to reduce or set the dislocation could add to the damage. Therefore, it is important to treat dislocations of the shoulder with gentle care.

Forearm

The two bones of the forearm (radius and ulna) lie side by side. The larger of the two, the **ulna,** is on the little finger side, and part of it forms the elbow. The flat, curved lower end of the humerus fits into a big notch at the upper end of the ulna to form the elbow joint. This hinge joint permits movement in one direction only. The **radius,** shorter and smaller than the ulna, is on the thumb side of the forearm **Figure 3-14** .

Wrist, Hand, and Fingers

The wrist is composed of eight small, irregularly shaped bones (carpals) united by ligaments. Tendons extending from the muscles of the forearm to the bones of the hand and fingers pass down the front and the back of the wrist close to the surface. Wrist lacerations could sever these tendons, resulting in total or partial immobility of the fingers.

Figure 3-12

The principal parts of the lower extremity include the thigh, leg, and foot. The principal parts of the leg include the tibia and fibula.

Figure 3-13

A. The surface landmarks of the foot and ankle include the medial malleolus, the calcaneus, and the phalanges. **B.** Soft tissue of the ankle.

The palm of the hand has five long bones (metacarpals). The 14 bones of the fingers (phalanges) give the hand its great flexibility. The thumb is the most important digit. A good thumb and one or two fingers make a far more useful hand than four fingers minus the thumb **Figure 3-15**.

Joints

A **joint** is where two or more bones meet or join. Some joints, such as those in the cranium, allow little, if any, movement of the bones. Other joints, such as the hip and the shoulder, allow a wide range of motion. In a typical joint, a layer of cartilage (gristle), which is softer than bone, acts as a pad or buffer. The bones of such a joint are held in place by firmly attached ligaments, which are bands of very dense, tough, but

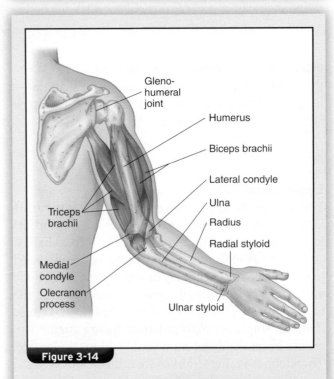

Figure 3-14

The principal bones in the arm and forearm include the humerus, the radius, and the ulna.

Figure 3-15

The principal bones in the wrist and hand include the carpals, the metacarpals, and the phalanges.

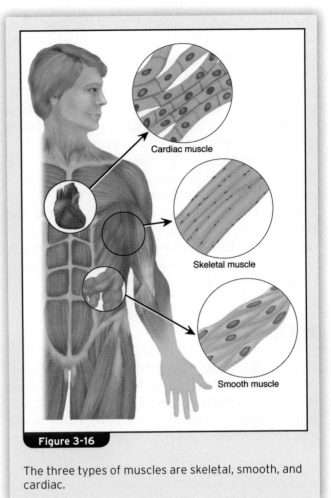

Figure 3-16

The three types of muscles are skeletal, smooth, and cardiac.

flexible connective tissue. Joints are enclosed in a capsule, a layer of thin, tough material, strengthened by the ligaments. The inner side of the capsule (synovial membrane) secretes a thick fluid (synovial fluid) that lubricates and protects the joint.

▶ The Muscular System

Body movement is due to work performed by muscles. Examples are walking, breathing, the beating of the heart, and the movements of the stomach and the intestines. What enables muscle tissue to perform work is its ability to contract—that is, to become shorter and thicker—when stimulated by a nerve impulse. The cells of a muscle, usually long and threadlike, are called fibers. Each muscle has countless bundles of closely packed, overlapping fibers bound together by connective tissue. The three kinds of muscles are skeletal muscle (voluntary), smooth muscle (involuntary), and cardiac muscle (heart). They differ in appearance and in the specific jobs they do **Figure 3-16**.

The **voluntary muscles,** which are under the control of a person's will, make possible all deliberate acts, including walking, chewing, swallowing, smiling, frowning, talking, and moving the eyeballs. Also called **skeletal muscles,** most voluntary muscles are attached by one or both ends to the skeleton by tendons. However, some muscles are attached to skin, cartilage, and special organs (such as the eyeball) or to other muscles, such as the tongue.

Muscles help to shape the body and to form its walls. Most skeletal muscles end in tough, whitish cords (tendons) that attach them to the bones they move. Tendons continue into the fascia, which covers the skeletal muscles. The fascia is much like the skin of a sausage in that it surrounds the muscle tissue. At either end of the muscle, the fascia extends beyond the muscle to attach to a bone. Tendons are covered with a synovial membrane, which secretes a lubricating substance, the synovial fluid. This makes it easier for the tendon to move when the muscle contracts or relaxes. Muscular contraction pulls the bone in the direction permitted by a joint.

When they are not working, muscles become comparatively slack. Normally, muscles never completely relax; some fibers are contracting all the time. They always have some tension (muscle tone). Loss of muscle tone can be a sign of nerve injury. Muscles can be injured in many ways. Overexerting a muscle can break fibers. Muscles can be bruised, crushed, cut, torn, or otherwise injured, with or without breaking the skin. Muscles injured in any of those ways are likely to become swollen, tender, painful, or weak.

A person has little or no control over the **smooth muscles** and usually is not conscious of them. Smooth muscles line the walls of tubelike structures such as the gastrointestinal tract, the urinary system, the blood vessels, and the bronchi of the lungs. Cardiac muscle is a specialized form of muscle found only in the heart. A continuous supply of oxygen and glucose is needed for cardiac muscle to work properly.

▶ The Skin

The skin covers the entire body, protecting the deep tissues from being injured, drying out, or being invaded by bacteria and other foreign bodies. The skin helps to regulate body temperature by aiding in the elimination of water and various salts. The skin senses heat, cold, touch, pressure, and pain and transmits that information to the brain and the spinal cord.

The skin consists of two layers: the outer layer (**epidermis**) and the inner layer (**dermis**) **Figure 3-17**. The epidermis varies in thickness in different parts of the body (the palms and the soles of the feet are thickest), and its dead cells are constantly worn off. The dermis has a rich supply of blood vessels and nerve endings. Hair grows from the dermis through openings called hair follicles. Sweat glands and oil glands in the dermis empty onto the surface of the epidermis through pores in the skin. Beneath the dermis is the subcutaneous layer (under the skin), which is well supplied with fat cells and blood vessels.

Sweat glands, which create perspiration, occur in nearly all parts of the skin. Sweat contains essentially the same minerals as blood plasma and urine, but it is more dilute. Normally, only traces of the waste products excreted in urine are in sweat. But when sweating is profuse or when the kidneys are diseased, the amounts of such wastes excreted in sweat could be considerable. Several mineral salts are removed from the body in sweat. Chief among those in quantity is sodium chloride (the same mineral as common table salt).

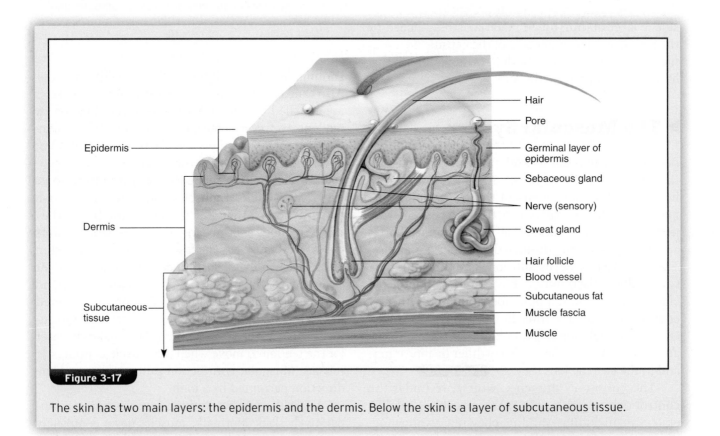

Figure 3-17

The skin has two main layers: the epidermis and the dermis. Below the skin is a layer of subcutaneous tissue.

▶ Ready for Review

- A first aider must be familiar with the basic structure and functions of the human body.
- The circulatory system is made up of the blood, heart, and blood vessels.
- The nervous system is a complex collection of nerve cells that coordinate the work of all parts of the human body.
- The skeletal system is the bony framework that shapes the body.
- The muscular system lets the body move.
- Skin covers the entire body and protects the deep tissues.

▶ Vital Vocabulary

abdomen The body cavity that contains the major organs of digestion and excretion. It is located below the diaphragm and above the pelvis.

Adam's apple The projection on the anterior surface of the neck, formed by the thyroid cartilage over the larynx.

alveoli The air sacs of the lungs in which the exchange of oxygen and carbon dioxide takes place.

aorta The principal artery leaving the left side of the heart and carrying freshly oxygenated blood to the body.

arteries A blood vessel, consisting of three layers of tissue and smooth muscle, that carries blood away from the heart.

blood The fluid that circulates through the heart, arteries, capillaries, and veins carrying nutrients and oxygen to the body cells and removing waste products such as carbon dioxide and various metabolic products for excretion.

bones The hard form of connective tissue that constitutes most of the skeleton in humans.

brachial artery The artery of the arm that, in turn, branches at the elbow into the radial and ulnar arteries. Used to determine an infant's pulse.

brain The soft, large mass of nerve tissue that is contained in the cranium.

brain stem The area of the brain between the spinal cord and cerebrum, surrounded by the cerebellum; controls functions that are necessary for life, such as respirations.

capillaries The small blood vessels through whose walls various substances pass into and out of the tissues and onto the cells.

carotid artery The major arteries that supply blood to the head and brain.

central nervous system (CNS) The brain and spinal cord.

cerebellum One of the three major subdivisions of the brain; coordinates the various activities of the brain, particularly fine body movements.

cerebrospinal fluid (CSF) A clear, watery solution similar to blood plasma.

cerebrum The largest part of the three subdivisions of the brain, made up of several lobes that control movement, hearing, balance, speech, visual perception, emotions, and personality.

circulatory system The arrangement of connected tubes, including the arteries, arterioles, capillaries, venules, and veins, that moves blood, oxygen, nutrients, carbon dioxide, and cellular waste throughout the body.

clavicle The collarbone.

cranium The area of the head above the ears and eyes; the skull. The cranium contains the brain.

dermis The inner layer of the skin, containing hair follicles, sweat glands, nerve endings, and blood vessels.

diaphragm A muscular dome that forms the undersurface of the thorax, separating the chest from the abdominal cavity. Contraction of the diaphragm brings air into the lungs. Relaxation allows air to be expelled from the lungs.

dorsalis pedis artery The artery on the anterior (top) surface of the foot between the first and second metatarsals.

epidermis The outer layer of the skin, which is made up of cells that are sealed together to form a watertight protective covering for the body.

esophagus A collapsible tube that extends from the pharynx to the stomach; contractions of the muscle in the wall of the esophagus propel food and liquids through it to the stomach.

femoral artery The principal artery of the thigh. It supplies blood to the lower abdominal wall, external genitalia, and legs. It can be palpated in the groin area.

prep kit

femur The thighbone; the longest and one of the strongest bones in the body.

floating ribs The 11th and 12th ribs, which do not attach to the sternum.

heart A hollow muscular organ that receives blood from the veins and propels it into the arteries.

humerus The supporting bone of the upper arm.

joint The place where two bones come into contact.

larynx The voice box.

ligament A band of the fibrous tissue that connects bones to bones. It supports and strengthens a joint.

nervous system The system that controls virtually all activities of the body, both voluntary and involuntary.

patella The kneecap; a specialized bone that lies within the tendon of the quadriceps muscle.

perfusion The circulation of oxygenated blood within an organ or tissue in adequate amounts to meet the cells' current needs.

plasma A sticky, yellow fluid that carries the blood cells and nutrients and transports cellular waste material to the organs of excretion.

platelets Tiny, disk-shaped elements that are much smaller than cells; they are essential in the initial formation of a blood clot, the mechanism that stops bleeding.

posterior tibial artery The artery just posterior to the medial malleolus; supplies blood to the foot.

pulse The wave of pressure created as the heart contracts and forces blood out the left ventricle and into the major arteries.

radial artery The major artery in the forearm; it is palpable at the wrist on the thumb side.

radius The bone on the thumb side of the forearm.

red blood cells Cells that carry oxygen to the body's tissues; also called erythrocytes.

respiratory system All the structures of the body that contribute to the process of breathing, consisting of the upper and lower airways and their component parts.

skeletal muscle Muscle that is attached to bones and usually crosses at least one joint; striated, or voluntary, muscle.

skeleton The framework that gives us our recognizable form; also designed to allow motion of the body and protection of vital organs.

smooth muscle Nonstriated, involuntary muscle; it constitutes the bulk of the gastrointestinal tract and is present in nearly every organ to regulate automatic activity.

spinal cord An extension of the brain, composed of virtually all the nerves carrying messages between the brain and the rest of the body. It lies inside of and is protected by the spinal canal.

tibia The shinbone; the larger of the two bones of the lower leg.

trachea The windpipe; the main trunk for air passing to and from the lungs.

ulna The inner bone of the forearm, on the side opposite the thumb.

vein Any blood vessel that carries blood from the tissues to the heart.

voluntary muscle Muscle that is under direct voluntary control of the brain and can be contracted or relaxed at will; skeletal or striated muscle.

white blood cells Blood cells that play a role in the body's immune defense mechanisms against infection.

xiphoid process The lowest part of the sternum.

▶ Assessment in Action

You are helping a friend with her human anatomy and physiology homework. Having taken the same class, you feel confident that you can help explain how the human body works. Your friend seems impressed. While explaining the different types of muscles, your friend clutches her throat and appears to be choking. You ask her if she is choking and can she talk to you. She shakes her head "no" and continues clutching her throat. You notice that she had been eating a hotdog.

Directions: Circle Yes if you agree with the statement; circle No if you disagree.

Yes   No   **1.** You shouldn't panic because she is young and with a little more time the hotdog will pass into the esophagus.

Yes   No   **2.** Because your friend is alert and responsive, she can survive without breathing for over ten minutes.

Yes No **3.** Her face begins to turn blue and she collapses to the floor. Her chest is not moving, which is a sign that she is not breathing.

Yes No **4.** If your friend is not breathing, her tissues and organs are not getting enough carbon dioxide.

▶ Check Your Knowledge

Directions: Circle Yes if you agree with the statement; circle No if you disagree.

Yes No **1.** A first aider does not have to understand how the human body works in order to effectively provide care.

Yes No **2.** The human body can store oxygen for hours.

Yes No **3.** Blood is the delivery system for cells throughout the body.

Yes No **4.** The heart is a pear-shaped, muscular organ.

Yes No **5.** Once neurons have been destroyed, the body can replace them.

Yes No **6.** The automatic nervous system consists of a group of nerves that control heart rate, digestion, sweating, and other automatic body processes.

Yes No **7.** The adult skeleton has 208 bones.

Yes No **8.** A joint is where two or more bones meet or join.

Yes No **9.** There are three kinds of muscle: skeletal, smooth, and cardiac.

Yes No **10.** Skin transmits information to the brain and helps regulate body temperature.

4

Finding Out What's Wrong

chapter
at a glance

▶ Victim Assessment Overview

During emergency situations when panic exists, knowing what to do and what not to do is crucial. A victim assessment is a sequence of actions that helps determine what is wrong and thus helps provide safe and appropriate first aid. Becoming familiar with the process of victim assessment will enable you to act quickly and decisively in hectic emergency situations. Victim assessment is an important first aid skill. It requires an understanding of each assessment step as well as decision-making skills.

Finding out what is wrong with a person will be influenced by whether the victim is suffering from an illness or an injury, whether the victim is responsive or unresponsive, and whether life-threatening conditions exist. A key point is to conduct a **primary check** first and to care for any problems you uncover before going on with the assessment.

Different problems and conditions require different approaches for determining what is wrong. Not all parts of an assessment apply to every victim, and the sequencing can vary depending on the victim's problem. Most victims do not require a complete assessment. For example, a victim who cut a finger while whittling a stick will not require a complete assessment, but a victim who slipped and fell 20 feet down a mountainside and cut a finger will, because other injuries might be present. **Table 4-1** and the flowchart give a preview of the sequence for the different types of victim you may encounter.

Table 4-1 Sequence of Victim Assessment

Injured Victim			Suddenly Ill Victim	
	Responsive			
Unresponsive	**With Significant COI**	**Without Significant COI**	**Unresponsive**	**Responsive**
• Primary check • Secondary check using the DOS parts of DOTS • SAMPLE history from others	• Primary check • Secondary check using DOTS • SAMPLE history	• Primary check • Examine chief complaint using DOTS • SAMPLE history	• Primary check • Secondary check using the DOS parts of DOTS • SAMPLE history from others	• Primary check • SAMPLE history • Examine chief complaint

COI = cause of injury; also known as mechanism of injury. DOTS = deformity, open wounds, tenderness, swelling. SAMPLE = symptoms, allergies, medications, pertinent history, last oral intake, and events leading up to the illness or injury

A victim assessment can provide important information about a problem and help you determine how to treat it and whether medical care is needed. If the victim requires medical care, pass what you found during the assessment to the emergency medical service (EMS) personnel or health care providers. Call 9-1-1 for any victim with a significant **cause of injury (COI)** or **nature of illness**, and for any unresponsive victim.

Q&A

Can a first aider make a diagnosis as to what is wrong?

No. Diagnosing a medical condition is best left to a physician. A layperson diagnosing a medical condition could be accused of practicing medicine without a license, which has legal consequences. However, a first aider can suspect what may be wrong based on the signs and symptoms found.

You should check the victim systematically. You can do this by performing these five steps:

1. Perform a scene size-up.
2. Perform a primary check.
3. Perform a secondary check, also known as a physical exam or head-to-toe exam.
4. Obtain the victim's SAMPLE history.
5. Perform a reassessment.

The **scene size-up** helps determine the safety of the scene and the general condition of the victim. It is followed by the primary check, in which the first aider identifies and treats immediate life-threatening conditions involving problems with the victim's breathing and severe bleeding. Victims with immediate life-threatening conditions can die within minutes unless their problems are quickly recognized and treated.

A **secondary check**, consisting of a physical examination, follows the primary check. These procedures can reveal information that will help identify the injury or illness, its severity, and what first aid is needed. Detailed information is gained about the victim's injury (eg, a painful ankle or bleeding nose) or chief complaint (eg, chest pain or itchy skin).

Performing the secondary check right after the primary check and before doing the **SAMPLE history** allows an injury to be found and cared for sooner than if the SAMPLE history comes before the secondary check. In some cases, especially when caring for a stranger, performing the SAMPLE history before the secondary check involves a conversation with the stranger, which may ease the victim's anxiety about having a first aider conduct a secondary check. Also, in cases of illness, performing the SAMPLE history before the secondary check can indicate which part of the secondary check should be performed first.

▶ Scene Size-up

Every time you encounter a victim, first check out the scene. The scene size-up determines the safety of the scene, the cause of the injury or nature of illness, and the number of victims.

Victim Assessment

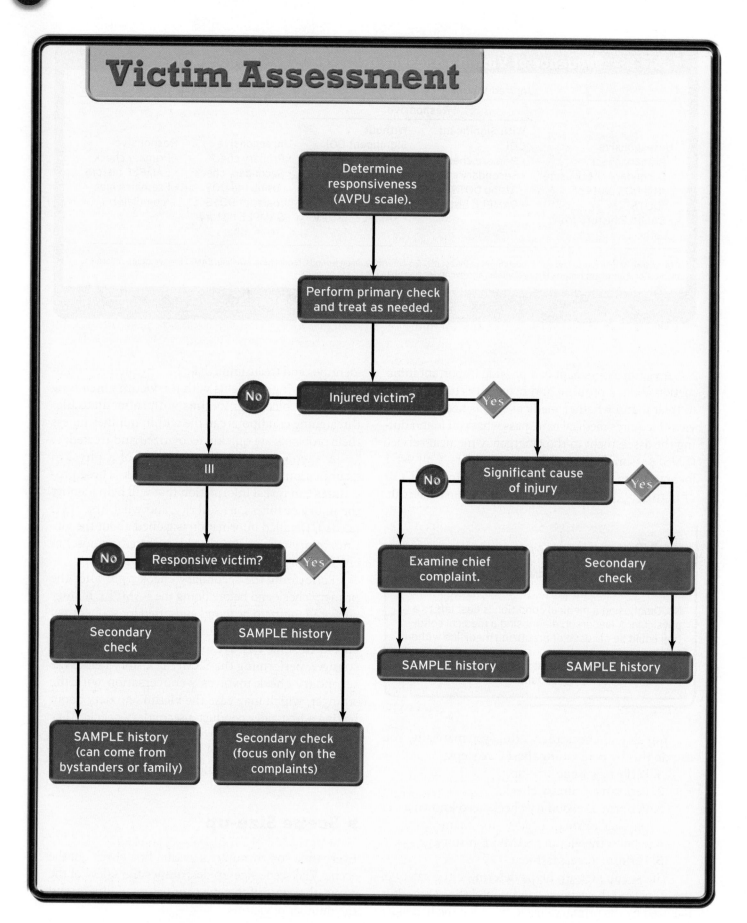

Without a scene size-up, a potentially hazardous situation could result in further injury to the victim or to you and bystanders. Hazards come in many different forms (eg, chemicals, electricity, water, fires, explosions, and carbon monoxide). Hazards exist at most motor vehicle crash scenes. Some scenes have the potential for violence—violent victims, distraught family members, angry bystanders, gangs, and unruly crowds. Be observant for weapons. If the scene appears hazardous, do not enter the area. You cannot help a victim if you become a victim yourself.

Reduce exposure to potentially dangerous body substances that can carry disease. Disease transmission is very rare; however, exam gloves should be worn and first aiders should assume that all victims are infected.

Determining whether the problem is an injury or an illness is also an important step. This gives you a starting point and determines the order of the assessment. If the scene size-up or primary check suggests serious illness or injury, call 9-1-1.

▶ Primary Check

The second part of a victim assessment sequence is always the primary check. The purpose of the primary check is to identify life-threatening conditions so you can immediately take action to treat the conditions. The primary check includes checking the victim's responsiveness, checking circulation, checking for breathing, and checking for severe bleeding.

First Impression of the Victim

While approaching the victim, form an immediate first impression of the victim. This has also been referred to as a general impression, look test, or gut reaction. Both the scene size-up and your first impression of the victim should help determine:

1. Does the victim appear to have an injury or an illness? If you are unable to determine whether the victim is ill or injured, treat the situation as though he or she were injured. Impressions can come from such things as the victim's position and the victim's breathing sounds.
2. Is the victim obviously responsive or unresponsive?

3. Is the victim obviously breathing adequately or normally? Talking?
4. Are there signs of obvious bleeding—blood spurting, blood-soaked clothing, blood pooled on the ground or floor?
5. Is there a chance of exposure to the victim's blood or other body fluids? If so, be sure to use standard precautions before making physical contact with the victim.
6. Is there any danger to you, the victim, or bystanders at the scene?

Check Responsiveness

Shortly after reaching the victim, you should have a good idea of whether the victim is responsive or unresponsive. If the victim is motionless, gently tap the victim's shoulder and ask loudly, "Are you okay?"

Beyond this point, how and in what order you conduct the checks will largely depend on the answer to the above question.

If the victim answers, moans, or moves, the victim is responsive. If the victim does not respond, call 9-1-1 to activate EMS. In the unresponsive victim, look for regular breathing by taking a quick look at the chest to see if it rises and falls. If you cannot see any chest movement and cannot hear any sounds (except occasional gasping) of air coming from the nose and mouth, this indicates the victim is not breathing. Do not mistake occasional gasping for breathing—it is not! Take immediate steps to begin CPR, starting with 30 chest compressions followed by two breaths (1 second each). See Chapter 5, *CPR*, for directions on how to perform CPR.

A victim's level of responsiveness can range from fully responsive (conscious) to unresponsive (unconscious). Not all responsive victims are fully alert, and they may respond to different levels of stimulation. The four-level **AVPU scale** can be used to describe the victim's responsiveness Table 4-2.

For an alert victim, begin by introducing yourself. Tell the victim that you are trained in first aid and ask permission to help. For an alert, responsive victim, you can evaluate the victim's ability to remember by asking:

- Person—What is your name?
- Place—Do you know where you are?
- Time—What is the month and year?
- Event—What happened?

If the victim can talk, breathing and heartbeat are present.

Table 4-2 AVPU Scale

A	Alert	The victim's eyes are open, and he or she can answer questions clearly. A victim who knows the month and year (time), where he or she is (place), and his or her own name is said to be "alert and oriented."
V	Responsive to verbal stimulus	The victim might not know the month of the year, where he or she is, or his or her name, but does respond in some meaningful way when spoken to.
P	Responsive only to painful stimulus	The eyes do not open, and the victim does not respond to questions. The victim moves or cries out in response to a painful stimulus such as pinching the muscle above the clavicle or firmly pinching the earlobe.
U	Unresponsive to any stimulus	The eyes do not open, and the victim does not respond to any stimulus.

FYI

Verbal First Aid: What to Say to a Victim

Use these guidelines for gaining rapport and calming alert and responsive injured and ill victims:

1. Avoid negative statements that could add to a victim's distress and anxiety.
2. Your first words to a victim are very important because they set the tone of your interaction.
3. Do not ask unnecessary questions unless it aids treatment or satisfies the victim's need to talk.
4. Tears and/or laughter can be normal. Let the victim know this if such responses seem to make him or her feel embarrassed.
5. Stress the positive. For example, instead of, "You will not have any pain," say, "The worst is over."
6. Do not deny the obvious. For example, instead of saying, "There is nothing wrong," say, "You've had quite a fall and probably don't feel too well, but we're going to look at you."
7. Use the victim's name while providing first aid.

For a motionless victim, tap his or her shoulder and ask, "Are you okay?" If there is no response, check for breathing.

For an unresponsive victim, the steps resemble the same steps used when beginning to perform cardiopulmonary resuscitation (CPR)—RAP-CAB—although most unresponsive victims do not need CPR (see Chapter 5, *CPR*) **Skill Drill 4-1** :

R For any motionless person, check responsiveness by gently tapping the victim's shoulder and shouting, "Are you okay?" Speak loudly enough to wake the victim if he or she is sleeping (**Step ❶**).

A If there is no response, call 9-1-1 (**Step ❷**).

P After calling to activate EMS, you should position the victim onto his or her back on a flat, firm surface. If the victim is breathing, place him or her in the recovery position and check for severe bleeding (**Step ❸**).

CAB Immediately begin CPR for adult victims who are unresponsive and not breathing or not breathing normally (only gasping) (**Step ❹**). If you are alone and the victim is a child or an infant, perform CPR for five cycles before calling 9-1-1. If a bystander is present for any victim, have him or her call 9-1-1 while you begin CPR. (See Chapter 5, *CPR*, for directions.)

An unresponsive, breathing victim can receive other first aid, especially to control severe bleeding. Providing care would be covered by implied consent. (Refer to Chapter 1, *Background Information*.)

The steps for an alert, responsive victim are RAP-ABC. A first aider is more likely to see this type of victim. Responsive victims rarely need the type of primary check used in unresponsive victims. However, a responsive victim may be developing an airway obstruction, may have severe bleeding, may be having a heart attack, or may be in the early stages of shock or some other serious condition. Each of these conditions is considered a medical emergency, and immediate care must be provided if you suspect

skill drill

4-1   Primary Check: RAP-CAB

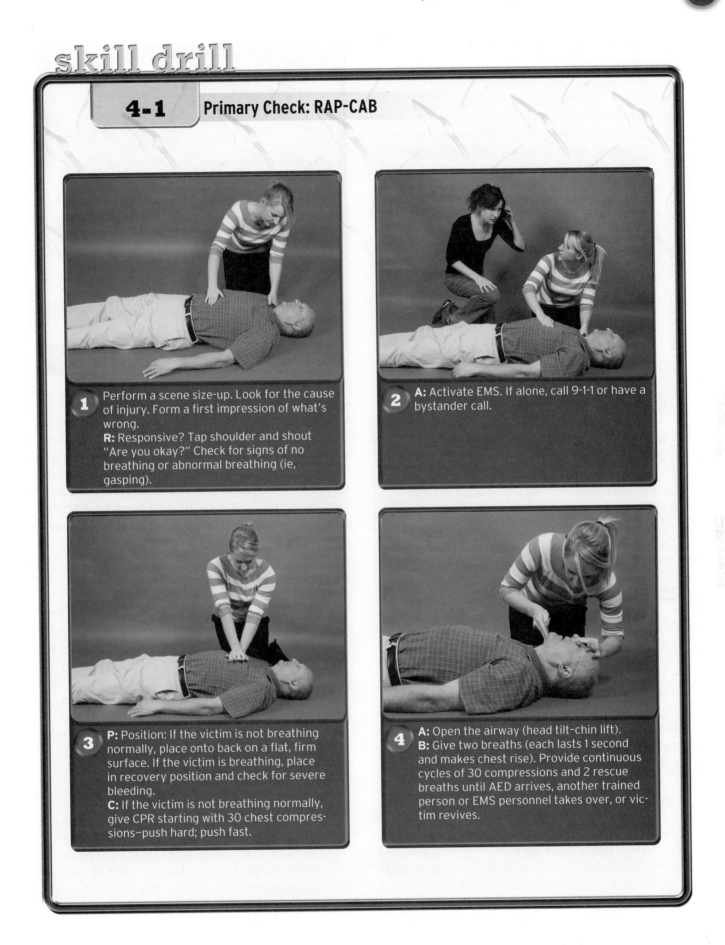

1 Perform a scene size-up. Look for the cause of injury. Form a first impression of what's wrong.
R: Responsive? Tap shoulder and shout "Are you okay?" Check for signs of no breathing or abnormal breathing (ie, gasping).

2 **A:** Activate EMS. If alone, call 9-1-1 or have a bystander call.

3 **P:** Position: If the victim is not breathing normally, place onto back on a flat, firm surface. If the victim is breathing, place in recovery position and check for severe bleeding.
C: If the victim is not breathing normally, give CPR starting with 30 chest compressions—push hard; push fast.

4 **A:** Open the airway (head tilt-chin lift).
B: Give two breaths (each lasts 1 second and makes chest rise). Provide continuous cycles of 30 compressions and 2 rescue breaths until AED arrives, another trained person or EMS personnel takes over, or victim revives.

any of them. Follow these steps to care for an alert, responsive victim:

R While approaching a responsive victim, make eye contact, introduce yourself as a trained first aider, and give your name. Next, ask if you can help—this is asking for the victim's consent to help. With permission from the victim, perform a victim assessment.

A If the victim appears to be severely injured or ill, activate EMS.

P Position the victim in a comfortable position (eg, lying down, tripod position, leaning against stable object).

A Make sure that the airway stays open.

B Check breathing—are there abnormal breathing sounds (eg, wheezing, gurgling) or is the victim breathing fast?

C Check circulation—is there severe bleeding?

Table 4-3 Breathing Sounds

Breathing Sound	Possible Cause
Snoring	Airway partially blocked (usually by tongue)
Gurgling (breaths passing through liquid)	Fluids in throat
Crowing (noisy creak or squeak)	Spasm of the larynx; foreign body
Wheezing	Spasm or partial obstruction in bronchi (asthma, emphysema)
Occasional gasping breaths (known as agonal respirations)	Breathing after the heart has stopped

Q&A

When should a first aider interrupt a primary check?

When a life-threatening condition is identified during the primary check, first aid should begin immediately. For example, if a victim has an obstructed airway, this should be treated before going through the other assessment steps. Once the life-threatening condition (eg, choking) has been cared for and/or corrected, the primary check of the victim should continue until completed.

Check Breathing

Check for adequate breathing by looking for chest rise and fall, listening for normal or abnormal breath sounds, and feeling for adequate air movement. Distinguish between effective and ineffective breathing efforts. Cyanosis and ashen (grey) skin are signs of inadequate oxygenation. See **Table 4-3** for breathing sounds that indicate a breathing problem.

Check for Severe Bleeding

Check for severe bleeding by quickly looking over the victim's entire body for blood (eg, blood-soaked clothing or blood pooling on the floor or the ground). This is not a head-to-toe examination, but a search for large amounts of blood around the victim or in the victim's clothing. In most cases, placing a sterile dressing over the wound and applying direct pressure with a hand or a pressure bandage controls the bleeding. Life-threatening external bleeding is rare, but when found, it must be controlled immediately or the victim can bleed to death. Avoid contact with the victim's blood whenever possible by using exam gloves or extra layers of dressings or cloth.

Position the Victim

Most victims should not be moved, especially if a spinal injury is suspected. The exceptions to this "rule of thumb" include:

- When the victim and first aider(s) are in an unsafe location.
- When an unresponsive victim is face down (prone position) and needs CPR, the victim should be turned to face up (supine position) on a firm, flat surface to be in a position to receive CPR.
- When the victim has difficulty breathing because of vomiting or secretions, or if the first aider is alone and must leave to get help. The victim can be placed in a modified High Arm IN Endangered Spine (HAINES) recovery position. It is best for the victim to rest on his or her left side (see section "Advantages of

the Left-Side Position"). While rolling the victim into the side position, keep the victim's nose and navel pointing in the same direction to avoid twisting the spine. Roll the victim onto the left side using the following steps:

1. Keeping the victim's left arm straight, extend it above the head with the upper part of the arm next to the head.
2. Bring the right arm across the chest and place the back of the victim's right hand against the left cheek; hold it there.
3. Hold the victim's hand against the cheek to support the head. Bend the victim's far leg at the knee and pull the bent leg to roll the victim toward you.
4. The victim's head remains on top of the left arm while rolling and the right hand stabilizes the head. The right bent knee prevents rolling.

- When signs of shock develop, place the victim on his or her back (supine position). Do not move the victim if suspected leg fractures or head or spine injuries exist.

Most victims with no suspected spine injuries may be placed in a position in which they are most comfortable. Victims with chest pain, nausea, or difficulty breathing fare better if in a half-sitting (semi-sitting) position at about a 45° angle. During an asthma attack, a victim may prefer the tripod position, which is sitting up, leaning forward with hands on knees and elbows out.

Advantages of the Left-Side Position

When placing a victim in either the recovery or the HAINES position, rolling him or her to the left side has several advantages:

- It keeps the airway open in an unresponsive, breathing victim.
- It delays vomiting by placing the esophagus above the stomach.
- It delays a poison's effects by retaining the poison in the stomach. A poison can be better handled in the stomach than in the small intestines.
- It relieves pressure on a pregnant woman's vena cava (the body's largest vein). Many pregnant women faint or at least feel dizzy if they lie supine because of the reduced blood flow.

▶ Secondary Check

A first aider should complete a secondary check following the primary check. Immediately treat any life-threatening problems found during a secondary check.

The goal of doing a hands-on secondary check is to identify any potentially life-threatening illness or injury needing first aid. A good secondary check is essential in discovering what is wrong. The adage of "find it; fix it" stresses the fact that you cannot provide first aid unless you know what is wrong. And, you will not know what is wrong until you do a victim assessment.

Q&A

Do I have to perform a complete victim assessment for every injured or suddenly ill victim?

No. Perform a primary check for every victim and acquire as much of each victim's SAMPLE history as you can. Performing a complete secondary check, which includes a head-to-toe physical exam, is crucial for the unresponsive, ill, or significantly injured victim. However, for the responsive ill person and the nonsignificantly injured victim, the secondary check focuses primarily on the victim's chief complaint.

Most of the victims a first aider will encounter require a secondary check of only the chief complaint, and a full secondary check (described below) is not needed. Nevertheless, first aiders should know how to perform one. In addition to the question, "What's wrong?" or "What happened to you?," another important question to ask of the victim who has been injured is "Do you hurt anywhere?" Many victims view a physical examination with apprehension and anxiety—they feel vulnerable and exposed. Maintain dignity throughout the assessment. Show compassion toward the victim and family members. If possible, the victim should be sitting or lying down.

Start by reconsidering the cause or mechanism of injury that you identified during the scene size-up. Ask the victim to describe what happened in detail, so that you can use the mechanism or cause of injury to predict possible injured areas—especially head, neck, spine, and internal injuries (see Chapter 2, *Action at*

Table 4-4 Significant Causes of Injury

- Falls of more than 15′ for adults, more than 10′ for children, or more than three times the victim's height
- Falls head-first from the victim's height or greater distance
- Vehicle collisions involving ejection, a roll-over, high speed, a pedestrian, a motorcycle, or a bicycle
- Head trauma with altered mental status (V, P, or U on AVPU scale)
- Penetrations of the head, chest, or abdomen (for example, stab or gunshot wounds)
- Major burn injury
- Death of an occupant in the same vehicle
- Pedestrian hit by a vehicle

Q&A

When might an assessment be unreliable?

Use caution when assessing any victim who has an altered mental status, a distracting painful injury (eg, femur fracture), or who has ingested alcohol or drugs.

an Emergency). This helps to determine which first aid procedures to use.

Determine whether the cause or mechanism of injury was significant Table 4-4. In addition to the significant causes of injury, assume that a victim with a head injury also has a spinal injury until proven otherwise. About 15% to 20% of head injury victims also have a spinal injury.

For a responsive victim, check for a spinal injury by asking the victim the following questions (refer to Skill Drill 12-1 in Chapter 12, *Head and Spinal Injuries*):

- Can you feel me squeezing your fingers and toes? (Before doing this, have the victim look away or close his or her eyes.) While you are squeezing, ask the victim which finger or toe you are squeezing.
- Can you wiggle your fingers and toes?
- Can you squeeze my hand, and can you push your foot against my hand?

For an unresponsive victim, check the spinal cord by stroking the bottom of the foot firmly toward the big toe with a key or similar blunt object. This is known as the Babinski reflex test. The normal response is an involuntary reflex that makes the big toe go down (except in infants, in whom it goes in the opposite direction). If the spinal cord or brain is injured, the toe will flex upward for both adults and children.

If you suspect a spinal injury, do not move the victim's head or neck. Stabilize the victim against any movement, and tell him or her not to move.

A secondary check assesses the victim's entire body from head to toe; you will note the victim's signs and symptoms:

- **Signs**—victim's conditions you can see, feel, hear, or smell.
- **Symptoms**—things the victim feels and is able to describe; known as the chief complaint.

To check a part of the body, look and feel (mnemonic is LAF) for the following signs and symptoms of injury: deformities, open wounds, tenderness, and swelling. The mnemonic **DOTS** is helpful for remembering the signs and symptoms of an injury Figure 4-1:

- D = Deformity—abnormal shape of the body part (compare with the opposite uninjured part). Deformities occur when bones are broken or joints are dislocated.
- O = Open wounds—the skin is broken and there is bleeding.
- T = Tenderness—sensitivity, discomfort, or pain when touched.
- S = Swelling—area looks larger than usual. Caused by excess fluid in the tissue. When possible, compare one side of the body with the other side (eg, if an ankle appears swollen, look at the other one).

Victim with a Significant Cause of Injury

This is a hands-on, full-body, head-to-toe assessment and should take no more than 2 minutes to complete. The victim may be responsive or unresponsive. Assume that an unresponsive victim has a spinal injury and stabilize the head and neck against movement. When a male examines a female, it is wise, if possible, to have another female present. Follow the steps in Skill Drill 4-2 to perform a secondary check:

1. **Check the head.** Use both hands to check the scalp for DOTS. A deformity may be a

D = deformity; O = open wounds; T = tenderness; S = swelling.

Figure 4-1

Examine an area by looking and feeling for: D = deformity; O = open wounds; T = tenderness; S = swelling.

bump or a depression. Do not move the victim's head during this procedure. Check the skin condition for temperature, color, and moisture.

2. **Check the eyes.** Compare the pupils, the dark part at the center of the eye. They should be the same size and react to light. The mnemonic PERRL helps remember what to look for **Figure 4-2**:
   - P = pupils
   - E = equal
   - R = round
   - R = react
   - L = light

   Use a flashlight to determine whether the pupils are reactive. If there is no flashlight, cover an eye with your hand and notice the pupil reaction when the eye is uncovered. Normally, the pupil constricts (gets smaller) within 1 second. No pupil reaction to light could mean death, coma, cataracts (in older persons), or an artificial eye. Pupil dilation happens within 30 to 60 seconds of cardiac arrest.

   Look for unequal pupils. A difference in the size of the two pupils is almost always a sign of a medical emergency, such as a stroke or a brain injury. However, the unequal condition occurs normally in 2% to 4% of the population. Also, an artificial eye may give the appearance of unequal pupils. Look at the inner eyelid surface—pink is normal in all healthy people regardless of skin pigmentation. A pale color may indicate poor blood circulation.

3. **Check the ears and nose** for clear or blood-tinged fluid. Check the nose for DOTS.

4. **Check the mouth** for swelling or objects (eg, broken teeth, dentures, chewing gum, vomit,

Figure 4-2

A. Constricted pupils. B. Dilated pupils. C. Unequal pupils.

food, and foreign objects), which could block the airway (**Step ❶**).

5. **Check the neck** for DOTS. Look for a medical identification necklace chain and tag (**Step ❷**).

6. **Check the chest** for DOTS. Warn the victim that you are going to apply pressure to the sides of the chest. Gently squeeze the chest inward and ask if doing so is painful. Pain from squeezing or compressing the sides may indicate a rib fracture (**Step ❸**).

7. **Check the abdomen** for DOTS. Feel the abdomen for tenderness by pushing gently downward in all four of the abdominal quadrants (divide the abdomen into four parts by two imaginary lines intersecting at right angles at the navel). If a chief complaint is abdominal pain, ask the victim to point to where it hurts. Do not push on the area that hurts. Begin on the opposite side from the spot, and press gently on each abdominal quadrant to see if it hurts. As you press on an area, ask the victim if it hurts. Feel for abnormal lumps and hardened areas. Do not push too deeply. The victim may "guard" an area if it is tender by tightening abdominal muscles or protecting that area with his or her hands. Anything protruding from the abdomen will be obvious, but be sure to check for penetrating objects (**Step ❹**).

8. **Check the pelvis** for DOTS. If the victim does not report pain, gently press inward on the tops of the hip bones and then, if there was no pain, press downward on the same bones. Warn the victim before pressing about possible tenderness (**Step ❺**).

9. **Check all four extremities** for DOTS. Use both hands to encircle an extremity and gently but firmly squeeze each part of the extremity for any sign of tenderness. Compare the two sides of the body with each other. Look for a medical identification bracelet on a wrist (**Step ❻**).

Check all four extremities for circulation, sensation, and movement (CSM):

- C = Circulation—for arms, feel for radial (on the wrist's thumb side) pulse, and for legs, feel the posterior tibial pulse behind the ankle bone (malleolus) on the inner (medial) side of the ankle.
- S = Sensation—pinch the end of fingers and toes (have victim close his or her eyes and tell you which finger or toe is being squeezed).
- M = Movement—have the victim wiggle fingers and toes.

10. **Check the back.** If no spinal injury is suspected, turn the victim onto his or her side and check for DOTS. You may have to turn the victim toward one side to check half of the back and then turn the victim the other direction to check the other half of the back (**Step ❼**).

If you suspect a neck or spinal injury and the victim's position is stable, tell the victim not to move while you are performing the check. If the victim is uncooperative or in an

skill drill

4-2   **Perform a Secondary Check**

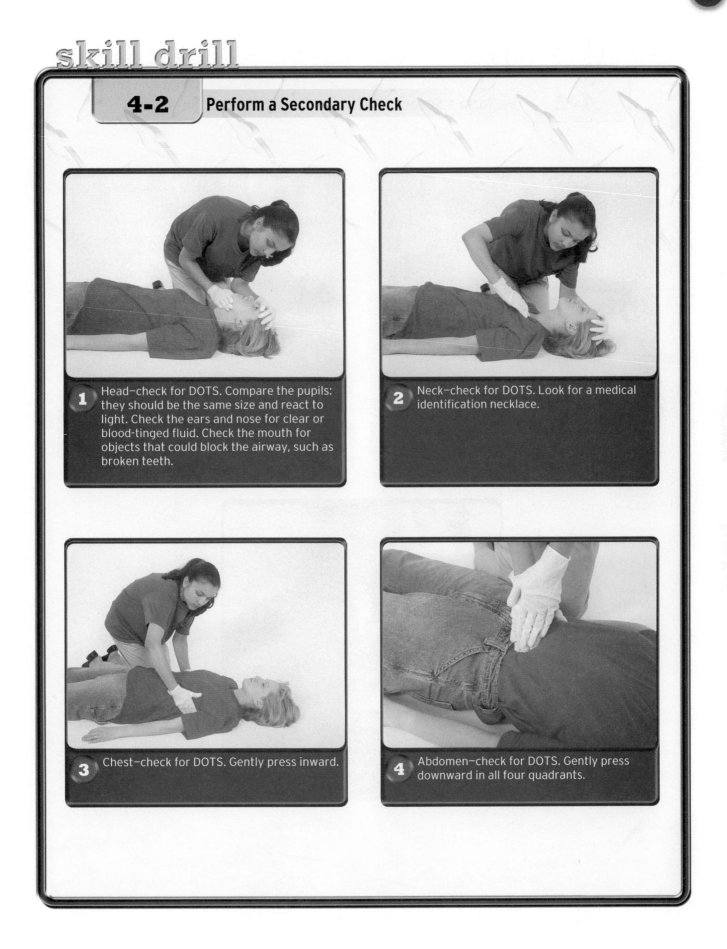

1 Head–check for DOTS. Compare the pupils: they should be the same size and react to light. Check the ears and nose for clear or blood-tinged fluid. Check the mouth for objects that could block the airway, such as broken teeth.

2 Neck–check for DOTS. Look for a medical identification necklace.

3 Chest–check for DOTS. Gently press inward.

4 Abdomen–check for DOTS. Gently press downward in all four quadrants.

4-2   Perform a Secondary Check—Continued

5a Pelvis—check for DOTS. Gently press inward on the tops of the hips.

5b Pelvis—check for DOTS. Gently press downward on the tops of the hips.

6 Extremities—check both arms and legs for DOTS.

7 Back—if no spinal injury is suspected, turn the victim on his or her side and check for DOTS.

unstable position, you may have to stop at that point and stabilize the victim's head and neck manually until more help arrives.

Victim with No Significant Cause of Injury

When a victim has no significant cause (mechanism) of injury, a full body physical exam from head to toe is not needed. Instead, focus the assessment on the chief complaints (the areas that the victim complains about). For most first aiders, this will be the more frequently performed type of assessment.

Special Considerations

Skin Condition

A quick check of the victim's skin can also provide information about the victim's condition. When assessing the head, check skin temperature, color, and moisture. Skin color, especially in light-skinned people, reflects the circulation under the skin as well as oxygen status **Table 4-5**. For those with dark complexions, changes might not be readily apparent but can be assessed by the appearance of the nail beds, the inside of the mouth, and the inner eyelids.

You can get a rough idea of skin temperature by putting the back of your hand or wrist on the victim's

Table 4-6 Skin Temperature

Skin Temperature/ Moisture	Possible Cause
Warm and dry	Normal
Hot and dry or moist	Excessive body heat (heat stroke, high fever)
Cool and moist (clammy)	Poor circulation, heat exhaustion, shock, acute stress reaction
Cold and moist	Body is losing heat
Cold and dry	Exposed to cold and has lost considerable heat (hypothermia)

forehead to determine whether the temperature is elevated or decreased. Dry skin is normal. Skin that is wet, moist, or excessively dry and hot suggests a problem **Table 4-6**.

Capillary Refill Test

Some health care providers use the capillary refill technique to check adequacy of blood circulation in an extremity. It can be performed by gently pressing a fingernail or toenail for a few seconds and then releasing the pressure **Figure 4-3**. When released, the blanched skin should return to its normal color within 2 seconds. (Saying "capillary refill" takes 2 seconds.) Anything more than 2 seconds indicates poor circulation, which needs medical care. Some medical experts question the capillary refill test's reliability in adults because of various factors (eg, exposure to cold, heavy tobacco use, medications, and preexisting medical conditions). It appears to be more accurate in children and infants.

Expose the Injury

Clothing might have to be removed to check for an injury and to give proper first aid. If you need to remove clothing, explain what you intend to do (and why) to the victim and any family members or bystanders. Remove as much clothing as necessary, try to maintain privacy, and prevent exposure to cold. Damage clothing only if necessary—cut along the seams **Figure 4-4**.

Table 4-5 Skin Color

Skin Color	Possible Cause
Pink	Normal color in nonpigmented areas regardless of skin complexion—lining of the eyelids, inside mouth, fingernail beds
Red (flushed)	Dilated blood vessels; excess circulation to that part of the body
White (pale)	Constricted blood vessels from blood loss, shock, hypothermia, emotional distress
Blue (cyanosis)	Lack of oxygen in the blood from breathing or heart problems
Yellow (jaundice)	Liver disease or failure

Figure 4-3

A. To test capillary refill, gently compress the fingertip until it blanches. **B.** Release the fingertip and count until it returns to its normal pink color.

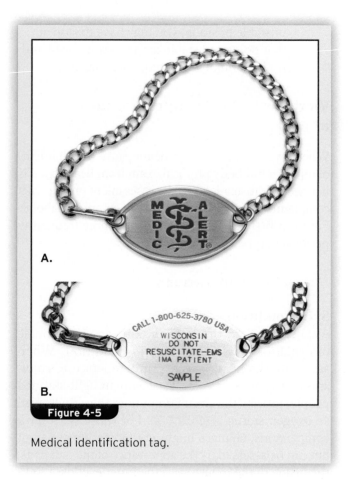

Figure 4-5

Medical identification tag.

Figure 4-4

Expose the injury. Remove as much clothing as necessary, while trying to maintain privacy.

Check for Medical Identification Tags

Look for a medical identification tag or for a medical information card in the victim's wallet or purse (this might be illegal in some states). It can be beneficial in identifying allergies, medications, or medical history **Figure 4-5**. A medical identification tag, worn as a necklace or as a bracelet, contains the wearer's medical problem(s) and a 24-hour telephone number that offers, in case of an emergency, access to the victim's medical history plus names of physicians and close relatives. These can be especially useful when the wearer is unresponsive or not old enough to answer questions. Necklaces and bracelets are durable, instantly recognizable, and less likely than cards to be separated from the victim in an emergency. Always look for victim identification in a wallet or purse in the presence of another person at the scene to protect you against later accusations should money or credit cards be missing.

Table 4-7 SAMPLE History

Description	Questions
S = Symptoms	What's wrong? Where do you hurt? (known as the chief complaint)
A = Allergies	Are you allergic to anything?
M = Medications	Are you taking any prescription or nonprescription medications? What are they for?
P = Past medical history	Have you had this problem before? Have you had recent medical problems?
L = Last oral intake	When did you last eat or drink anything? What was it? How much?
E = Events leading up to the illness or injury	Injury: How did you get hurt? Illness: What led to this problem?

▶ SAMPLE History

The information in a SAMPLE history could help you identify what is wrong with the victim and can indicate the needed first aid. It is called a SAMPLE history because the letters in SAMPLE stand for the elements of the history Table 4-7 .

In the best of circumstances, the victim will be able to answer all questions about his or her chief complaint and medical history. In other cases, this information may be obtained from family, friends, bystanders, medical identification jewelry, or other medical information sources.

▶ What to Do Until Medical Help Is Available

The primary and secondary checks and SAMPLE history are done quickly so that injuries and illnesses can be identified and given first aid. After the most serious problems have been cared for, regularly recheck an alert victim who has a serious injury or illness every 15 minutes, and at least every 5 minutes for an unresponsive victim or one having breathing difficulties, major blood loss, or who has experienced a significant cause of injury. When in doubt, keep checking the victim every 5 minutes or as frequently as possible.

▶ Triage: What to Do With Multiple Victims

You might encounter emergency situations in which there are two or more victims. This is often the case in multiple-car collisions or disasters. After making a quick scene size-up, decide who must be cared for and transported first. This process of prioritizing victims is called **triage**.

Various systems have been used to establish priorities. To find those needing immediate care for life-threatening conditions, tell all victims who can get up and walk to move to a specific area. Victims who can get up and walk rarely have life-threatening injuries. These victims are known as "the walking wounded." Do not force a victim to move if he or she complains of pain.

Find the life-threatened victims by performing only the primary check on all remaining victims. Go to motionless victims first. You must move rapidly (spend less than 60 seconds with each victim) from one victim to the next until all have been checked. Classify victims according to the following care and transportation priorities:

1. **Immediate care.** Victims who have life-threatening injuries but can be saved.
   a. Breathing difficulties (abnormal breath sounds or not breathing)
   b. Severe bleeding
   c. Severe burns
   d. Signs of shock
   e. Open chest or abdominal injuries

2. **Delayed care.** Victims who do not fit into the immediate or "walking wounded" categories. Care and transportation can be delayed up to 1 hour.
3. **Walking wounded.** Victims with minor injuries. Care and transportation can be delayed up to 3 hours.
4. **Dead.** Victims who are obviously dead, or unlikely to survive.

Recheck victims regularly for changes in their condition. Only after those with immediate life-threatening conditions receive care should those with less serious conditions be given care. You will usually be relieved from triage responsibility when more highly trained emergency personnel arrive on the scene. You might then be asked to provide first aid, to help move victims, or to help with ambulance or helicopter transportation.

▶ Ready for Review

- Victim assessment is a sequence of actions that helps determine what is wrong and thus ensures safe and appropriate first aid.
- Every time you encounter a victim, first check out the scene.
- Victim assessment will be influenced by whether the victim is suffering from an illness or an injury, whether the victim is responsive or unresponsive, and whether life-threatening conditions are present.
- The primary check determines whether there are life-threatening problems requiring quick care.
- The goal of a hands-on secondary check is to identify immediately any potentially life-threatening illness or injury.
- Look for medical identification tags on the victim.
- The information in a SAMPLE history can help you identify what is wrong with the victim and can indicate the needed first aid.
- Triage is the process of prioritizing victims.

▶ Vital Vocabulary

AVPU scale A method of assessing a victim's level of responsiveness; used mainly during the primary check. It stands for alert, responsive to verbal stimulus, responsive only to pain, and unresponsive.

cause of injury (COI) The force that causes an injury.

DOTS A mnemonic for assessment in which each area of the body is evaluated for deformities, open wounds, tenderness, and swelling.

first impression The part of the victim assessment that helps identify any immediately or potentially life-threatening conditions.

nature of illness The general type of illness a victim is experiencing.

primary check A step of the victim assessment process in which a first aider checks for life-threatening injuries and gives care for any that are found.

SAMPLE history A brief history of a victim's condition to determine symptoms, allergies, medications, pertinent past history, last oral intake, and event leading to the illness/injury.

scene size-up A quick assessment of the scene and the surroundings for safety issues, the cause of injury or nature of illness, and the number of victims; completed before starting first aid.

secondary check Part of the victim assessment process in which a detailed, area-by-area exam is performed on victims whose problems cannot be readily identified or when more specific information is needed about a problem.

sign Evidence of an injury or disease that can be seen, heard, or felt.

symptom What a victim tells a first aider about what he or she feels.

triage A system of placing priorities for first aid and/or transportation in cases when two or more people are injured or suddenly ill.

▶ Assessment in Action

You are in a crowded mall doing some last-minute holiday shopping. You hear someone yelling for help at a nearby store. You are the first to arrive on the scene. Bystanders begin to approach and ask what is going on. The person who called for help witnessed the victim collapse.

Directions: Circle Yes if you agree with the statement; circle No if you disagree.

Yes No **1.** The first thing you should do is conduct a secondary check.

Yes No **2.** Your primary check of the victim includes identifying and treating immediate life-threatening conditions such as problems with the victim's breathing and severe bleeding.

Yes No **3.** When conducting the secondary check, use the AVPU scale to determine physical injuries.

Yes No **4.** The victim is responsive and alert. Ask permission from him before beginning first aid.

Yes No **5.** The victim asks you to stay until medical help arrives. You should continue to do regular checks of the victim every 15 minutes until medical help arrives.

▶ Check Your Knowledge

Directions: Circle Yes if you agree with the statement; circle No if you disagree.

Yes No **1.** The purpose of a primary check is to find life-threatening conditions.

Yes No **2.** A quiet, motionless victim could indicate a breathing problem.

Yes No **3.** Most injured victims require a complete secondary check.

Yes No **4.** For a secondary check, you usually begin at the head and work down the body.

Yes No **5.** If the victim is not breathing, give two breaths before giving chest compressions.

Yes No **6.** The mnemonic DOTS helps in remembering what information to obtain about the victim's history that could be useful.

Yes No **7.** For all injured and suddenly ill persons, look for a medical identification tag during a secondary check.

Yes No **8.** The mnemonic SAMPLE can remind you how to examine an area for signs of an injury.

Yes No **9.** If there is more than one victim, go to the quiet, motionless victim first.

Yes No **10.** A gurgling sound heard while checking for breathing indicates possible fluid in the throat.

CPR

5

▶ Heart Attack and Cardiac Arrest

A **heart attack** occurs when heart muscle tissue dies because its blood supply is severely reduced or stopped. This often occurs because of a clot in one or more coronary arteries. The signs of a heart attack and the steps for caring for a heart attack are discussed in detail in Chapter 6, *Automated External Defibrillation*.

   If damage to the heart muscle is too severe, the victim's heart can stop beating—a condition known as **cardiac arrest**. Sudden cardiac arrest is a leading cause of death in the United States.

▶ Caring for Cardiac Arrest

Few victims experiencing sudden cardiac arrest outside of a hospital survive unless a rapid sequence of events takes place. One way of describing the ideal sequence of care that should take place when a cardiac arrest occurs is to think about the links in a chain. Each link is dependent on the others for strength and success. In this way, the links form a **chain of survival**.

   The five events (links) that must occur rapidly and in an integrated manner during cardiac arrest are as follows:

1. *Recognition and Action* Recognizing the early warning signs of cardiac arrest and immediately calling 9-1-1 to activate emergency medical services (EMS).

2. *CPR* The chest compressions delivered during **cardiopulmonary resuscitation (CPR)** circulate blood to the heart and brain. Effective chest compressions are critical to buying time until a defibrillator and EMS personnel are available.

3. *Defibrillation* Administering a shock to the heart can restore the heartbeat in some victims. Time is a critical factor. The earlier the shock, the better the chance of success.

4. *Advanced Care* Paramedics provide advanced cardiac life support to victims of sudden cardiac arrest. This includes providing IV fluids, medications, advanced airway devices, and rapid transportation to the hospital.

5. *Post-Arrest Care* The hospital can provide life-saving medications, surgical procedures, and advanced medical care to enable the victim of sudden cardiac arrest to survive and recover.

FYI

Risk Factors of Cardiovascular Disease

Several factors contribute to an increased risk of developing heart disease. Risk factors you cannot change are as follows:

- **Heredity:** Tendencies appear in family lines.
- **Gender:** Men have a greater risk. After menopause, the death rate from heart disease in women increases. Coronary heart disease is the leading cause of death in American men and women.
- **Age:** Over 80% of those who die of heart disease are 65 years or older.

Risk factors you can change are as follows:

- **Tobacco smoking:** Smokers have a two to four times greater chance of developing heart disease than nonsmokers.
- **High blood pressure:** This condition increases the heart's workload.
- **High cholesterol:** Too much cholesterol can cause a buildup in the walls of the arteries.
- **Diabetes:** This condition affects blood cholesterol and triglyceride levels.
- **Overweight and obesity:** Excess body fat, especially around the waist, increases the likelihood of developing heart disease. Being overweight affects blood pressure and cholesterol and places an added strain on the heart.

▶ Performing CPR

When a victim's heart stops beating, he or she needs CPR, defibrillation, and EMS professionals quickly. CPR consists of moving blood to the heart and brain by giving **chest compressions** and providing periodic breaths to place oxygen into the victim's lungs. CPR techniques are similar for infants (birth to 1 year), children (1 year to puberty), and adults (puberty and older), with just slight variations.

Q&A

For CPR purposes, what defines an adult, child, and infant victim?

- Infants are those less than 1 year of age.
- A child ranges from 1 year to puberty. (Puberty can be recognized by hair in the armpits of males and breast development in females.)
- Adults include those at puberty and older.

Check for Responsiveness and Breathing

In a motionless victim, check for responsiveness by tapping the victim's shoulder and asking if he or she is okay. If the victim does not respond (ie, answers, moves, or moans), he or she is said to be unresponsive.

At the same time you check for responsiveness, you should look at the victim to see whether he or she is breathing. If the victim is not breathing or is only gasping, EMS professionals are needed. Ask a bystander to call 9-1-1. If you are alone with an adult victim and a phone is nearby, call 9-1-1 yourself. If you are alone with a child or infant, give CPR for five cycles of 30 compressions and two breaths (2 minutes); then call 9-1-1.

Give Chest Compressions

Chest compressions are the most important step in CPR and, whenever possible, should be performed on a firm, flat surface. Perform chest compressions with two hands for an adult, one or two hands for a child, and two fingers for an infant. Effective compressions require rescuers to push hard and push fast. The chest of an adult should be compressed at least 2″; the chest of a child about 2″; and the chest of an infant about 1½″. The desired hand position for chest compressions is in the center of the chest (lower half of the sternum [breast bone]) **Figure 5-1**.

Give compressions at a rate of at least 100 compressions per minute for adults, children, and infants. The 100-compression rate is not the actual number of compressions given in a minute; it is the speed of compressions. Give 30 compressions in about 18 seconds and then give two rescue breaths. Continue CPR until an automated external defibrillator (AED) becomes available, the victim shows signs of life, EMS personnel take over, or you are too tired to continue. Interruptions in compressions should be kept to a minimum. If other rescuers are available, they can rotate performing chest compressions after every five cycles of 30 compressions and two breaths (2 minutes) or after an AED delivers a shock.

Give Rescue Breaths

Tilt the victim's head back and lift the chin to open the airway **Figure 5-2**. This moves the tongue away from the back of the throat. Lay rescuers should use this

Figure 5-1

The hand position for chest compressions is in the center of the chest.

Figure 5-2

Tilt the victim's head back and lift the chin to open the airway.

Rescue Breaths

Other methods of rescue breathing are as follows:
- Mouth-to-breathing device
- Mouth-to-nose method
- Mouth-to-stoma method

Mouth-to-Breathing Device
A breathing device is placed in the victim's mouth or over the victim's mouth and nose as a precaution against disease transmission. There are several different types of barrier devices **Figure 5-3**.

Mouth-to-Nose Method
If you cannot open the victim's mouth, the victim's mouth is severely injured, or you cannot make a good seal with the victim's mouth (for example, because there are no teeth), use the mouth-to-nose method. With the head tilted back, push up on the victim's chin to close the mouth. Make a seal with your mouth over the victim's nose and provide rescue breaths.

Mouth-to-Stoma Method
Some diseases of the vocal cords may result in surgical removal of the larynx. People who have this surgery breathe through a small permanent opening in the neck called a stoma. To perform mouth-to-stoma breathing, close the victim's mouth and nose and breathe through the opening in the neck.

Figure 5-3

Barrier devices.

method for all victims—even for those with a possible spinal injury. With the airway open, pinch the victim's nose and make a tight seal over the victim's mouth with your mouth. Give one breath lasting 1 second, take a normal breath for yourself, and then give the victim another breath lasting 1 second. Each rescue breath should make the victim's chest rise. Rescue breaths can cause stomach distention. Minimize this problem by limiting the force of your breath—you need only to make the victim's chest gently rise.

Adult CPR

To perform adult CPR, follow the steps in **Skill Drill 5-1**.

Child CPR

To perform CPR on a child, follow the steps in **Skill Drill 5-2**.

Infant CPR

To perform CPR on an infant, follow the steps in **Skill Drill 5-3**.

▶ Airway Obstruction

People can choke on all kinds of objects. Foods such as candy, peanuts, and grapes are major offenders because of their shapes and consistencies. Nonfood choking deaths are often caused by balloons, balls and marbles, toys, and coins inhaled by children and infants.

Recognizing Airway Obstruction

An object lodged in the airway can cause a mild or severe **airway obstruction**. In a mild airway obstruction, good air exchange is present. The victim is able to make forceful coughing efforts in an attempt to relieve the obstruction. The victim should be encouraged to cough.

A victim with a severe airway obstruction will have poor air exchange. The signs of a severe airway obstruction include the following:

- Breathing becomes more difficult
- Weak and ineffective cough
- Inability to speak or breathe
- Skin, fingernail beds, and the inside of the mouth appear bluish gray (indicating cyanosis)

Choking victims may clutch their necks to communicate that they are choking **Figure 5-4**. This motion is known as the universal distress signal for choking. The victim becomes panicked and desperate.

Figure 5-4

The universal sign of choking.

Caring for Airway Obstruction

For a responsive adult or child with a severe airway obstruction, ask the victim "Are you choking?" If the victim is unable to respond, but nods yes, provide care for the victim. Move behind the victim and reach around the victim's waist with both arms. Place a fist with the thumb side against the victim's abdomen, just above the navel. Grasp the fist with your other hand and press into the abdomen with quick inward and upward thrusts (Heimlich maneuver). Continue thrusts until the object is removed or the victim becomes unresponsive. If a rescuer is unable to encircle an obese victim's abdomen, chest thrusts should be applied. For a choking pregnant woman in the late stages of pregnancy, the rescuer should use chest thrusts instead of abdominal thrusts.

To relieve airway obstruction in a responsive adult or child who cannot speak, breathe, or cough, follow the steps in **Skill Drill 5-4**.

For a responsive infant with a severe airway obstruction, give back blows and chest compressions instead of abdominal thrusts to relieve the obstruction. Support the infant's head and neck and lay the infant face down on your forearm, then lower your arm to your leg. Give five back blows between the infant's shoulder blades with the heel of your hand. While supporting the back of the infant's head, roll the infant face up and give five chest compressions with two fingers on the infant's sternum in the same location used for CPR. Repeat these steps until the object is removed or the infant becomes unresponsive.

To relieve airway obstruction in a responsive infant who cannot cry, breathe, or cough, follow the steps in **Skill Drill 5-5**.

skill drill

5-1 Adult CPR

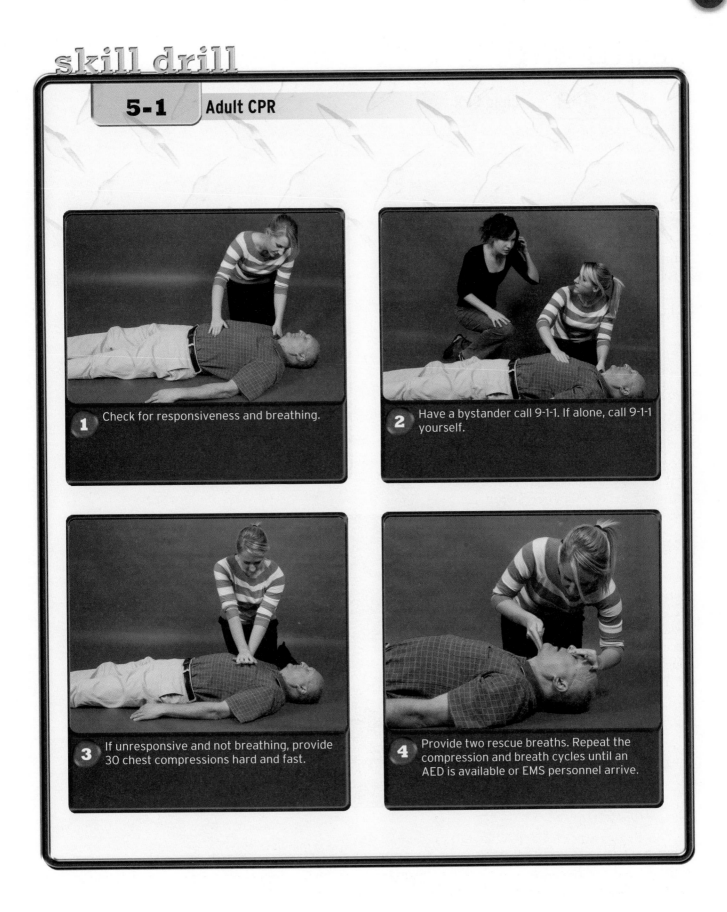

1 Check for responsiveness and breathing.

2 Have a bystander call 9-1-1. If alone, call 9-1-1 yourself.

3 If unresponsive and not breathing, provide 30 chest compressions hard and fast.

4 Provide two rescue breaths. Repeat the compression and breath cycles until an AED is available or EMS personnel arrive.

skill drill

5-2 Child CPR

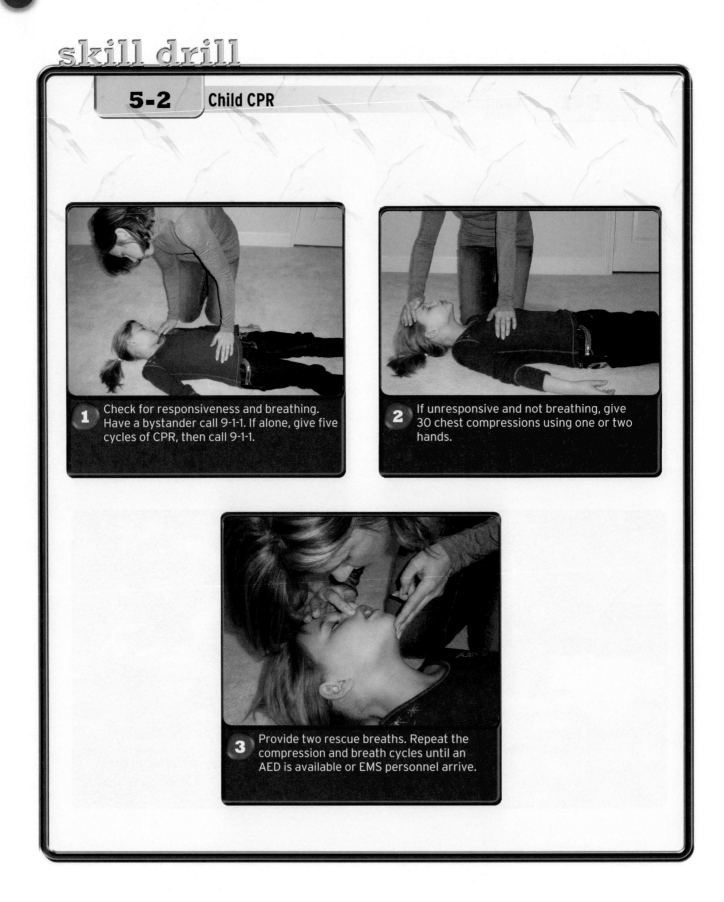

1 Check for responsiveness and breathing. Have a bystander call 9-1-1. If alone, give five cycles of CPR, then call 9-1-1.

2 If unresponsive and not breathing, give 30 chest compressions using one or two hands.

3 Provide two rescue breaths. Repeat the compression and breath cycles until an AED is available or EMS personnel arrive.

skill drill

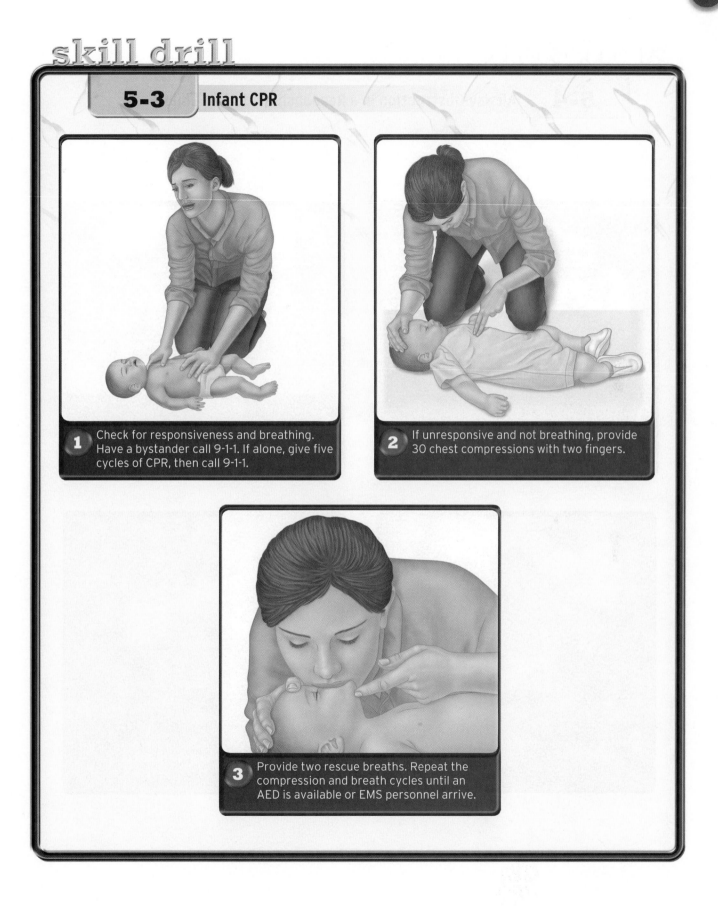

5-3 Infant CPR

1 Check for responsiveness and breathing. Have a bystander call 9-1-1. If alone, give five cycles of CPR, then call 9-1-1.

2 If unresponsive and not breathing, provide 30 chest compressions with two fingers.

3 Provide two rescue breaths. Repeat the compression and breath cycles until an AED is available or EMS personnel arrive.

skill drill

5-4 Airway Obstruction in a Responsive Adult or Child

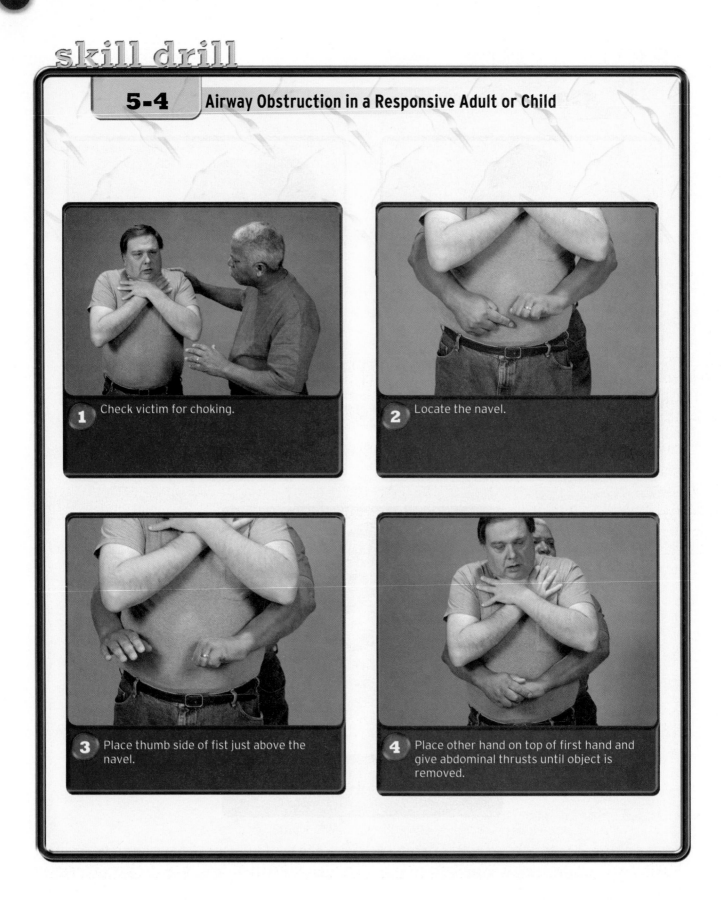

1 Check victim for choking.

2 Locate the navel.

3 Place thumb side of fist just above the navel.

4 Place other hand on top of first hand and give abdominal thrusts until object is removed.

skill drill

5-5   Airway Obstruction in a Responsive Infant

1 Support the infant's head, neck, and back. Give five back blows.

2 Give five chest compressions.

CPR and Airway Obstruction Review

CPR
These steps are the same for all victims regardless of age:
1. Check for responsiveness and look for signs of breathing and gasping.
   - If the victim is unresponsive and has normal breathing, place the victim in the recovery position, and have someone call 9-1-1.
   - If the victim is unresponsive and has abnormal breathing (not breathing or only gasping), have someone call 9-1-1, and retrieve an AED if available. Perform Steps 2 through 5.
2. Provide chest compressions:
   - Give 30 chest compressions in the center of the victim's chest.
3. Open the airway:
   - Tilt the victim's head back and lift the chin.
4. Give 2 breaths:
   - Each breath lasts 1 second to produce visible chest rise.
5. Continue CPR until an AED is available, EMS personnel take over, or the victim starts to move.

Airway Obstruction
For responsive adults and children (anyone older than 1 year):
1. Check for choking.
2. Provide abdominal thrusts (Heimlich maneuver).

For responsive infants (birth to 1 year):
1. Support the infant's head, neck, and back.
2. Alternate five back blows followed by five chest compressions repeatedly.

If a choking victim becomes unresponsive, immediately call 9-1-1 and begin CPR. Each time the airway is opened during CPR, the rescuer should look for an object in the victim's mouth and, if seen, remove it.

Q&A

What are the types of upper airway obstruction?

- **Tongue.** Unconsciousness produces relaxation of soft tissues, and the tongue can fall into the airway. "Swallowing one's tongue" is impossible, but the widespread belief that it can happen is explained by slippage of the relaxed tongue into the airway. The tongue is the most common cause of airway obstruction.

- **Foreign body.** People, especially children, inhale all kinds of objects. Foods such as hot dogs, candy, peanuts, and grapes are major offenders because of their shapes and consistencies. Meat is the main cause of choking in adults. Balloons are the top cause of nonfood choking deaths in children, followed by balls, marbles, toys, and coins. Unconscious victims' airways can also be obstructed by a foreign body such as vomit and teeth.

- **Swelling.** Severe allergic reactions (anaphylaxis) and irritants (eg, smoke, chemicals) can cause swelling. Even a nonallergic person who is stung inside the throat by a bee, yellow jacket, or other flying insect can experience swelling in the airway.

- **Spasm.** Water that is suddenly inhaled can cause a spasm in the throat.

- **Vomit.** Many people vomit when they are at or near death. Whenever performing CPR, expect vomit before or during CPR.

FYI

The Tongue and Airway Obstruction

Airway obstruction in an unresponsive victim lying on his or her back is usually the result of the tongue relaxing in the back of the mouth, restricting air movement. Opening the airway with the head tilt–chin lift method may be all that is needed to correct this problem.

Q&A

Why change the sequence from A-B-C to C-A-B?

Chest compressions are critical to resuscitating a cardiac arrest victim. The A-B-C sequence involved opening the airway, giving rescue breaths, and perhaps getting and placing a mouth-to-barrier device. This delayed the giving of chest compressions. The C-A-B shortens the time for giving the first chest compressions. Giving chest compressions first may also encourage rescuers to begin CPR, because most victims of out-of-hospital cardiac arrest do not receive any bystander CPR.

Q&A

Why isn't the pulse checked?

Studies show that lay rescuers as well as health care providers take too long to check for a pulse and have difficulty determining whether a pulse is present. Taking too long delays giving chest compressions.

Lay Rescuer Adult CPR

Use the mnemonic **RAP-CAB** to remember what to do. Start as soon as possible!

R: Responsive? Tap shoulder and shout, "Are you OK?" Check for breathing and gasping.	
If ...	Then ...
Unresponsive and gasping or not breathing	Go to next step (A). Gasping is a sign of cardiac arrest.
Unresponsive and breathing normally	Place victim in recovery position (on victim's side with lower arm in front of body). For a suspected spinal injury, extend arm above head and roll body to the side so victim's head rests on extended arm.

A: Activate EMS. Call 9-1-1.	
If ...	Then ...
Alone	Immediately call 9-1-1 (EMS) and get AED, if available. Then, return to the victim to attach and use AED.
Second rescuer is available	While one calls 9-1-1 and gets an AED, if available, the other goes to steps (P) and (C).

P: Position victim on back, on a flat, firm surface.

C: Chest compressions. Push hard and fast.

Where to place hands?	How deep?	How fast?	How many?
Place the heel of your hand in center of chest with the other hand on top and fingers interlaced.	Push down on chest at least 2″. Allow chest to recoil completely before the next compression.	Push chest at rate of at least 100 pushes per minute (the same beat of the Bee Gee's song, "Stayin' Alive").	Give 30 compressions without interruption unless AED arrives. (AED should be used immediately.)

A: Airway open. Open the victim's airway using the head tilt–chin lift method for all victims.

B: Breaths. Pinch the victim's nose and make an airtight mouth-to-mouth seal. Use a CPR mask if available. Give two breaths (1 second each) that make chest rise.

If ...	Then ...
Two breaths make chest rise	Begin CPR: • 30 compressions (push hard and fast). • Two breaths (1 second each). Take a regular breath, not a deep breath, between the two breaths. • Continue 30:2 compression-breath ratio until AED arrives and is ready to use, or until trained person or EMS provider takes over. • Do not stop to check for breathing.
First breath does not make chest rise; the airway may be blocked.	Retilt head, give a second breath: • If second breath does not make chest rise, begin CPR (30 compressions and two breaths). Each time the airway is opened during CPR, look for an object in the victim's mouth and, if found, remove it.

Quick Review of Lay Rescuer Basic Life Support Using the RAP-CAB Steps

Steps/Action	Adults (at or above puberty)	Child (1 year to puberty)	Infant (<1 year)
R = Responsive?			
Technique	Tap shoulder and shout "Are you Ok?" If the victim does not answer, move, or moan, he/she is unresponsive.		
Breathing?	If not breathing or only gasping, CPR is needed. If normal breathing is seen, no CPR is needed; place in recovery position and monitor breathing.		
A = Activate Emergency Medical Service (EMS) and get AED (if nearby and accessible; use as soon as possible)			
When	If one rescuer: Call immediately If two rescuers: One calls immediately	If one rescuer: Call after five cycles (2 minutes) of CPR If two rescuers: One calls immediately	
Who to call	In a community: Call 9-1-1 In a facility or institution: Call its emergency number		
P = Position on back (on firm, flat surface)			
C = Chest compressions			
Where to place hand	Center of chest		Two fingers, with one touching and below nipple line
Technique: • Push hard and fast • Allow complete recoil	Two hands: Heel of one hand on breastbone; other hand on top	One hand: Heel of one hand only Two hands: Heel of one hand with second on top	Two fingers
Depth	At least 2" (5 cm)	About 2" (5 cm)	At least 1½" (4 cm)
Rate	At least 100 per minute (same beat as the Bee Gee's song, "Stayin' Alive")		
Ratio of chest compressions to breaths	30:2		
A = Airway open			
Technique	Head tilt-chin lift		

Steps/Action	Adults (at or above puberty)	Child (1 year to puberty)	Infant (<1 year)
B = Breaths			

Technique	• Pinch nose and make airtight mouth-to-mouth seal
	• Give two breaths:
	  • Each breath lasting 1 second
	  • Blow enough to make chest rise
	• If first breath does not cause chest to rise, retilt head and give second breath. If second breath does not make chest rise, begin CPR (30 compressions and two breaths). Each time the airway is opened, look for an object in mouth and, if seen, remove it.
			• Cover the infant's mouth and nose with your mouth, making an airtight seal. If this does not work, try either mouth-to-mouth or mouth-to-nose
			• Same procedures as for an adult and child.

Continue CPR until:
1. Victim begins breathing
2. Other rescuer(s) (ie, trained lay person, EMS personnel) take over
3. AED arrives and is used
4. Rescuer is physically exhausted and unable to continue

Defibrillation

• Use AED as soon as possible.
• Expose chest, turn on AED, attach appropriate pads.
• Follow voice directions.

If no shock advised	Resume CPR immediately (five sets of 30 compressions and two breaths)
If shock advised	Do not touch victim; give one shock. Or, shock as advised by AED. Resume immediately 30 compressions and two breaths.

prep kit

chest compressions Depressing the chest and allowing it to return to its normal position as part of CPR.

CPR Cardiopulmonary resuscitation; the act of providing chest compressions and rescue breaths for a victim in cardiac arrest.

heart attack Death of a part of the heart muscle.

▶ Ready for Review

- A heart attack occurs when heart muscle tissue dies because the blood supply is severely reduced or stopped.
- The five links in the chain of survival are: recognition and action, CPR, defibrillation, advanced care, and post-arrest care.
- CPR consists of moving blood to the heart and brain by giving chest compressions and breathing oxygen into a victim's lungs.
- The signs of a severe airway obstruction include difficult breathing, weak and ineffective cough, inability to speak or breathe, and signs of cyanosis.

▶ Vital Vocabulary

airway obstruction A blockage, often the result of a foreign body, in which air flow to the lungs is reduced or completely blocked.

cardiac arrest Stoppage of the heartbeat.

chain of survival A concept involving five critical links to help improve survival from cardiac arrest.

▶ Assessment in Action

You are having dinner in a very crowded restaurant with your family on New Year's Eve. An elderly man is pushing a piano into the restaurant as part of the entertainment that evening. As he passes your table, he clutches his chest and falls to the floor. He is not moving.

Directions: Circle Yes if you agree with the statement; circle No if you disagree.

Yes　No　**1.** If he is not breathing or is breathing abnormally, you should next call 9-1-1.

Yes　No　**2.** The man must be choking since he is in a restaurant.

Yes　No　**3.** Perform abdominal thrusts.

Yes　No　**4.** Perform cycles of 30 chest compressions and 2 breaths.

Yes　No　**5.** Check for breathing before giving any breaths to the victim.

Yes　No　**6.** Continue CPR until an AED becomes available or EMS personnel arrive.

▶ Check Your Knowledge

Directions: Circle Yes if you agree with the statement; circle No if you disagree.

Yes   No   **1.** Gasping is not considered breathing.

Yes   No   **2.** After you determine that an adult victim is unresponsive, the next step is for someone to call 9-1-1.

Yes   No   **3.** Tilting the head back and lifting the chin helps move the tongue and open the airway.

Yes   No   **4.** If you determine that a victim is not breathing, begin chest compressions.

Yes   No   **5.** Do not start chest compressions until you have checked for a pulse.

Yes   No   **6.** For all victims (adult, child, infant) needing CPR, give 30 compressions followed by two breaths.

Yes   No   **7.** Use two fingers when performing CPR on an infant.

Yes   No   **8.** A sign of choking is that the victim is unable to speak or cough.

Yes   No   **9.** To give abdominal thrusts to a responsive choking victim, place your fist below the victim's navel.

Yes   No   **10.** When giving abdominal thrusts to a responsive choking victim, repeat the thrusts until the object is removed or the victim becomes unresponsive.

Automated External Defibrillation

6

▶ Public Access Defibrillation

A victim's chance of survival dramatically improves through early cardiopulmonary resuscitation (CPR) and early <u>defibrillation</u> with the use of an <u>**automated external defibrillator (AED)**</u>. To be effective, defibrillation must be used in the first few minutes following cardiac arrest. The implementation of state public access defibrillation (PAD) laws and the Food and Drug Administration's (FDA) approval of "home use" AEDs have made this important care step available to many rescuers in many places, including the following :

- Airports and airplanes
- Stadiums
- Health clubs
- Golf courses
- Schools
- Government buildings
- Offices
- Homes
- Shopping centers/malls

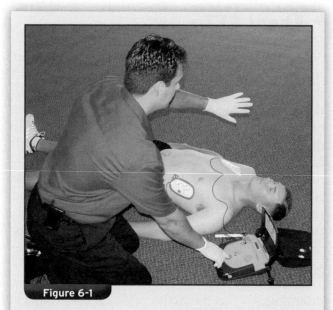

Figure 6-1

AEDs are available in many places for use by trained rescuers.

▶ How the Heart Works

The heart is an organ with four hollow chambers. The two chambers on the right side receive blood from the body and send it to the lungs for oxygen. The two chambers on the left side of the heart receive freshly oxygenated blood from the lungs and send it back out to the body **Figure 6-2**.

The heart has a unique electrical system that controls the rate at which the heart beats and the amount of work the heart performs. In the right upper chamber of the heart, there is a collection of special pacemaker cells. These cells emit electrical impulses about 60 to 100 times a minute that cause the other heart muscle cells to contract in a coordinated manner.

Because the heart contracts approximately every second, it needs an abundant supply of oxygen, which it gets through the coronary arteries. These arteries run along the outside of the heart muscle and branch into smaller vessels. These arteries sometimes become diseased (atherosclerosis), resulting in a lack of oxygen to the pacemaker cells, which can cause abnormal electrical activity in the heart.

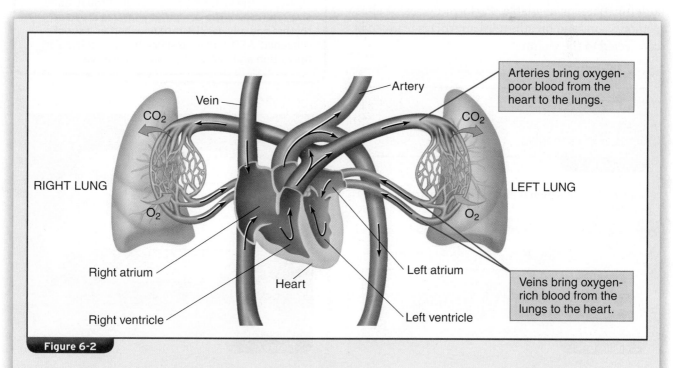

Vein

Artery

CO_2

RIGHT LUNG

O_2

Arteries bring oxygen-poor blood from the heart to the lungs.

CO_2

LEFT LUNG

O_2

Right atrium

Heart

Left atrium

Right ventricle

Left ventricle

Veins bring oxygen-rich blood from the lungs to the heart.

Figure 6-2

The right side of the heart receives blood from the body and sends it to the lungs. The left side of the heart receives the oxygenated blood and sends it to the body.

When Normal Electrical Activity Is Interrupted

Ventricular fibrillation (also known as *V-fib*) is the most common abnormal heart rhythm in cases of sudden cardiac arrest in adults **Figure 6-3**.

The organized wave of electrical impulses that cause the heart muscle to contract and relax in a regular fashion is lost when the heart is in ventricular fibrillation. As a result, the lower chambers of the heart quiver and cannot pump blood, so circulation is lost (no pulse).

A second, potentially life-threatening, electrical problem is ventricular tachycardia (*V-tach*), in which the heart beats too fast to pump blood effectively **Figure 6-4**.

▶ Care for Cardiac Arrest

When the heart stops beating, the blood stops circulating, cutting off all oxygen and nourishment to the entire body. In this situation, time is a crucial factor. For every minute that defibrillation is delayed, the victim's chance of survival decreases by 7% to 10% **Figure 6-5**.

CPR is the initial care for cardiac arrest until a defibrillator is available. Perform cycles of chest compressions and breaths until an AED is ready to be connected to the victim.

▶ About AEDs

An AED is an electronic device that analyzes the heart rhythm and if necessary (such as in cardiac arrest) delivers an electric shock, known as defibrillation, to the heart. The purpose of this shock is to correct one of the abnormal electrical disturbances previously discussed and to reestablish a heart rhythm that will result in normal electrical and pumping function.

All AEDs are attached to the victim by a cable connected to two adhesive pads (electrodes) placed on the victim's chest. The pad and cable system sends the electrical signal from the heart into the device for analysis and delivers the electric shock to the victim when needed **Figure 6-6**.

AEDs have built-in rhythm analysis systems that determine whether the victim needs a shock. This system enables first aiders and other rescuers to deliver early defibrillation with only minimal training.

AEDs also record the victim's heart rhythm (known as an electrocardiogram, or ECG), shock data,

Q&A

How does an AED work?

A microprocessor inside the defibrillator interprets (analyzes) the victim's heart rhythm through adhesive electrodes. The computer analyzes the heart rhythm and advises the rescuer whether a shock is needed. AEDs advise a shock to only ventricular fibrillation and fast ventricular tachycardia.

Figure 6-3

Ventricular fibrillation is disorganized electrical activity.

Figure 6-4

Ventricular tachycardia is very rapid electrical activity.

Figure 6-5

A victim's chance of survival decreases with every minute that passes without proper care.

Figure 6-6

Two adhesive pads are placed on the victim's chest and connected by a cable to the AED.

Figure 6-7

AEDs store data, including heart rhythms and shocks.

and other information about the device's performance (for example, the date, time, and number of shocks supplied) **Figure 6-7**.

Common Elements of AEDs

Many different AED models exist. The principles for use are the same for each, but the displays, controls, and options vary slightly. You will need to know how to use your specific AED. All AEDs have the following elements in common:

- Power on/off mechanism
- Cable and pads (electrodes)
- Analysis capability

- Defibrillation capability
- Prompts to guide you
- Battery operation for portability

▶ Using an AED

Once you have determined the need for the AED (victim unresponsive and not breathing), the basic operation of all AED models follows the sequence in **Skill Drill 6-1**.

1. Some AEDs power on by pressing an on/off button. Others power on when opening the AED case lid. Once the power is on, the AED will quickly go through some internal checks and will then begin to provide voice and screen prompts **(Step ❶)**.

2. Expose the victim's chest. The skin must be fairly dry so that the pads will adhere and conduct electricity properly. If necessary, dry the skin with a towel. Because excessive chest hair may also interfere with adhesion and electrical conduction, you may need to shave quickly the area where the pads are to be placed.

3. Remove the backing from the pads and apply them firmly to the victim's bare chest according to the diagram on the pads **(Step ❷)**. One pad is placed to the right of the breastbone, just below the collarbone and above the right nipple. The second pad is placed on the left side of the chest, left of the nipple and above the lower rib margin.

4. Make sure the cable is attached to the AED, and stand clear for analysis of the heart's electrical activity **(Step ❸)**. No one should be in contact with the victim at this time, or later if a shock is indicated.

Q&A

Will I get zapped if a victim is shocked in the rain or near water?

It is remotely possible to get shocked or to shock bystanders if there is standing water around and under the victim. Try to move the victim to a dry area and cut off wet clothing. Also be sure that the skin has been dried off so that the electrode pads will stick to the skin. No one should be touching any part of the victim while the device emits an electrical current.

skill drill

6-1   Using an AED

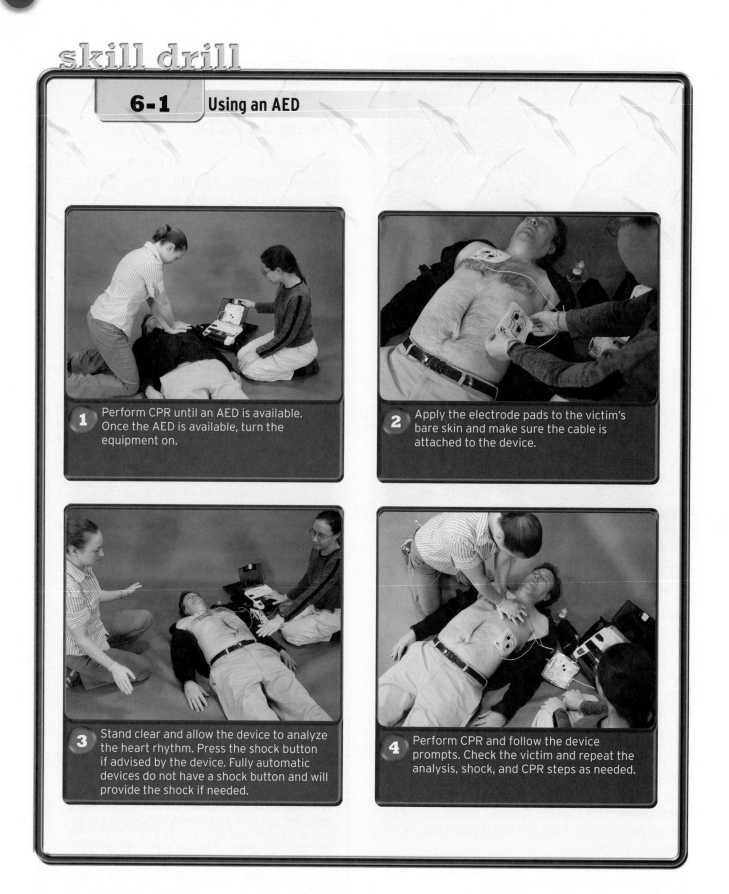

1 Perform CPR until an AED is available. Once the AED is available, turn the equipment on.

2 Apply the electrode pads to the victim's bare skin and make sure the cable is attached to the device.

3 Stand clear and allow the device to analyze the heart rhythm. Press the shock button if advised by the device. Fully automatic devices do not have a shock button and will provide the shock if needed.

4 Perform CPR and follow the device prompts. Check the victim and repeat the analysis, shock, and CPR steps as needed.

5. Verify that no one is in contact with the victim. The AED will advise of the need to shock and, depending on the device, will either advise the rescuer to push a button to administer the shock, or will deliver the shock automatically. Begin CPR immediately following the shock and follow the prompts that include reanalyzing the rhythm **(Step ❹)**. If the shock worked, the victim may begin to regain signs of life. Continue providing care until EMS personnel arrive and take over.

▶ Special Considerations

There are several special situations that you should be aware of when using an AED. These include the following:

- Water
- Children
- Medication patches
- Implanted devices

Water

Because water conducts electricity, it may provide an energy pathway between the AED and the rescuer or bystanders. Remove the victim from free-standing water. Quickly dry the chest before applying the pads. The risk to the rescuers and bystanders is very low if the chest is dry and the pads are secured to the chest.

Children

Cardiac arrest in children is usually caused by an airway or breathing problem, rather than a primary heart problem as in adults. AEDs can deliver energy levels appropriate for children aged 1 year or older. If your AED has special pediatric pads and cable, use these for the child **Figure 6-8**. If the pediatric equipment is not available, use the adult equipment.

AED Use on an Infant

For infants (children younger than 1 year), a manual defibrillator can be used. If a manual defibrillator is not available, an AED with a pediatric dose attenuation can be used. If neither is available, an AED without a dose attenuator may be used.

Figure 6-8

If your AED has pediatric pads, use them according to the manufacturer's instructions.

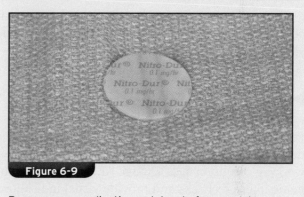

Figure 6-9

Remove any medication patches before applying AED pads.

Medication Patches

Some people wear an adhesive patch containing medication (such as nitroglycerin, nicotine, or pain medication) that is absorbed through the skin. Because these patches may block the delivery of energy from the pads to the heart, they need to be removed and the skin wiped dry before attaching the AED pads **Figure 6-9**.

Implanted Devices

Implanted pacemakers and defibrillators are small devices placed underneath the skin of people with certain types of heart disease **Figure 6-10**. These devices can often be seen or felt when the chest is exposed. Avoid placing the pads directly over these devices whenever possible. If an implanted defibrillator is

Figure 6-10

Implanted defibrillator.

Figure 6-11

Periodic inspection of your AED supplies can ensure that all items are in working condition.

discharging, you may see the victim twitching periodically. Allow the implanted unit to stop before using your AED.

▶ AED Maintenance

Periodic inspection of your AED can ensure that the device has the necessary supplies and is in proper working condition **Figure 6-11**. AEDs conduct automatic internal checks and provide visual indications that the unit is ready and functioning properly. You do not need to turn the device on daily to check it as part of any inspection. Doing so will only wear down the battery.

AED supplies should include items such as the following:

- Two sets of electrode pads with expiration dates that are not expired
- An extra battery
- Razor
- Hand towel

Other items that should be considered are a breathing device (for example, a mask or shield) and exam gloves.

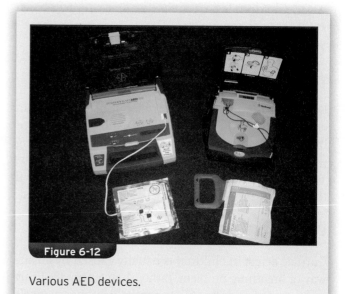

Figure 6-12

Various AED devices.

▶ AED Manufacturers

AED devices and related supplies are available from different manufacturers **Figure 6-12**.

▶ Emergency Care Wrap-up

Condition	What to Look For	What to Do
Cardiac arrest	• Unresponsiveness	1. Perform CPR until an AED is available. 2. Turn on the AED. 3. Apply the pads. 4. Analyze the heart rhythm. 5. Administer a shock if needed. 6. Perform CPR for five cycles (2 minutes). 7. Reanalyze and follow prompts.

AED Skill Checklist

Student's Name _____ Date _____

Skills	Satisfactory	Unsatisfactory
Check for Scene Safety	○	○

Primary check and care:
If two rescuers are involved, one assesses and performs CPR while the other applies the AED.

Skills	Satisfactory	Unsatisfactory
• Establish unresponsiveness and breathing status (not breathing or is gasping).	○	○
• Begin 30 chest compressions (regardless of the compression number, interrupt compressions to apply an AED when it arrives).	○	○
• Open airway.	○	○
• Give two breaths (1 second each).	○	○
• Continue cycles of 30 compressions and two breaths until an AED becomes available.	○	○

Defibrillation:

Skills	Satisfactory	Unsatisfactory
• Turn AED power on.	○	○
• Ensure skin surface is dry.	○	○
• Apply electrode pads correctly.	○	○
• Ensure electrode cable is plugged in.	○	○
• Stand clear while analyzing.	○	○
• If shock is indicated:	○	○
a. Remain clear.	○	○
b. Deliver shock.	○	○
c. Perform 2 minutes of CPR.	○	○
d. Reanalyze.	○	○
• If shock is indicated, repeat steps a through d.	○	○
• If no shock is indicated:	○	○
a. Check victim for breathing.	○	○
b. If victim is not breathing, perform 2 minutes of CPR and reanalyze.	○	○

Pass _____   Fail _____

▶ Ready for Review

- A victim's chances for survival are dramatically improved through early CPR and early defibrillation.
- Because the heart contracts approximately every second, it needs an abundant supply of oxygen.
- CPR is the initial care for cardiac arrest until a defibrillator is available.
- An AED is an electronic device that analyzes the heart rhythm and delivers an electrical shock to the heart of a person in cardiac arrest.
- There are several special situations to be aware of when using an AED, including: water, children, medication patches, and implanted devices.
- Periodic inspection of the AED can ensure that the device has the necessary supplies and is in proper working condition.

▶ Vital Vocabulary

<u>automated external defibrillator (AED)</u> Device capable of analyzing the heart rhythm and providing a shock.

<u>defibrillation</u> The electrical shock administered by an AED to reestablish a normal heart rhythm.

▶ Assessment in Action

Your workplace has recently implemented an AED program. You and several other employees have been trained to locate and use an AED. While at work, a coworker collapses. She is around 50 years old and you know she has a history of heart problems. You tell a coworker to call 9-1-1 and to bring the AED.

Directions: Circle Yes if you agree with the statement; circle No if you disagree.

Yes   No   **1.** You should establish unresponsiveness before starting anything else.

Yes   No   **2.** Chest compressions should begin as soon as possible and stop only to apply the AED pads to the chest or to give two breaths.

Yes   No   **3.** AED pads can be applied over the top of the victim's blouse.

Yes   No   **4.** The AED will alert you about improper pad placement and connection.

Yes   No   **5.** You should deliver a shock even if the AED has not alerted you to do so.

▶ Check Your Knowledge

Directions: Circle Yes if you agree with the statement; circle No if you disagree.

Yes   No   **1.** The earlier defibrillation occurs, the better the victim's chance of survival.

Yes   No   **2.** An AED is to be applied only to a victim who is unresponsive and not breathing.

Yes   No   **3.** CPR is not needed if you are sure an AED will be available in 3 to 4 minutes.

Yes   No   **4.** AEDs require the operator to know how to interpret heart rhythms.

Yes   No   **5.** Because all AEDs are different, the basic steps of operation are also different.

Yes   No   **6.** The AED pads (electrodes) need to be attached to a dry chest.

Yes   No   **7.** Two electrode pads are placed on the left side of the victim's chest.

Yes   No   **8.** Batteries and pads have expiration dates of which you should be aware.

Yes   No   **9.** An AED can still be used if an implanted pacemaker is present.

Yes   No   **10.** You need to turn the AED on daily as part of a routine inspection.

Shock

Shock

Perfusion is when adequate blood and oxygen are provided to all cells in different tissues and organs in the body. Shock occurs when the body's tissues do not receive enough oxygen-rich blood. Do not confuse this with electric shock or being shocked, as in being scared or surprised. Shock (hypoperfusion) describes a state of collapse and failure of the cardiovascular system in which blood circulation decreases and eventually ceases. Shock can be associated with a wide variety of conditions—from a heart attack to a severe allergic reaction.

▶ Causes of Shock

Understanding the basic physiologic causes of shock will better prepare you to treat it. The damage caused by shock depends on which body part is deprived of oxygen and for how long. For example, without oxygen, the brain will be irreparably damaged in 4 to 6 minutes, the abdominal organs in 45 to 90 minutes, and the skin and muscle cells in 3 to 6 hours.

To understand shock, think of the circulatory system as having three components: a working pump (the heart), a network of pipes (the blood vessels), and an adequate amount of fluid (the blood) pumped through the pipes. Damage to any of these components can deprive tissues of blood and produce the condition known as shock. These three parts can be referred to as the perfusion triangle Figure 7-1 . When a victim is in shock, one or more of the three sides is not working properly.

Figure 7-1

Perfusion triangle.

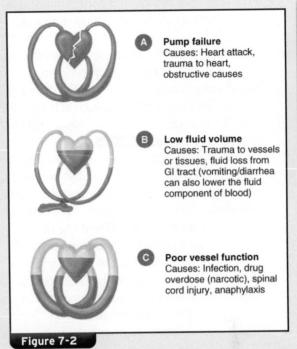

Figure 7-2

There are three basic causes of shock and impaired tissue function. **A.** Pump failure occurs when the heart is damaged by disease, injury, or obstructive causes. The heart may not generate enough energy to move the blood through the system. **B.** Low fluid volume, often a result of bleeding, leads to inadequate perfusion. **C.** The blood vessels can dilate excessively so that the blood within them, even though it is of normal volume, is inadequate to fill the system and provide efficient perfusion.

Causes of shock can be both cardiovascular and noncardiovascular. The noncardiovascular causes of shock are respiratory insufficiency, psychogenic shock, and **anaphylaxis,** an extreme allergic reaction to a foreign substance. There are three major cardiovascular causes of shock **Figure 7-2** :

- *Poor pump function.* If damaged by disease or injury, the heart might not generate sufficient energy to move blood through the system (for example, cardiogenic shock).
- *Blood or fluid loss from blood vessels.* If enough blood or plasma is lost, the volume of fluid left in the vascular system is inadequate to perfuse all tissues and organs (for example, hemorrhagic shock).
- *Poor vessel function.* With widespread vessel dilation, the normal volume of blood will be insufficient to fill the system and provide efficient perfusion (for example, neurogenic shock).

Cardiovascular Causes of Shock

- *Pump failure.* Cardiogenic shock is caused by inadequate function of the heart, or pump failure. Circulation requires the constant pumping action of a normal heart muscle. Many diseases can cause destruction or inflammation of this muscle. The heart can adapt somewhat to these problems, but if too much muscle damage occurs, as sometimes happens in a heart attack, the heart no longer functions well. The major effect is the backup of blood into the lungs. The resulting buildup of fluid in the lungs is called pulmonary edema.
- *Content failure.* In injuries, shock is most often the result of fluid or blood loss. This type of shock is called hypovolemic (low-volume) shock or hemorrhagic shock. The loss can be due to internal or external bleeding. Hypovolemic shock also occurs with severe thermal burns. Plasma, the fluid portion of the blood, leaks from the circulatory system into burned tissues adjacent to the injury. Dehydration aggravates shock. In all these circumstances, the common factor is an insufficient volume of blood within the vascular system to provide adequate perfusion to the tissues.

- *Poor vessel function.* Spinal cord damage can injure the part of the nervous system that controls blood vessel size and muscle tone. Neurogenic shock can result. Cut off from their impulses to contract, muscles in the blood vessels dilate (relax) widely, increasing the size and capacity of the vascular system. The blood in the body can no longer fill the enlarged vessels **Figure 7-3** .

- *Combined vessel and content failure.* Septic shock is seen in victims who have severe bacterial infections that produce toxins (poisons). The toxins damage the vessel walls, causing them to become leaky and making them unable to contract well. Widespread vessel dilation, combined with the loss of plasma through injured vessel walls, results in shock. Septic shock is almost always a complication of a serious illness, injury, or surgery. Septic shock also occurs with anaphylaxis.

Noncardiovascular Cause of Shock

- *Respiratory insufficiency.* A severe chest injury or an airway obstruction can make a victim unable to breathe adequately. Insufficient oxygen in the blood can produce shock as rapidly as vascular causes, even when cardiovascular function is normal. Circulation of nonoxygenated blood will not benefit the victim.

- *Anaphylactic shock.* Anaphylaxis, or anaphylactic shock, occurs when the immune system reacts violently to a substance to which it has already been sensitized. Severe allergic reactions commonly follow exposure by one of these:
  - Medications (penicillin and related drugs, aspirin, sulfa drugs)
  - Food (shellfish, nuts—especially peanuts, eggs)
  - Insect stings (honeybee, wasp, yellow jacket, hornet, fire ant)

Anaphylactic reactions can develop in minutes or even seconds after contact with the substance to which a victim is sensitized. The signs of such allergic reactions are distinct from those of other forms of shock. **Table 7-1** shows the signs and symptoms of anaphylactic shock.

In anaphylactic shock, although there is no loss of blood, no vascular damage, and only a slight possibility of cardiac muscular injury, the widespread vascular dilation causes poor oxygenation and poor perfusion of tissues, which can easily cause death.

- *Psychogenic shock.* Psychogenic shock is a sudden nervous system reaction that produces a

Spinal cord damage →
Dilated vessels
Absence of sweating
Loss of body temperature control

Normal vessel   Dilated vessel

Figure 7-3

Neurogenic shock.

Table 7-1 Signs and Symptoms of Anaphylactic Shock

Skin
- Flushing, itching, or burning, especially over the face and upper chest
- Hives, which can spread over large areas of the body
- Swelling, especially of the face, tongue, and lips
- Bluish lips (cyanosis)

Circulatory system
- Weak pulse (you might be barely able to feel it)
- Dizziness
- Fainting and unresponsiveness

Respiratory system
- Sneezing or itching in the nostrils
- Tightness in the chest, with a persistent, dry cough
- Breathing difficulty
- Secretions of fluid and mucus into the throat and lungs
- Wheezing (forced expirations during breathing)
- Breathing stops

temporary vascular dilation, resulting in fainting, or syncope. Blood pools in the dilated vessels, reducing the blood supply to the brain, and the victim becomes unresponsive. Causes of fainting (psychogenic shock) include fear, bad news, or unpleasant sights (often the sight of blood).

▶ The Progression of Shock

Although shock itself cannot be seen, you can see its signs and symptoms progress **Table 7-2**. The early stage of hemorrhagic (blood loss) shock, when the body can still compensate for blood loss, is called compensated shock. The late stage, when blood pressure is falling, is decompensated shock. The final stage, when shock is terminal, is called irreversible shock. Even transfusion will not save the victim's life at this point.

FYI

Red Flags for Shock

Shock is seen in both injured and suddenly ill victims. Anticipate and expect shock if a victim has any of these conditions:

- Massive external or internal bleeding
- Multiple severe fractures
- Abdominal or chest injury
- A severe infection
- Sign of a heart attack
- Anaphylaxis

▶ Care for Shock

Because every injury affects the circulatory system to some degree, first aiders should automatically treat injured victims for shock. Shock is one of the most common causes of death in an injured victim. Even if an injured victim does not have signs or symptoms of shock, first aiders should care for shock. You can prevent shock from getting worse; first aiders cannot reverse it.

General Care for Shock

1. Monitor breathing and, if absent, begin CPR.
2. Control all obvious external bleeding.

Table 7-2 Progression of Shock

Compensated Shock

- Agitation
- Anxiety
- Restlessness
- Feeling of impending doom
- Altered mental status
- Weak, rapid, or absent pulse
- Clammy (pale, cool, moist) skin
- Paleness, with cyanosis about the lips
- Shallow, rapid breathing
- Shortness of breath
- Nausea or vomiting
- Capillary refill longer than 2 seconds in infants and children
- Thirst

Decompensated Shock

- Difficulty breathing
- Ashen, mottled, or cyanotic skin
- Dull eyes, dilated pupils

Q&A

What is the optimal position for a person in shock? Does elevating the legs improve outcome?

Most victims should not be moved. However, first aiders are often taught to raise the feet of a suspected victim of shock in theory to return blood volume to the victim's central circulation, thus raising cardiac output and blood pressure. While the evidence is mixed on the effects of leg elevation, no studies demonstrate improved victim outcome in the medical literature.

The elevation of the legs for a victim suffering potential pelvic or lower extremities injuries may not be apparent to a first aider and the elevation of the legs may cause a greater harm. Therefore, the legs should not be raised if a leg is injured or if moving an injured leg causes pain.

Additionally, raising the feet 6 to 12 inches can be beneficial in some cases (eg, fainting, dehydration, and heat exhaustion).

3. Place the victim on his or her back (supine position). Those having a heart attack or those with lung disease breathe easier in a half-sitting position **Figure 7-4**.

Figure 7-4A

Figure 7-4C

Figure 7-4B

Figure 7-4D

Shock positions. **A.** For a victim with head injury, elevate the head (if spinal injury is not suspected). **B.** Position an unresponsive or stroke victim in the recovery position. **C.** Use a half-sitting position for victims with breathing difficulties, chest injuries, or a heart attack. **D.** Keep the victim flat if a spinal injury or leg fracture is suspected.

CAUTION

DO NOT place victims with breathing difficulties, chest injuries, penetrating eye injuries, or heart attacks on their backs. Place them in a half-sitting position to help breathing.

DO NOT give the victim anything to eat or drink. It could cause nausea and vomiting. It could also cause complications if surgery is needed.

DO NOT lift the foot of a bed or stretcher—breathing will be affected, and the blood flow from the brain could be impeded and lead to brain swelling.

DO NOT raise the legs of a victim with head injuries, stroke, chest injuries, breathing difficulty, or those of a victim in whom a heart attack is suspected.

DO NOT use external heat sources (such as hot water bottles or heating pads).

4. Do not move the victim if there are suspected fractures or head, spine, or torso injuries. Loosen tight clothing at the neck, chest, and waist.
5. Splint any bone or joint injuries to minimize pain and bleeding. This also prevents further damage to tissues.
6. Keep the victim warm. Place blankets under and over the victim. Do not use external heat sources (for example, hot water bottles or heating pads).

7. Handle the victim gently.
8. Seek immediate medical care. Depending on the problem, it might require calling 9-1-1 or transporting a victim using a private vehicle if EMS is not available.

Care for Anaphylaxis

1. Call 9-1-1 immediately.
2. Monitor breathing and, if absent, begin CPR.

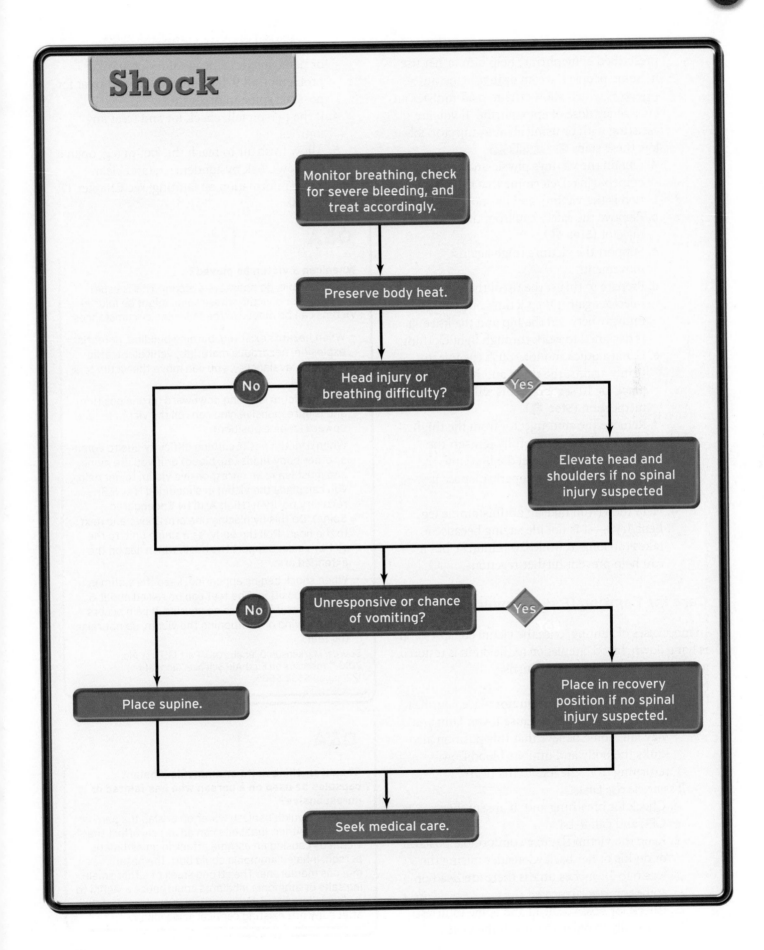

Shock

Monitor breathing, check for severe bleeding, and treat accordingly.

Preserve body heat.

Head injury or breathing difficulty?

No

Yes → Elevate head and shoulders if no spinal injury suspected

Unresponsive or chance of vomiting?

No → Place supine.

Yes → Place in recovery position if no spinal injury suspected.

Seek medical care.

3. If the victim has his or her own physician-prescribed epinephrine, help him or her use it. Some people have an **epinephrine auto-injector**, which allows them to administer an emergency dose of epinephrine. If you are assisting with or using an auto-injector, follow these steps `Skill Drill 7-1`:

   a. Obtain the victim's physician-prescribed epinephrine. Determine that the prescription is the victim's and has not expired.

   b. Remove the safety cap from the auto-injector (**Step ❶**).

   c. Support the victim's thigh against movement.

   d. Prepare to thrust the tip of the auto-injector against the victim's outer thigh, midway between the hip and the knee. It is designed to work through light clothing.

   e. Using a quick motion, push the injector firmly against the thigh and hold it in place for 10 seconds. This will inject the medication (**Step ❷**).

   f. Remove the auto-injector from the thigh. Using one hand, carefully reinsert the used auto-injector, needle first, into the carrying tube and properly dispose it (**Step ❸**).

4. Help the victim take an antihistamine (eg, Benadryl)—it is not life saving because it takes too long to work (20 minutes), but it can help prevent further reactions.

Care for Fainting (Psychogenic Shock)

In most cases of fainting, once the victim collapses and is lying down, blood circulation to the brain is restored and responsiveness usually returns.

If you feel faint:

- Lie down or sit down. **Do not** place your head between your knees because if you faint you may fall. Some believe that this position also kinks the body and inhibits blood flow returning from the legs to the heart.

If someone else faints:

1. Check for breathing and, if absent, begin CPR and call 9-1-1.

2. Keep the victim flat in a comfortable position or on his or her back. Consider raising the legs 6 to 12 inches unless there are head or spine injuries suspected.

3. Check for possible head and spine injuries, especially in older victims. If the victim is unable to walk without weakness, dizziness, or pain, suspect a head injury or another problem. Call 9-1-1 immediately and treat for possible spine injury.

4. If the person fell, check for and treat any injuries.

5. Allow fresh air to reach the victim (eg, open a window). Ask bystanders to stand clear.

For more information on fainting, see Chapter 17, *Sudden Illness.*

Q&A

When can a victim be moved?

When possible, do not move a victim. This is especially true for a victim whose spine might be injured. Victims can be moved in the following circumstances:

- When hazards exist (eg, burning building, potential explosion, hazardous materials, vehicular traffic, landslide, avalanche), you can move the victim to a safer area.

- When a victim is facing downward (prone position) and is unresponsive, you can roll the victim to face upward (supine position).

- When a victim has breathing difficulty due to vomit or other body fluids (eg, blood) or if you are alone and must leave an unresponsive victim to get help, you can place the victim in a modified HAINES recovery position (**H**igh **A**rm **IN E**ndangered **S**pine). Do this by placing one arm above and next to the head. Roll the body, as a single unit, to the victim's side. Support the head, which lies on the extended arm.

- When shock begins appearing, keep the victim in a supine position. The feet can be raised about 6 to 12 inches if there are no injuries. If pain occurs while moving or positioning the victim, do not raise the feet.

Source: Markenson D, et.al. 2010. Part 13: First Aid: 2010 Consensus on First Aid Science. *Circulation.* 122(suppl):S532-S605.

Q&A

Should smelling salts or ammonia inhalant capsules be used on a person who has fainted or is unresponsive?

No. You shouldn't splash water on or slap the person's face either. Inhalants can adversely affect the victim by causing an asthma attack in an asthmatic person. Inhaled ammonia could burn the nasal mucous membrane. The strong smell of either smelling salts or ammonia inhalants could cause a victim to suddenly jerk his or her head, which could adversely affect any pre-existing cervical spine injury.

skill drill

7-1   Using an Epinephrine Auto-Injector

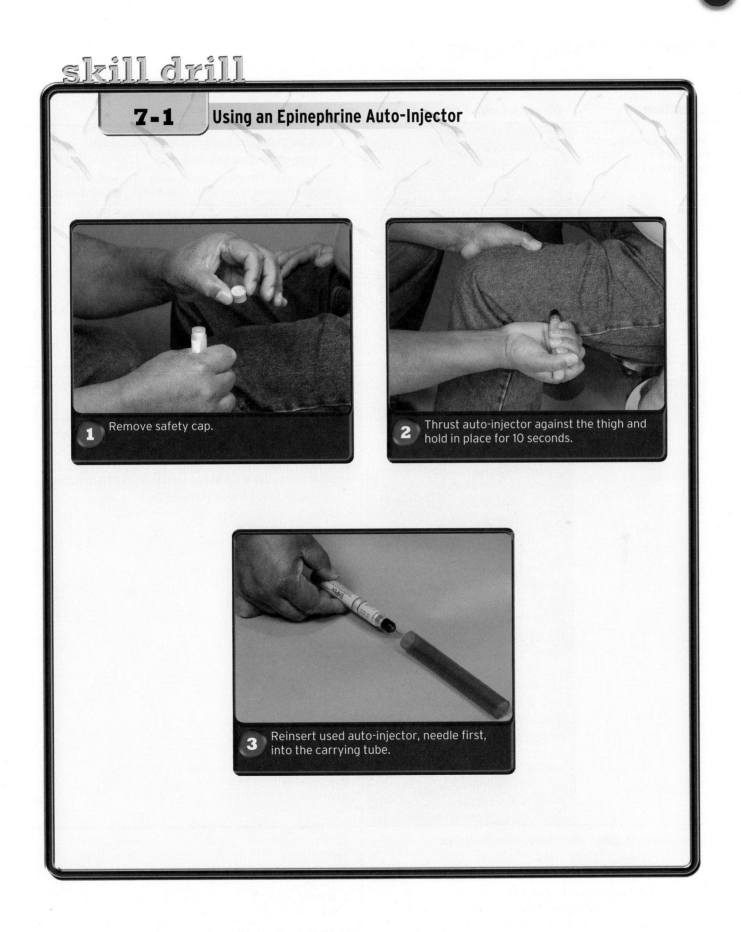

1 Remove safety cap.

2 Thrust auto-injector against the thigh and hold in place for 10 seconds.

3 Reinsert used auto-injector, needle first, into the carrying tube.

▶ Emergency Care Wrap-up

Condition	What to Look For	What to Do
Shock (cardiogenic, hemorrhagic, septic, neurogenic)	• Agitation • Anxiety • Restlessness • Feeling of impending doom • Altered mental status • Weak, rapid, or absent pulse • Clammy (pale, cool, moist) skin* • Paleness, with cyanosis about the lips • Shallow, rapid breathing • Shortness of breath • Nausea or vomiting	1. Monitor breathing and provide care if needed. 2. Control all obvious bleeding. 3. Place the victim on his or her back. (Those having a heart attack or those with lung disease breathe easier in a half-sitting position). 4. Do not move the victim if there are suspected fractures or head, spine, or torso injuries. 5. Splint any bone or joint injuries. 6. Place blankets under and over the victim. 7. Handle the victim gently. 8. Seek medical care by calling 9-1-1 if signs of shock are present.
Anaphylaxis	**Skin** • Flushing, itching, or burning, especially over the face and upper chest • Hives, which can spread over large areas of the body • Swelling, especially of the face, tongue, and lips • Bluish lips (cyanosis) **Circulatory system** • Weak pulse (you might be barely able to feel it) • Dizziness • Fainting and unresponsiveness **Respiratory system** • Sneezing or itching in the nostrils • Tightness in the chest, with a persistent dry cough • Breathing difficulty • Secretions of fluid and mucus into the throat and lungs • Wheezing (forced expirations during breathing) • Breathing stops	1. Call 9-1-1 immediately. 2. Monitor breathing, and if necessary, give CPR. 3. If the victim has his or her own prescribed epinephrine, help the victim use it. If you are assisting with or using an auto-injector, follow the container's instructions. 4. Give an antihistamine (such as Benadryl)—it is not life saving because it takes too long to work (20 minutes), but can prevent further reactions.

*Victims of neurogenic shock have warm, pink skin.

▶ Ready for Review

- Shock is a state of collapse and failure of the cardiovascular system in which blood circulation decreases and eventually ceases.
- The damage caused by shock depends on which body part is deprived of oxygen and for how long.
- Causes of shock can be both cardiovascular and noncardiovascular.
- Anaphylaxis occurs when the immune system reacts violently to a substance to which it has already been sensitized.
- Although shock itself cannot be seen, you can see its signs and symptoms progress.
- First aiders should automatically treat victims for shock.

▶ Vital Vocabulary

anaphylaxis A life-threatening allergic reaction.

epinephrine auto-injector Prescribed device used to administer an emergency dose of epinephrine to a victim experiencing anaphylaxis.

shock Inadequate tissue oxygenation resulting from serious injury or illness.

▶ Assessment in Action

You are walking up a popular canyon trail on a cool fall afternoon. You hear someone call for help further up the trail, near a cliff. You jog up the trail and find a hiker bent over another person at the base of a cliff. The hiker says the person lying motionless fell about 20 feet while climbing the cliff with no ropes or harness. There are no obvious signs of injury. The victim appears to be breathing and no serious bleeding is seen.

Directions: Circle Yes if you agree with the statement; circle No if you disagree.

Yes No 1. You should suspect spinal injury.

Yes No 2. You should preserve the victim's body heat, but do not use external heat sources.

Yes No 3. You should offer the victim something to eat and drink.

Yes No 4. There is no need to seek medical care for this situation.

▶ Check Your Knowledge

Directions: Circle Yes if you agree with the statement; circle No if you disagree.

Yes No 1. Place *all* severely injured victims in the recovery position.

Yes No 2. Prevent body heat loss by putting blankets under and over the victim.

Yes No 3. A shock victim with possible spinal injuries should be placed in a seated position.

Yes No 4. A shock victim with breathing difficulty or chest injury should be placed on his or her back.

Yes No 5. Anxiety and restlessness are signs of shock.

Yes No 6. An epinephrine auto-injector requires a doctor's prescription.

Yes No 7. All severely injured or ill victims should be treated for shock.

Yes No 8. Treat severely injured victims for shock even if there are no signs of it.

Yes No 9. Anaphylaxis is a life-threatening breathing emergency.

Yes No 10. Victims in shock have hot skin.

Bleeding

Bleeding

The average-size adult has 5 to 6 quarts (10–12 pints) of blood and can safely donate a pint. However, rapid blood loss of 1 quart or more can lead to shock and death. A child who loses 1 pint of blood is in extreme danger.

▶ External Bleeding

External bleeding refers to blood coming from an open wound. The term <u>hemorrhage</u> refers to a large amount of bleeding in a short time. External bleeding can be classified into three types according to the type of blood vessel that is damaged: an artery, vein, or capillary **Figure 8-1**. In arterial bleeding, blood spurts (up to several feet) from the wound. <u>Arterial bleeding</u> is the most serious type of bleeding because a large amount of blood can be lost in a very short period of time. Arterial bleeding also is less likely to clot because blood can clot only when it is flowing slowly or not at all. Arterial bleeding is dangerous and must be controlled. Unless a very large artery has been cut, however, it is unlikely that a person will bleed to death before the flow can be controlled.

In <u>venous bleeding</u>, blood from a vein flows steadily or gushes. Venous bleeding is easier to control than arterial bleeding. Most veins collapse when cut. Bleeding from deep veins, however, can be as mas-

Figure 8-1

Capillary, venous, and arterial bleeding.

sive and as hard to control as arterial bleeding. In <u>capillary bleeding</u>, the most common type of bleeding, blood oozes from capillaries. It usually is not serious and can be controlled easily. Quite often, this type of bleeding will clot and stop by itself. Each type of blood vessel—artery, vein, or capillary—contains blood of a different shade of red. An inexperienced person may have difficulty detecting the color difference but would still be able to identify the type of bleeding by its flow. The body naturally responds to bleeding in the following ways:

- *Blood vessel spasm.* Arteries contain small amounts of muscle tissue in their walls. If a blood vessel is completely severed, it draws back into the tissue, constricts its diameter, and slows the bleeding dramatically. If an artery is only partially cut across its diameter, however, constriction is incomplete. The vessel may not contract and the loss of blood may not slow as dramatically.
- *Clotting.* Special elements in blood, called *platelets,* form a clot. Clotting serves as a protective covering for a wound until the tissues

CAUTION

DO NOT come in contact with blood with your bare hands. Protect yourself with exam gloves, extra gauze pads, or clean cloths, or have the victim apply the direct pressure. If you must use your bare hands, do so only as a last resort. After the bleeding has stopped and the wound has been cared for, vigorously wash your hands with soap and water.

DO NOT use direct pressure on an eye injury, a wound with an embedded object, or a skull fracture.

DO NOT remove a blood-soaked dressing. Doing so can pull off clots that have already formed. Apply another dressing on top and continue putting pressure over the wound.

underneath can repair themselves. In a healthy person, initial clot formation normally takes about 10 minutes. Clotting time is longer in people who have lost a great deal of blood over a prolonged period of time, are taking aspirin or anticoagulants, are anemic, or have hemophilia or severe liver disease.

Care for External Bleeding

Regardless of the type of bleeding or the type of wound, the first aid is the same. First, and most important, you must control the bleeding **Skill Drill 8-1** :

1. Protect yourself against disease by wearing exam gloves. If they are not available, use several layers of gauze pads, clean cloths, plastic wrap, a plastic bag, or waterproof material. If those are unavailable, you can have the victim apply pressure on the wound with his or her hand.
2. Expose the wound by removing or cutting the victim's clothing to find the source of the bleeding (**Step ❶**).
3. Place a sterile gauze pad or a clean cloth such as a handkerchief, washcloth, or towel over the entire wound and apply direct pressure with your fingers for small wounds and with the palm of your hand for large wounds (**Step ❷**). Hold steady, firm, and uninterrupted pressure on the wound for at least 5 minutes. The gauze or cloth allows you to apply even pressure. Direct pressure stops most bleeding. Applying direct pressure to the wound compresses the sides of the torn vessel and helps the body's natural clotting mechanisms work. Be sure the pressure remains constant, is not too light, and is applied to the bleeding source. Do not remove blood-soaked dressings; simply add new dressings over the old ones.
4. To free you to attend to other injuries or victims, use a pressure bandage to hold the dressing on the wound. Wrap a roller gauze bandage tightly over the dressing and above and below the wound site (**Step ❸**). Do not wrap it so tightly that it cuts off circulation.
5. When direct pressure cannot be applied, such as in the case of a protruding bone, skull fracture, or embedded object, use a doughnut-shaped (ring) pad to control bleeding. To make a ring pad, wrap one end of a

skill drill

8-1   Care for External Bleeding

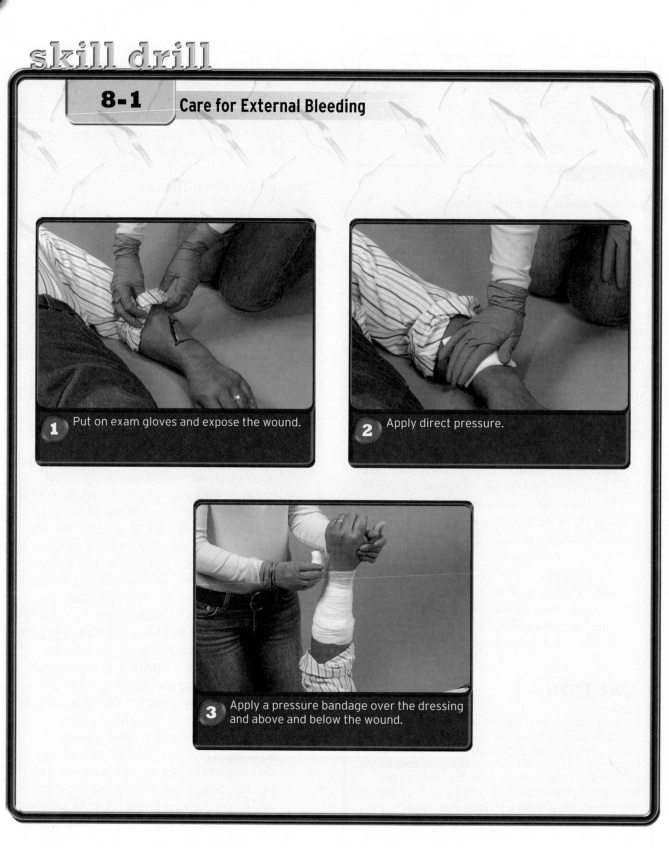

1. Put on exam gloves and expose the wound.

2. Apply direct pressure.

3. Apply a pressure bandage over the dressing and above and below the wound.

narrow bandage (roller or cravat) several times around your four fingers to form a loop. Pass the other end of the bandage through the loop and wrap it around and around until the entire bandage is used and a ring has been made.

When bleeding stops, use procedures found in Chapter 9, *Wounds*, for wound care.

Some people panic when they see even the smallest amount of blood. The sight of more than a couple of tablespoonfuls of blood generally is enough to frighten victims and bystanders. Take time to reassure the victim that everything possible is being done. Do not belittle the victim's concerns.

Q&A

While attempting to control severe bleeding on an arm or leg, should the injured part be elevated and pressure points be used?

Studies show that bleeding can be stopped by manual (direct) pressure applied over gauze pads. It is the single most effective method for controlling bleeding. Studies found that an elastic adhesive bandage applied over gauze pads is best for maintaining a hands-free stopping of bleeding. No evidence exists that pressure points eliminated distal pulses–blood flow continued. No evidence exists that elevation of a bleeding part has any role in stopping bleeding.

CAUTION

DO NOT apply a pressure bandage so tightly that it cuts off circulation. Check the radial pulse if the bandage is on an arm; for a leg, check the pulse between the inside ankle bone knob and the Achilles tendon (posterior tibial). Pulses are hard to feel. Other signs that the dressing is too tight are increasing pain, numbness or tingling, loss of color in the skin, loss of muscle function.

▶ Internal Bleeding

Internal bleeding occurs when the skin is not broken and blood is not seen. It can be difficult to detect and can be life threatening. A person with bleeding stomach ulcers, a lacerated liver, or a ruptured spleen may lose a considerable amount of blood into the abdomen with no outward sign of bleeding other than the presence of shock. Broken bones can also cause serious internal blood loss. A broken femur can easily result in a loss of 1 or more quarts of blood.

Recognizing Internal Bleeding

The signs of internal bleeding may be seen in either injured or suddenly ill victims:

- Bright red blood from the mouth or rectum or blood in the urine
- Nonmenstrual vaginal bleeding
- Vomited blood; may be bright red, dark red, or look like coffee grounds
- Black, foul-smelling, tarry stools
- Pain, tenderness, bruising, or swelling
- Broken ribs, bruises over the lower chest, or a rigid abdomen

Q&A

What are the largest artery and the largest vein in the human body?

The aorta is the largest artery in the human body. In adults, it is about the size of a garden hose. Its internal diameter is 1" (2.5 cm) and its wall is about 0.079" (0.2 cm) thick.

The largest vein in the human body is the inferior vena cava, the vein that returns blood from the lower half of the body back to the heart.

Care for Internal Bleeding

For severe internal bleeding, follow these steps:

1. Monitor breathing.
2. Expect vomiting. If vomiting occurs, keep the victim lying on his or her left side to allow drainage and to prevent inhalation (aspiration) of vomitus.
3. Treat for shock and cover the victim with a coat or blanket for warmth. See Chapter 7, *Shock*, for when to use other body positions.

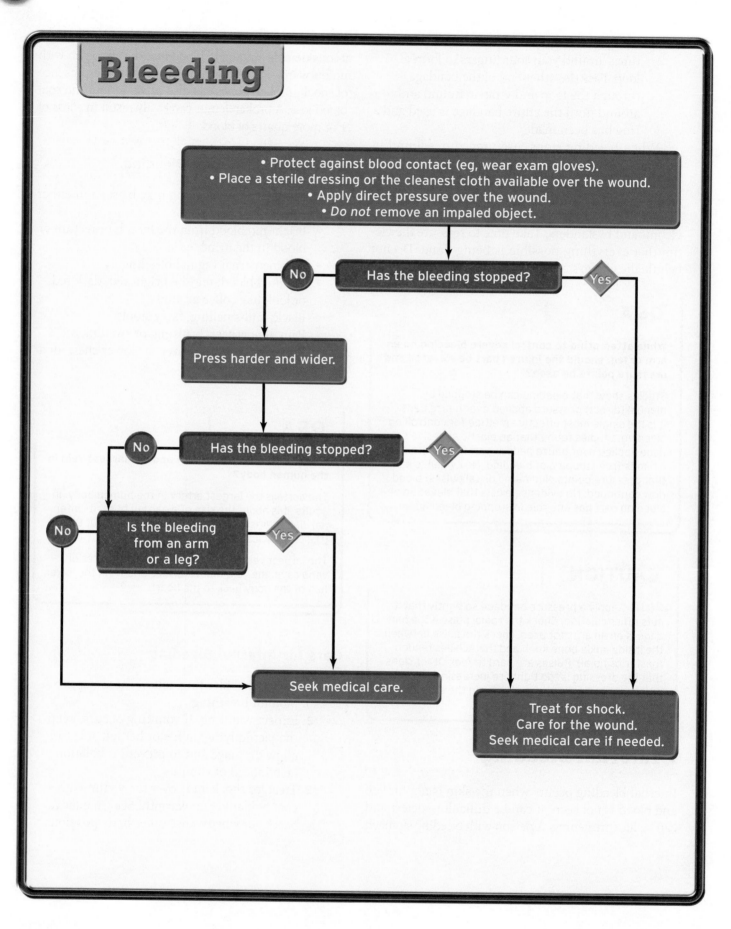

Bleeding

- Protect against blood contact (eg, wear exam gloves).
- Place a sterile dressing or the cleanest cloth available over the wound.
- Apply direct pressure over the wound.
- *Do not* remove an impaled object.

No ← **Has the bleeding stopped?** → Yes

Press harder and wider.

No ← **Has the bleeding stopped?** → Yes

No ← **Is the bleeding from an arm or a leg?** → Yes

Seek medical care.

Treat for shock.
Care for the wound.
Seek medical care if needed.

4. Treat suspected internal bleeding in an extremity by applying a splint.
5. Seek immediate medical care.

CAUTION

DO NOT give a victim anything to eat or drink. It could cause nausea and vomiting, which could result in aspiration. Food or liquids could also cause complications if surgery is needed.

Bruises are a form of internal bleeding, but are not life threatening. To treat bruises:

1. Apply an ice pack over the injury for 20 minutes.
2. If an arm or a leg is involved, apply an elastic bandage for compression. Several layers of gauze pads or other cloth could be placed between the bandage and the injury to concentrate the compression to a specific location.

▶ Emergency Care Wrap-up

Condition	What to Look For	What to Do
Bleeding	External bleeding	1. Protect against blood contact. 2. Place sterile dressing over wound and apply pressure. 3. Apply a pressure bandage.

	Internal bleeding	Minor internal bleeding (bruise):
		  Use RICE procedures (see Chapter 15, *Extremity Injuries*):
		    R = Rest
		    I = Ice
		    C = Compress the area with an elastic bandage.
		    E = Elevate the injured extremity.
		Serious internal bleeding:
		  Call 9-1-1.
		  Treat for shock.
		  If vomiting occurs, roll the victim onto his or her side.

▶ Ready for Review

- Rapid blood loss of 1 quart or more can lead to shock and death.
- External bleeding can be classified into three types according to the type of blood vessel that is damaged: artery, vein, or capillary.
- Regardless of the type of bleeding or the type of wound, the first aid is the same. First, and most important, you must control the bleeding.

▶ Vital Vocabulary

arterial bleeding Bleeding from an artery; this type of bleeding tends to spurt with each heartbeat.

capillary bleeding Bleeding that oozes from a wound steadily but slowly.

hemorrhage A large amount of bleeding in a short time.

venous bleeding Bleeding from a vein; this type of bleeding tends to flow steadily.

▶ Assessment in Action

You are enjoying a bike ride on a paved trail with your friend. As she rounds the next bend, her bike tires slide out on the gravel and she falls to the ground. She gets up but has a large scrape on her knee and part of her lower leg. Blood is oozing from the wound.

Directions: Circle Yes if you agree with the statement; circle No if you disagree.

Yes   No   **1.** This victim is experiencing capillary bleeding.

Yes   No   **2.** This type of bleeding is the most common type.

Yes   No   **3.** This type of bleeding is difficult to control and usually does not clot and stop by itself.

Yes   No   **4.** Direct pressure will control this type of bleeding.

prep kit

▶ Check Your Knowledge

Directions: Circle Yes if you agree with the statement; circle No if you disagree.

Yes   No   **1.** Most cases of bleeding require more than direct pressure to stop the bleeding.

Yes   No   **2.** Remove any blood-soaked dressings before applying additional ones.

Yes   No   **3.** Applying a pressure bandage over a wound can allow you to attend to another injury or another injured victim.

Yes   No   **4.** If a bleeding arm wound is not controlled through direct pressure, apply pressure to the brachial artery.

Yes   No   **5.** Dressings are placed directly on a wound.

Yes   No   **6.** Internal bleeding is normal.

Yes   No   **7.** Dressings should be sterile or as clean as possible.

Yes   No   **8.** Clotting is the body's way of stopping bleeding.

Yes   No   **9.** If the victim feels sick to the stomach and may vomit, roll him or her onto the left side.

Yes   No   **10.** It is important to remove impaled objects because they could be driven in deeper.

9 Wounds

▶ Open Wounds

An open wound is a break in the skin's surface resulting in external bleeding. It may allow bacteria to enter the body, causing an infection. There are several types of open wounds. Recognizing the type of wound helps you give proper first aid. With an <u>abrasion</u>, the top layer of skin is removed, with little or no blood loss **Figure 9-1**. Abrasions tend to be painful because the nerve endings often are abraded along with the skin. Ground-in debris may be present. This type of wound can be serious if it covers a large area or becomes embedded with foreign matter. Other names for an abrasion are *scrape*, *road rash*, and *scuff*.

A <u>laceration</u> is cut skin with jagged, irregular edges **Figure 9-2**. This type of wound is usually caused by a forceful tearing away of skin tissue. <u>Incisions</u> tend to have smooth edges and resemble a surgical or paper cut **Figure 9-3**. The amount of bleeding depends on the depth, the location, and the size of the wound. <u>Punctures</u> are usually deep, narrow wounds in the skin and underlying organs such as a stab wound from a nail or a knife **Figure 9-4**. The entrance is usually small, and the risk of infection is high. The object causing the injury may remain impaled in the wound.

With an <u>avulsion</u>, a piece of skin and/or underlying tissue is torn loose and is hanging from the body or completely removed. This type of wound can bleed heavily. If the flap is still attached, lay it flat and realign it into its normal position. Avulsions most often involve ears, fingers, and hands **Figure 9-5**. An <u>amputation</u> involves the cutting or tearing off of a body part, such as a finger, toe, hand, foot, arm, or leg.

chapter *at a glance*

- ▶ **Open Wounds**
- ▶ **Amputations**
- ▶ **Blisters**
- ▶ **Impaled (Embedded) Objects**
- ▶ **Closed Wounds**
- ▶ **Wounds That Require Medical Care**
- ▶ **Gunshot Wounds**

Figure 9-1

Abrasion.

Figure 9-2

Laceration.

Figure 9-3

Incision.

Figure 9-4

Puncture.

Figure 9-5

Avulsion.

Care for Open Wounds

1. Protect yourself against disease by wearing exam gloves. If they are not available, use several layers of gauze pads, clean cloths, plastic wrap or bags, or waterproof material. If none of these are available, you can have the victim apply pressure with his or her hand. Your bare hand should be used only as a last resort.

2. Expose the wound by removing or cutting away the clothing to find the source of the bleeding.

3. Control the bleeding by using direct pressure and, if needed, other methods described in Chapter 8, *Bleeding*.

Q&A

Is a dirty wound the same as a contaminated wound?

No. For example, road rash, resulting from road gravel, has a low bacterial count. In contrast, wounds that occur in a barnyard or are exposed to soil contaminated with fecal material have a high bacterial count and are contaminated.

Figure 9-6

Irrigate a wound with water under pressure.

FYI

Wound Irrigation

A study compared the effectiveness of tap water with saline solution for irrigating simple skin lacerations to remove bacteria. The results showed no significant difference between bacterial counts in wounds irrigated with normal saline and those irrigated with tap water. The removal of bacteria from a wound depends more on the mechanical effects (speed and pressure) than on the type of solution. Tap water has these advantages over saline—it is readily available; it is more continuous and, therefore, takes less time; it is less expensive; and it does not require other materials such as sterile syringes or splash guards. Other irrigation solutions with antibacterial properties and detergents have an anticellular effect that impairs wound healing and/or resistance to infection. Irrigation pressures more than the 20 to 30 psi range are discouraged because the higher pressure can damage tissue.

Source: Moscati R, Mayrose J, Fincher L, Jehle D. 1996. Comparison of normal saline with tap water for wound irrigation. *Am J Emerg Med* 164(4):379-381.

Cleaning a Wound

A victim's wound should be cleaned to help prevent infection. Wound cleaning usually restarts the bleeding by disturbing the clot, but it should be done anyway for shallow wounds. For wounds with a high risk for infection, leave the pressure bandage in place because medical personnel will clean the wound.

1. Scrub your hands vigorously with soap and water. Put on exam gloves, if available.
2. Expose the wound.
3. Clean the wound.
   - *For a shallow wound:*
     - Wash inside the wound with soap and water.
     - Flush the wound with water (use water that is clean enough to drink) . Run water directly into the wound and allow the water to run over the wound and out, thus carrying the dirty particles away from the wound. Flushing with water needs pressure (at least 5 to 8 psi) to cleanse the tissue adequately. Water from a faucet provides sufficient pressure and quantity. Pouring water through the wound will not generate enough force for adequate cleaning. Irrigation with water is the most important factor in preventing infection.
   - *For a wound with a high risk for infection* (such as an animal bite, a very dirty or ragged wound, or a puncture), clean the wound and then seek medical care for additional wound cleaning. If you are in a remote setting (more than 1 hour from medical care), clean the wound as best you can.
4. Remove small objects not flushed out with sterile tweezers, if available. A dirty abrasion

FYI

High-Risk Wounds

These types of wounds have a high potential for infection:

- Bite wounds
- Very dirty, contaminated wounds
- Crushing, ragged wounds
- Wounds over injured bone, joint, or tendon
- Puncture wounds

CAUTION

DO NOT irrigate a wound with full-strength iodine preparations such as povidone iodine (10%) or isopropyl alcohol (70%). They kill body cells as well as bacteria and are painful. Also, some people are allergic to iodine.

DO NOT use hydrogen peroxide. It does not kill bacteria well, it adversely affects capillary blood flow, and it extends wound healing.

DO NOT use antibiotic ointment on wounds that require sutures or on puncture wounds (the ointment may prevent drainage). Use an antibiotic ointment only on abrasions and shallow wounds.

DO NOT soak a wound to clean it. No evidence supports the effectiveness of soaking.

DO NOT close gaping wounds with tape such as butterfly tape. Infection is more likely when bacteria are trapped in the wound. If a wound requires closure, this should be done by medical personnel. Extremity wounds are best sutured within 6 hours of the injury.

DO NOT breathe or blow on a wound or the dressing.

or other wound that is not properly cleaned will leave a "tattoo" on the victim's skin.

5. If bleeding restarts, apply direct pressure over the wound.

Covering a Wound

1. If the wound is small and does not require sutures, cover it with a thin layer of antibiotic ointment. These ointments can kill many bacteria and rarely cause allergic reactions. No physician prescription is needed.

FYI

Wound Care: What the Medical Literature Says

- Soaking wounds is not effective.
- The benefit of scrubbing wounds is debatable.
- Irrigating wounds requires a minimum pressure of 5 to 8 psi for tissue cleansing.
- Not closing a wound (for example, with butterfly bandages, elastic skin closures), especially a dirty wound, reduces the risk of infection.
- Applying antiseptic solutions such as Merthiolate, Mercurochrome, iodine, isopropyl alcohol, and hydrogen peroxide can injure wounded tissues.
- Applying an antibiotic ointment such as Neosporin or Polysporin reduces the risk of infection in shallow wounds or abrasions.

Source: Howell JM, Chisholm CD. 1992. Outpatient wound preparation and care: a national survey. *Ann Emerg Med* 21(8):976-981.

2. Cover a small or large wound with a sterile dressing. Do not close gaping or dirty wounds with tape or butterfly bandages. Bacteria may remain, leading to a greater chance of infection. Large, deep, or contaminated wounds should be managed by a medical professional.
3. If a wound bleeds after a dressing has been applied and the dressing becomes stuck, leave it on as long as the wound is healing. Pulling the scab loose to change the dressing retards healing and increases the chance of infection. If you must remove a dressing that is sticking, soak it in warm water to help soften the scab and make removal easier.
4. If a dressing becomes wet or dirty, change it. Dirt and moisture are both breeding grounds for bacteria.

Dressings and bandages are two different kinds of first aid supplies. A **dressing** is applied over a wound to control bleeding and prevent contamination. A **bandage** holds the dressing in place. Dressings should be sterile or as clean as possible; bandages need not be.

When to Seek Medical Care

High-risk wounds should receive medical care. Examples of high-risk wounds include those with embedded foreign material (such as gravel), animal and human bites, puncture wounds, and ragged wounds. Large or deep wounds should receive medical care. Any wound where edges do not come together spontaneously should receive medical care. Any wounds that have visible bone, joint, muscle, fat, or tendons and wounds that may have entered a joint or body cavity should receive medical care. A particularly high-risk wound is the "fight bite," a wound over the knuckle caused by punching a person in the teeth. Sutures, if needed, are best placed within 6 to 8 hours after the injury. Anyone who has not had a tetanus vaccination within 10 years (5 years in the case of a dirty wound) should seek medical attention within 72 hours to update his or her tetanus inoculation status.

Figure 9-7

Infected wound.

Q&A

When should wounds be closed by a physician?

Generally, a wound should be closed by one of several options (eg, sutures, staples, topical skin adhesives) when: (1) the edges of the skin do not fall together and/or (2) the cut is more than an inch long and is deep. Closing the wound speeds the healing process, lessens the risk of infection, and lessens scarring.

If sutures are needed, they should be made by a physician within 6 to 8 hours of the injury.

Wound Infection

Any wound, large or small, can become infected. Once an infection begins, damage can be extensive, so prevention is the best way to avoid the problem. A wound should be cleaned using the procedures described earlier in this chapter.

It is important to know how to recognize and treat an infected wound **Figure 9-7**. The signs and symptoms of infection include the following:

- Swelling and redness around the wound
- A sensation of warmth
- Throbbing pain
- Pus discharge
- Fever
- Swelling of lymph nodes
- One or more red streaks leading from the wound toward the heart

The appearance of one or more red streaks leading from the wound toward the heart is a serious sign that the infection is spreading and could cause death. If chills and fever develop, the infection has reached the circulatory system. Seek immediate medical care.

Factors that increase the likelihood for wound infection include the following:

- Dirty and foreign material left in the wound
- Ragged or crushed tissue
- Injury to an underlying bone, joint, or tendon
- Bite wounds (human or animal)
- Hand and foot wounds
- Puncture wounds or other wounds that cannot drain

FYI

Using Topical Antibiotics to Improve Wound Healing

The use of topical triple-antibiotics significantly decreases infection rates in minor wounds that are contaminated. Topical antibiotics are effective for minor wounds, but not for major wounds.

Many studies support the use of topical antibiotics on wounds that are clean. Topical bacitracin zinc (Bacitracin); a triple ointment of neomycin sulfate, bacitracin zinc, and polymyxin B sulfate (Neosporin); and silver sulfadiazine (Silvadene) were compared with petrolatum as a control in patients with minor wounds. Wound infection rates were 17.6% for petrolatum, 5.5% for Bacitracin, 4.5% for Neosporin, and 12.1% for Silvadene.

Source: Diehr S, Hamp A, Jamieson B. 2007. *The Journal of Family Practice*. 56(2):140-144.

In the early stages of an infection, a physician may allow a wound to be treated at home. Such home treatment would include the following:

- Keeping the area clean
- Soaking the wound in warm water or applying warm, wet packs
- Elevating the infected portion of the body
- Applying antibiotic ointment
- Changing the dressings daily
- Seeking medical care if the infection persists or becomes worse

Tetanus

Tetanus is also called *lockjaw* because of its best-known symptom, tightening of the jaw muscles. Tetanus is caused by a toxin produced by a bacterium. The bacterium, which is found throughout the world, forms a spore that can survive for years in a variety of environments. The World Health Organization reports that tetanus causes at least 500,000—perhaps even up to 1 million—deaths each year.

FYI

Tetanus Prevalence

Despite the wide availability of immunization against tetanus in the United States, many people are inadequately protected against this uncommon but often lethal disease. Protection was found in only 70% of people studied, with levels of immunity varying widely.

About 50 cases of tetanus occur in the United States each year, principally among elderly people and people who never received a primary series of vaccinations. Adults should have booster shots for tetanus every 10 years.

Source: Gergen PJ, McQuillan GM, Kiely M, Ezzati-Rice TM, Sutter RW, Virella G. 1995. A population-based serologic survey of immunity to tetanus in the United States. *N Engl J Med* 332(12):761-766.

Millions of adults in the United States have let their tetanus immunizations lapse; a smaller number have never been vaccinated. In addition, antibody levels in immunized children decline over time; one fifth of youngsters ages 10 to 16 years do not have protective levels. Tetanus is not communicable from one person to another.

The tetanus bacterium by itself does not cause tetanus. When it enters a wound, such as a puncture wound that contains little oxygen, the bacterium can produce a powerful, poisonous toxin. The toxin travels through the nervous system to the brain and the spinal cord. It then causes contractions of certain muscle groups, particularly in the jaw. There is no known antidote to the toxin once it enters the nervous system.

It is not just stepping on a rusty nail that can bring on the disease. Tetanus bacteria are commonly found in soil, street dust, organic garden fertilizers, and pet feces, and even minor cuts can introduce them into the bloodstream.

A tetanus vaccination can completely prevent the disease. Everyone needs an initial series of vaccinations to prepare the immune system to defend against the toxin, but then a booster shot only every 5 to 10 years is sufficient to maintain immunity.

The guidelines for tetanus immunization boosters are as follows:

- Anyone with a wound who has never been immunized against tetanus should be given a tetanus vaccine and booster immediately.
- A victim who was once immunized but has not received a tetanus booster within the last 10 years should receive a booster.

FYI

Myths About Wound Care

Myth: Wounds should be kept dry.

Fact: Healing is faster and infection rates are lower when wounds are kept moist. Keep them moist by applying an antibiotic ointment and a dressing.

Myth: Redness is a sign of an infected wound.

Fact: Although redness *can* signal an infected wound, it does indicate an inflammatory reaction. When you see it, check the other signs and symptoms of infection: fever and pus coming from the wound.

Myth: Saline solution should be used instead of tap water to irrigate a wound.

Fact: Saline solution is no more effective in preventing wound infections than tap water.

Myth: Don't cover a cut—let it "breathe."

Fact: If a cut is not covered, it dries out and scabs over. Scabs hinder healing. Keep a cut moist and prevent a scab from forming. Apply an antibiotic ointment and cover with a dressing.

- A victim with a dirty wound who has not had a booster within the past 5 years should receive a booster.
- Tetanus immunization shots must be given within 72 hours of the injury to be effective.

▶ Amputations

In many cases, an amputated extremity can be successfully replanted (reattached). It is generally attempted for only upper extremities.

Types of Amputations

Amputations usually involve fingers, hands, and arms rather than legs. Amputations are classified according to the type of injury:

- A **guillotine amputation** is a clean-cut, complete detachment **Figure 9-8**. Examples would include a finger cut off with an ax or an arm severed with a power tool.
- A **crushing amputation** occurs when an extremity separates by being crushed or mashed off, such as when a hand is caught in a roller machine.
- **Degloving** is when the skin is peeled off, much as you would take off a glove.

In a crushing amputation, the most common type, the chance of reattachment is poor. In a guillotine type, the chance of reattachment is much better because it is clean cut. Many amputations can be replanted by an experienced surgeon, and time is a

Figure 9-8

Guillotine amputation.

critical element in success. Function may be nearly normal in some cases.

A complete amputation may not involve heavy blood loss because blood vessels tend to go into spasms, recede into the injured body parts, and shrink in diameter, resulting in a surprisingly small amount of blood loss. More blood is seen in a partial amputation.

Care for Amputation

1. Control the bleeding with direct pressure. Apply a dry dressing or bulky cloths. Be sure to protect yourself against disease by following standard precautions. If bleeding cannot be controlled with direct pressure, a tourniquet may be required to prevent shock or death from blood loss.
2. Treat the victim for shock.
3. Recover the amputated part and, whenever possible, take it with the victim to the hospital. In multicasualty cases, in reduced lighting conditions, or when untrained people transport the victim, however, someone may be requested to locate and take the severed body part to the hospital after the victim's departure.
4. To care for the amputated body part **Figure 9-9**:
   - Do not clean the amputated portion.
   - Wrap the amputated part with dry, sterile gauze or other clean cloth.
   - Put the wrapped amputated part in a plastic bag or other waterproof container.
   - Place the bag or container with the wrapped part on a bed of ice. Keep the amputated part cool, but do not freeze.
5. Seek medical care immediately.

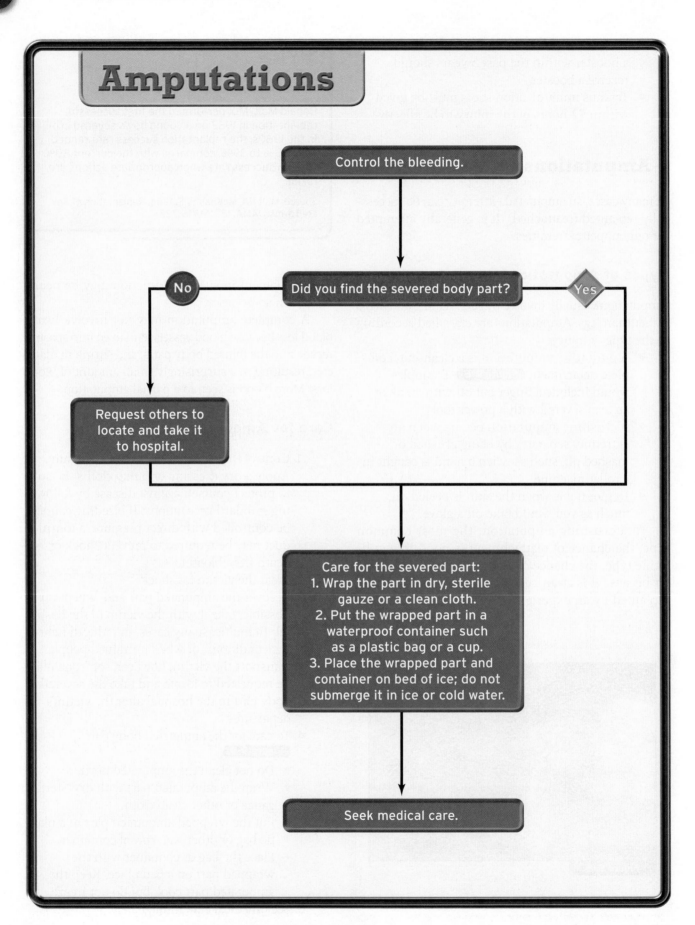

Amputations

Control the bleeding.

Did you find the severed body part?

No → Request others to locate and take it to hospital.

Yes

Care for the severed part:
1. Wrap the part in dry, sterile gauze or a clean cloth.
2. Put the wrapped part in a waterproof container such as a plastic bag or a cup.
3. Place the wrapped part and container on bed of ice; do not submerge it in ice or cold water.

Seek medical care.

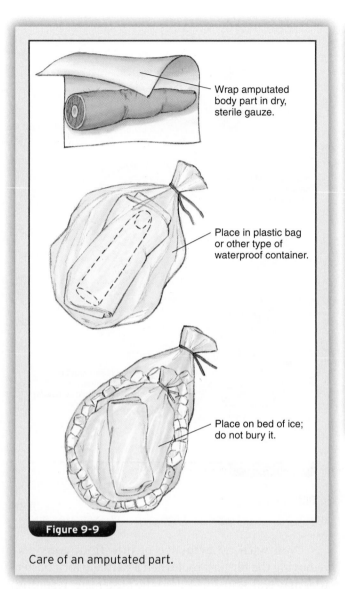

Wrap amputated body part in dry, sterile gauze.

Place in plastic bag or other type of waterproof container.

Place on bed of ice; do not bury it.

Figure 9-9

Care of an amputated part.

CAUTION

DO NOT try to decide whether a body part is salvageable or too small to save—leave that decision to a physician.

DO NOT wrap an amputated part in a wet dressing or cloth. Using a wet wrap on the part can cause waterlogging and tissue softening, which will make reattachment more difficult.

DO NOT bury an amputated part in ice—place it on ice. Reattaching frostbitten parts is usually unsuccessful.

DO NOT use dry ice.

DO NOT cut a skin "bridge," a tendon, or other structure that is connecting a partially attached part to the rest of the body. Instead, reposition the part in the normal position, wrap the part in a dry, sterile dressing or clean cloth, and place an ice pack on it.

Figure 9-10

Friction blister.

▶ Blisters

A blister is a collection of fluid in a "bubble" under the outer layer of skin. (Note: This section applies only to friction blisters and does not apply to blisters from burns, frostbite, drug reactions, insect or snake bites, or contact with a poisonous plant.)

Repeated rubbing of a small area of the skin will produce a blister **Figure 9-10**. Blisters are so common that many people assume they are a fact of life. However, blisters are avoidable, and life for many people could be more comfortable if they knew how to treat and prevent blisters.

Rubbing—as between a sock and a foot—causes stress on the skin's surface because the underlying supporting tissue remains stationary. The stress separates the skin into two layers, and the resulting space fills with fluid. The fluid may collect under or within the skin's outer layer, the epidermis. Because of differences in skin, blister formation varies considerably from person to person.

Care for Blisters

When caring for a friction blister, try to (1) avoid the risk of infection, (2) minimize the victim's pain and

FYI

Preventing Blisters

Keeping the skin lubricated and protected will reduce the potential for blister formation. Applying duct or adhesive tape to problem areas, such as around a big toe, can help reduce blister formation by allowing the sock to rub against the tape instead of directly against the skin.

Wearing proper clothing also can prevent blisters. For example, acrylic socks are considered superior to cotton socks in avoiding foot blisters because they are made in layers that are designed to absorb friction. Synthetic socks such as acrylic wick better than cotton. Avoid tube socks made of any material because their less precise fit tends to cause more friction than regular, fitted socks. Wear gloves to protect the skin on your hands.

Anything that can be done to keep the skin dry can also reduce blister formation. Moist skin is more susceptible to blisters than either very dry or very wet skin. One method is to wear socks that wick moisture from the skin. The application of antiperspirants to the feet has been shown to reduce the formation of serious blisters.

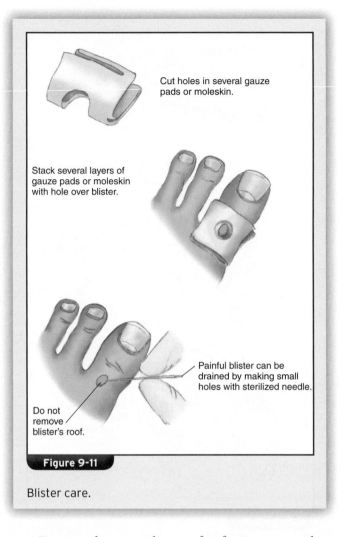

Cut holes in several gauze pads or moleskin.

Stack several layers of gauze pads or moleskin with hole over blister.

Painful blister can be drained by making small holes with sterilized needle.

Do not remove blister's roof.

Figure 9-11

Blister care.

discomfort, (3) limit the blister's development, and (4) promote a fast recovery. The best care for a particular blister is determined mainly by its size and location.

If an area on the skin becomes a "hot spot" (painful, red area), snugly apply a piece of tape (adhesive or duct). You could also cut a hole in several pieces of moleskin or molefoam in layered stacks around the blister, make a doughnut-shaped pad, and apply it over the blister.

If a blister on a foot is closed and not very painful, a conservative approach is to tape the blister with duct tape or waterproof adhesive tape. The tape must remain on the blister for several days; removing it may tear off the blister's "roof" and expose unprotected skin. Unfortunately, the tape may become damp and contaminated and have to be replaced, risking a tear. Small blisters, especially on weight-bearing areas, generally respond better if left intact.

With a few exceptions, the blister's roof (which is the best and most comfortable "dressing") should be removed only when an infection is present. Once a blister has been opened, the area should be washed with soap to prevent further infection. For 10 to 14 days, or until new skin forms, a protective bandage or other cover should be used.

Even with no evidence of infection, consider removing the blister's roof when a partially torn blister roof may tear skin adjacent to the blister site, resulting in an even larger open wound. In such cases, use sterilized scissors to remove the loose skin of the blister's roof up to the edge of the normal tissue. Treat it the same as for an open blister. Rubbing alcohol is effective for sterilizing instruments such as needles or scissors.

If a blister on the foot is open or a very painful closed blister affects walking or running:

1. Clean the area with soap and water.
2. Drain all fluid out of the blister by making several small holes at the base of the blister with a sterilized needle. Press the fluid out. Do not remove the roof of a blister unless it is torn and it may tear adjacent skin, or if there is an infection.
3. Apply several layers of moleskin or molefoam cut in a doughnut shape on top of each other **Figure 9-11**. Another option is to apply a commercial callus or corn pad over the blister.

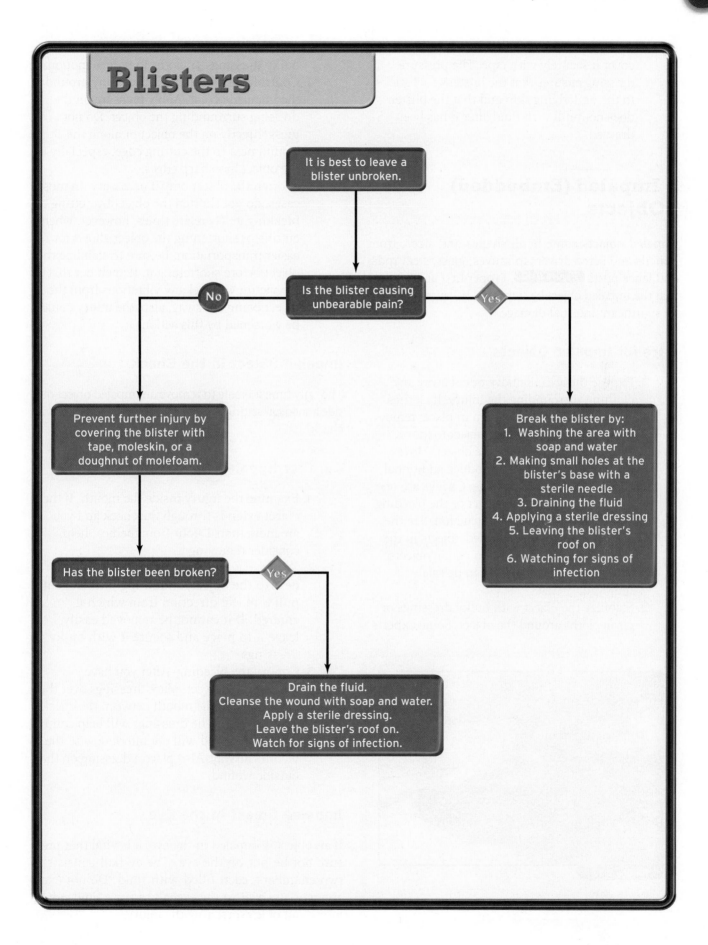

Blisters

It is best to leave a blister unbroken.

Is the blister causing unbearable pain?

No → Prevent further injury by covering the blister with tape, moleskin, or a doughnut of molefoam.

Has the blister been broken?

Yes → Drain the fluid.
Cleanse the wound with soap and water.
Apply a sterile dressing.
Leave the blister's roof on.
Watch for signs of infection.

Yes → Break the blister by:
1. Washing the area with soap and water
2. Making small holes at the blister's base with a sterile needle
3. Draining the fluid
4. Applying a sterile dressing
5. Leaving the blister's roof on
6. Watching for signs of infection

4. Apply antibiotic ointment in the hole and cover it securely with tape. The pressure dressing ensures that the blister's roof sticks to the underlying skin and that the blister does not refill with fluid after it has been drained.

▶ Impaled (Embedded) Objects

Impaled objects come in all shapes and sizes, from pencils and screwdrivers to knives, glass, steel rods, and fence posts **Figure 9-12**. Proper first aid requires that the impaled object be stabilized because there can be significant internal damage.

Care for Impaled Objects

1. Expose the area. Remove or cut away any clothing surrounding the injury. If clothes cover the object, leave them in place; removing them could cause the object to move.
2. Do not remove or move the object. Movement of any kind could produce additional bleeding and tissue damage. Cheeks are one exception because the object or the bleeding could cause an airway obstruction. See the following section on impaled objects in the cheek for more information. Small objects such as slivers (splinters) can be safely removed.
3. Stabilize the object with bulky dressings or clean cloths around the object. Some experts

Figure 9-12

Impaled object.

suggest securing 75% of the object with bulky dressings or cloths to reduce motion.
4. Control any bleeding with pressure around the impaled object. Apply pressure on the dressing surrounding the object. Do not press directly on the object or along the wound next to the cutting edge, especially if the object has sharp edges.
5. Shorten the object only if necessary. In most cases, do not shorten the object by cutting or breaking it. There are times, however, when cutting or shortening the object allows for easier transportation. Be sure to stabilize the object before shortening it. Remember that the victim will feel any vibrations from the object being cut away; also, the injury could be worsened by this action.

Impaled Object in the Cheek

The only time it is safe to remove an impaled object outside a medical setting is when the object is in the victim's cheek.

Care for Impaled Object in the Cheek

1. Examine the injury inside the mouth. If the object extends through the cheek and you are more than 1 hour from medical help, consider removing it.
2. To remove the object: Place two fingers next to the object, straddling it; then gently pull it in the direction from which it entered. If it cannot be removed easily, leave it in place and secure it with bulky dressings.
3. Control the bleeding. After you have removed the object, place dressings over the wound inside the mouth between the cheek and the teeth. The dressings will help control the bleeding and will not interfere with the victim's airway. Also place a dressing on the outside wound.

Impaled Object in the Eye

If an object is impaled in the eye, it is vital that pressure not be put on the eye. The eyeball consists of two chambers, each filled with fluid. Do not exert any pressure against the eyeball because fluid can be forced out of it, worsening the injury.

Care for Impaled Object in the Eye

1. Stabilize the object. Use bulky dressings or clean cloths to stabilize a long, protruding object. You can place a protective paper cup or cardboard folded into a cone over the affected eye to prevent bumping of the object. For short objects, surround the eye—without touching the object—with a doughnut-shaped (ring) pad held in place with a roller bandage.
2. Cover the undamaged eye. Most experts suggest that the undamaged eye should be covered to prevent sympathetic eye movement (that is, the injured eye moves when the undamaged eye does, thus aggravating the injury). Remember that the victim is unable to see when both eyes are covered and may be anxious. Make sure you explain to the victim everything you are doing.
3. Seek immediate medical care.

Care for Slivers

Small slivers of wood, glass, thorns, or metal can be painful and irritating and they also can cause infection. Because of their size, these slivers (also called *splinters*) can usually be easily removed with tweezers. Sometimes, it is necessary to tease one end of the object with a sterile needle to place it in a better position for removal with tweezers. After you have removed the sliver, clean the area with soap and water and apply an adhesive bandage.

Cactus Spines

Cacti are a part of the desert environment, and they also are used as ornamental plants. Infection from cactus-spine punctures is rare. Removing cactus spines is time consuming because they usually are acquired in groupings, are difficult to see, and are designed by nature to resist removal. Usually spines can easily, yet tediously, be removed with tweezers.

Another method for removing a large number of cactus spines is to coat the area with a thin layer of white woodworking glue or rubber cement and allow it to dry for at least 30 minutes. Slowly roll up the dried glue from the margins. Applying the glue in strips rather than puddles will make the rolling procedure go more smoothly. A single layer of gauze gently pressed onto the still-damp glue helps to remove it after it has dried. The combination of using tweezers and glue will remove most of the spines.

Using adhesive tape, duct tape, or cellophane tape, although quick and easy, removes only about 30% of the spines, even after multiple attempts. Do not use super glue (or other similar products) to remove cactus spines. Not only does it fail to roll up when applied to the skin, but it also welds the spines to the skin. In addition, there is the risk that the skin will permanently bond to anything it touches.

Care for Fishhooks

Tape an embedded fishhook in place and do *not* try to remove it if injury to a nearby body part such as the eye or an underlying structure such as a blood vessel or nerve is possible or if the victim (such as a young child) is uncooperative.

If the point of a fishhook has penetrated the skin but the barb has not, remove the fishhook by backing it out. Then treat the wound like a puncture wound. Seek medical advice for a possible tetanus shot.

If the hook's barb has entered the skin, follow these procedures:

1. If medical care is near, transport the victim and have a physician remove the hook.
2. If you are in a remote area, far from medical care, remove the hook using either the pliers method or the string-jerk method.

Use extreme care with the pliers method of fishhook removal because it can produce further severe injury if the hook is pushed into blood vessels, nerves, or tendons. Use pliers with tempered jaws that can cut through a hook **Figure 9-13**. The proper kind of pliers is often unavailable, or sometimes the barb is buried too deep to be pushed through. Test the pliers by first cutting a similar fishhook.

1. Use cold or use hard pressure around the hook to provide temporary numbness.
2. Push the embedded hook further in, in a shallow curve, until the point and the barb come out through the skin.
3. Cut off the barb, then back the hook out the way it came in.
4. After removing the hook, treat the wound and seek medical attention for a possible tetanus shot.

A better method to remove a fishhook is the string-jerk method.

1. Loop a piece of fishline over the bend or curve of the embedded hook **Figure 9-14**.
2. Stabilize the part of the victim's body in which the hook is embedded.

Figure 9-14

Fishhook removal; string-jerk method.

Figure 9-13

Fishhook removal; pliers method.

3. Use cold or use hard pressure around the hook to provide temporary numbness.
4. With one hand, press down on the hook's shank and eye while the other hand sharply jerks the fishline that is over the hook's bend or curve. The jerk movement should be parallel to the skin's surface. The hook will neatly come out of the same hole it entered, causing little pain.

5. After removing the hook, care for the wound and seek medical care for a possible tetanus shot.

▶ Closed Wounds

A closed wound happens when a blunt object strikes the body. In other words, the skin is not broken, but tissue and blood vessels beneath the skin's surface are crushed, causing bleeding within a confined area. There are three types of closed wounds:

1. *Bruises and contusions* occur when blood collects under the skin in the injured area. The victim will experience pain and swelling (immediately or within 24 to 48 hours). As blood accumulates, a black-and-blue mark may appear.
2. A *hematoma* is a clot of blood under the skin. There may be a lump or bluish discoloration.
3. *Crush injuries* are caused by extreme forces, which can injure vital organs and bones without breaking open the skin. Crush injuries may indicate an underlying problem such as a fracture. Signs and symptoms include discoloration, swelling, pain, and loss of use.

Care for Closed Wounds

1. Control bleeding by applying an ice pack over the area for no more than 20 minutes. Place a cloth between the ice pack and the skin to prevent frostbite.

2. If the injury involves a limb, apply an elastic bandage for compression. A splint may help make the victim more comfortable. See Chapter 10, *Bandaging Wounds*.

3. Check for a possible fracture.

4. Elevate an injured extremity above the victim's heart level to decrease the pain and swelling.

▶ Wounds That Require Medical Care

At some point, you will probably have to decide whether medical care is needed for a wounded victim. As a guideline, seek medical care for the following conditions as offered by the American College of Emergency Physicians:

- Wounds that will not stop bleeding after 15 minutes of applying direct pressure
- Long or deep cuts that need stitches
- Cuts over a joint
- Cuts that may impair function of a body area such as an eyelid or lip
- Cuts that remove all of the layers of the skin; such as those from slicing off the tip of a finger
- Cuts from an animal or human bite
- Cuts that have damaged or may have damaged underlying nerves, tendons, or joints
- Cuts over a possible broken bone
- Cuts caused by a crushing injury
- Cuts with an object embedded in them
- Cuts caused by a metal object or a puncture wound

Call 9-1-1 immediately if:

- Bleeding from a cut does not slow during the first 15 minutes of steady pressure
- Signs of shock occur
- Breathing is difficult because of a cut to the neck or chest
- A deep cut to the abdomen causes moderate to severe pain
- A cut occurs to the eyeball
- A cut amputates or partially amputates an extremity

Sutures

If sutures (stitches) are needed, they usually should be placed by a physician within 6 to 8 hours of the injury. Suturing wounds allows faster healing, reduces infection, and lessens scarring. Some wounds do not usually require sutures:

- Wounds in which the skin's cut edges tend to fall together
- Shallow cuts less than 1 inch long

Rather than close a gaping wound with butterfly bandages or elastic skin closures, cover the wound with sterile gauze. Closing the wound might trap bacteria inside, resulting in an infection. In most cases, a physician can be reached in time for sutures to be placed; if not, a wound without sutures will still heal but with scars. Scar tissue can be attended to later by a plastic surgeon.

▶ Gunshot Wounds

Guns are abundant in the United States; it is estimated that about one half of all American homes have a firearm. There are two general types of firearms: low velocity, such as most civilian firearms, and high velocity, such as military weapons. Shotguns have low velocity but create severe tissue damage.

A bullet causes injury in the following ways, depending on its velocity, or speed:

- *Laceration and crushing.* When the bullet penetrates the body, it crushes tissue and forces it apart. That is the main effect of low-velocity bullets. The crushing and laceration caused by the passage of the bullet usually are not serious unless vital organs or major blood vessels are injured. The bullet damages only the tissues that it contacts directly, and the wound is comparable to that caused by weapons such as knives.
- *Shock waves and temporary cavitation.* When a bullet penetrates the body, a shock wave exerts outward pressure from the bullet's path. The shock wave pushes tissues away and creates a temporary cavity that can be as much as 30 times the diameter of the bullet. As the cavity forms, a negative pressure develops inside, creating a vacuum. The vacuum then draws debris in with it. Temporary cavitation occurs only with high-velocity bullets and is the main reason for their immensely destructive effect. The cavitation lasts only a millisecond but can damage muscles, nerves, blood vessels, and bone.

In a *penetrating* wound, there is a bullet entry point but no exit. In a *perforating* wound, there are

Q&A

How do the physical characteristics of the bullet affect injury to the victim?

- The larger the size of the bullet, the greater the damage (eg, .22 versus .45 caliber).
- A hollow-point bullet widens when it hits tissues, causing a wider path of destruction.
- A bullet that tumbles around damages more tissue.
- Soft-nose bullets or bullets with vertical cuts in the nose break apart on impact, spreading fragments in a wider path and causing more tissue and organ damage. A shotgun blast also causes fragmentation.

both entry and exit points. The exit wound of a high-velocity bullet is usually larger than the entrance wound; the exit wound from a low-velocity bullet is about the same size as the entry wound **Figure 9-15**.

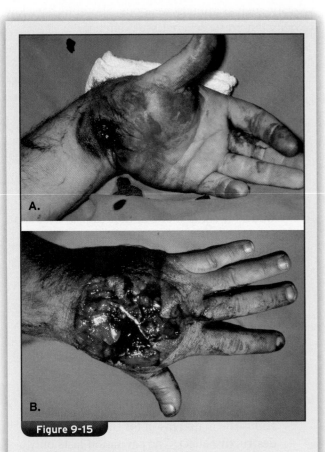

Figure 9-15

Gunshot wounds. **A.** An entrance wound from a gunshot may have burns around the edges. **B.** An exit wound is sometimes larger and results in greater damage to soft tissues.

If the bullet was fired at very close range, the entrance wound may be larger than the exit wound because the gases from the gun's muzzle contribute to the surface-tissue damage.

Bullets sometimes hit hard tissue such as bones and may bounce around in the body cavities, causing a great deal of damage to tissue and organs. Moreover, bone chips can ricochet to other body areas and cause damage. Because a split or misshapen bullet tumbles and exerts its force over a larger area, it does more damage than a smooth bullet going in a straight line does.

Care for Gunshot Wounds

Regardless of the type of gunshot wound, initial care is roughly the same as for any other wound.

1. Monitor the victim's breathing.
2. Expose the wound(s). Make sure to look at all the skin, including hidden areas.
3. Control the bleeding with direct pressure.
4. Apply dry, sterile dressings to the wound(s) and bandage them securely in place.
5. Treat the victim for shock.
6. Keep the victim calm and quiet.
7. Seek immediate medical care.

CAUTION

DO NOT try to remove material from a gunshot wound. The hospital emergency department personnel will clean the wound.

Legal Aspects

Because interactions with victims of gunshot wounds will involve contact with law enforcement agencies and possibly have you testifying in court, carefully observe the scene and the victim. Keep an accurate record of your observations. Preserve possible evidence, such as cartridge casings or shells, for the police. Do not touch or move anything unless absolutely necessary to treat the victim. All gunshot wounds must be reported to the police regardless of whether they are intentional (suicide, assault, murder, self-defense) or unintentional.

▶ Emergency Care Wrap-up

Condition	What to Look For	What to Do
Open wound	• Break in the skin's surface • External bleeding	1. Wash with soap and water. 2. Flush with running water under pressure. 3. Remove remaining small object(s). 4. If the bleeding restarts, apply pressure on the wound. 5. Apply antibiotic ointment if wound is shallow. 6. Cover with sterile or clean dressing. 7. For wounds with a high risk for infection, seek medical care for cleaning, possible tetanus booster, and closing.
Amputation	• Body part (eg, finger, toe, hand, foot, arm, leg) completely cut or torn off the body	1. Call 9-1-1. 2. Control bleeding. 3. Care for shock. 4. Recover amputated part(s) and wrap in sterile or clean dressing. 5. Place wrapped part(s) in a plastic bag or waterproof container. 6. Keep part(s) cool.
Embedded (impaled) object	• Foreign object penetrating a body part	1. Do not remove object. 2. Stabilize the object with bulky dressings or clean cloths. 3. Control bleeding with pressure around the object.

prep kit

▶ Ready for Review

- An open wound is a break in the skin's surface resulting in external bleeding.
- Knowing what type of open wound the victim has will help you in providing first aid.
- In many cases, an amputated extremity can be successfully replanted.
- A blister is a collection of fluid in a bubble under the outer layer of skin.
- Proper first aid of an impaled object requires that the object be stabilized because significant internal damage can occur.
- A closed wound happens when a blunt object strikes the body. Although the skin remains unbroken, the tissue and blood vessels beneath the skin's surface are crushed, causing bleeding within a confined area.
- Wounds that require medical care include:
  - Wounds that will not stop bleeding after 15 minutes of applying direct pressure
  - Long or deep cuts that need stitches
  - Cuts over a joint
  - Cuts that may impair function of a body area such as an eyelid or lip
  - Cuts that remove all of the layers of the skin such as those from slicing off the tip of a finger
  - Cuts from an animal or human bite
  - Cuts that have damaged or may have damaged underlying nerves, tendons, or joints
  - Cuts over a possible broken bone
  - Cuts caused by a crushing injury
  - Cuts with an object embedded in them
  - Cuts caused by a metal object or a puncture wound
- Call 9-1-1 immediately if:
  - Bleeding from a cut does not slow during the first 15 minutes of steady pressure
  - Signs of shock occur
  - Breathing is difficult because of a cut to the neck or chest
- A deep cut to the abdomen causes moderate to severe pain
- A cut occurs to the eyeball
- A cut amputates or partially amputates an extremity
- Guns are abundant in the United States, thus raising the risk of an accidental gunshot wound.

▶ Vital Vocabulary

abrasion An injury consisting of the loss of the partial thickness of skin from rubbing or scraping on a hard, rough surface.

amputation Complete removal of an appendage.

avulsion An injury that leaves a piece of skin or other tissue either partially or completely torn away from the body.

bandage Used to cover a dressing to keep it in place on the wound and to apply pressure to help control bleeding.

crushing amputation An extremity separates by being crushed or mashed off.

degloving The skin is peeled off the extremity.

dressing A sterile gauze pad or clean cloth covering that is placed over an open wound.

guillotine amputation A clean-cut, complete detachment of an extremity.

incisions Wounds usually made deliberately in connection with surgery; clean-cut as opposed to a laceration.

laceration A wound made by the tearing or cutting of body tissues.

punctures Deep, narrow wounds in the skin and underlying organs.

▶ Assessment in Action

You are helping your mother prepare for a barbeque on a Saturday afternoon. She is slicing tomatoes with a very dull kitchen knife. She is startled by something and cuts into her finger. The wound is bleeding and you can see the bone in the wound.

Directions: Circle Yes if you agree with the statement; circle No if you disagree.

Yes   No   **1.** This type of wound is called an avulsion.

Yes   No   **2.** You should not be concerned about infection because she was using a clean knife.

Yes   No   **3.** You should cover the wound with a sterile dressing but do not close the wound with tape or butterfly bandages.

Yes   No   **4.** You decide to take her to the emergency department for possible sutures. However, both you and your mother want to wait until the next day because you don't want to miss the barbeque.

▶ Check Your Knowledge

Directions: Circle Yes if you agree with the statement; circle No if you disagree.

Yes   No   **1.** An open wound may allow bacteria to enter the body, causing an infection.

Yes   No   **2.** A laceration is cut skin with smooth, straight edges.

Yes   No   **3.** A dressing is applied over a wound to control bleeding and prevent contamination.

Yes   No   **4.** A bandage is also applied over a wound to hold a dressing in place.

Yes   No   **5.** Any wound can become infected.

Yes   No   **6.** The signs and symptoms of an infection include swelling and redness around the wound, throbbing pain, and a lack of fever.

Yes   No   **7.** A bite wound is more likely to become infected.

Yes   No   **8.** Impaled objects should be removed immediately.

Yes   No   **9.** Tetanus is communicable from one person to another.

Yes   No   **10.** In many cases, an amputated extremity can be successfully reattached.

Bandaging Wounds

chapter
at a glance

Dressings

A dressing covers an open wound; it touches the wound. Whenever possible, a dressing should be:

- Sterile. If a sterile dressing is not available, use a clean cloth, handkerchief, washcloth, or towel.
- Larger than the wound.
- Thick, soft, and compressible so pressure is evenly distributed over the wound.
- Lint free.

The purposes of using a dressing are to:

- Control bleeding.
- Prevent infection and contamination.
- Absorb blood and wound drainage.
- Protect the wound from further injury.

▶ Types of Dressings

Use commercial dressings whenever possible. Dressings used in most first aid situations are commercially prepared, but dressings may need to be improvised.

- <u>Gauze pads</u> are used for small wounds. They come in separately wrapped packages of various sizes (for example, 2″

Figure 10-1

Gauze pads.

Figure 10-2

Adhesive strips.

Figure 10-3

Trauma dressings

they usually are not sterile **Figure 10-3**.

- When commercial sterile dressings are not available, an improvised dressing should be as clean, absorbent, soft, and free of lint as possible (for example, a handkerchief or a towel). Use the cleanest cloth available, or, in some conditions and if time allows, sterilize a cloth by ironing it for several minutes.

CAUTION

DO NOT use fluffy cotton or cotton balls as a dressing. Cotton fibers can get in the wound and be difficult to remove.

DO NOT remove a blood-soaked dressing until the bleeding stops. Cover it with a new dressing.

DO NOT pull off a dressing stuck to a wound. If it needs to be removed, soak it off in warm water.

by 2″; 4″ by 4″) and are sterile, unless the package is broken. Some gauze pads have a special coating to keep them from sticking to the wound and are especially helpful for burns or wounds secreting fluids **Figure 10-1**.

- **Adhesive strips** (for example, Band-Aids) are used for small cuts and abrasions and are a combination of a sterile dressing and a bandage **Figure 10-2**.
- **Trauma dressings** are made of large, thick, absorbent, sterile materials. Individually wrapped sanitary napkins can serve as a dressing because of their bulk and absorbency, but

Applying a Sterile Dressing

1. If possible, wash your hands and wear exam gloves.
2. Use a dressing large enough to extend beyond the edges of the wound. Hold the dressing by a corner. Place the dressing directly over the wound. Do not slide it on.
3. Cover the dressing with one of the types of bandages.

CAUTION

DO NOT touch any part of the wound or any part of the dressing that will be in contact with the wound.

Bandages

A bandage should be clean but need not be sterile. A bandage can be used to:

- Hold a dressing in place over an open wound
- Apply direct pressure over a dressing to control bleeding
- Prevent or reduce swelling
- Provide support and stability for an extremity or joint

Remember, bandages should be applied firmly enough to keep dressings and splints in place but not so tightly that they will reinjure the body part or impede blood circulation. The signs that a bandage is too tight include:

- Blue tinge of the fingernails or toenails
- Blue or pale skin
- Tingling or loss of sensation
- Coldness of the extremity
- Inability to move the fingers or toes
- A pulse could be felt before bandaging, but not after

CAUTION

DO NOT apply a bandage directly over a wound. Put a sterile dressing on first.

DO NOT bandage so tightly as to restrict blood circulation. Always check the extremity's pulse. If you cannot feel the pulse, loosen the bandage. Always check for signs that the bandage is too tight.

DO NOT bandage so loosely that the dressing will slip. This is the most common bandaging error. Bandages tend to stretch after a short time.

DO NOT leave loose ends. They might get caught on something or loosen.

DO NOT cover the victim's fingers or toes unless they are injured. They need to be observed for color changes that would indicate impaired circulation.

DO NOT use elastic bandages over a wound. There is a tendency to apply them too tightly.

DO NOT apply a circular bandage around a victim's neck; strangulation may occur.

DO NOT start a roller bandage above the wound. Instead, start below the wound and work upward.

A square knot is preferred because it is neat, holds well, and can be easily untied. However, the type of knot is not important. If the knot or the bandage is likely to cause the victim discomfort, a pad should be placed between the knot or bandage and the body.

▶ Types of Bandages

These are the basic types of bandages:

- <u>Roller bandages</u> come in various widths, lengths, and types of material. For best results, use different widths for different body areas:
  - 1-inch width for fingers
  - 2-inch width for wrists, hands, and feet
  - 3-inch width for ankles, elbows, and arms
  - 4-inch width for knees and legs
- <u>Self-adhering, conforming bandages</u> **Figure 10-4** come as rolls of slightly elastic, gauzelike material in various widths. Their self-adherent quality makes them easy to use.
- <u>Gauze rollers</u> are cotton and nonelastic. They come in various widths (1, 2, and 3 inches) and usually are 10 yards long. When commercial roller bandages are unavailable, you can improvise bandages from belts, neckties, or strips of cloth torn from a sheet or other similar material.

Figure 10-4

Self-adhering conforming bandages and gauze bandages of various sizes.

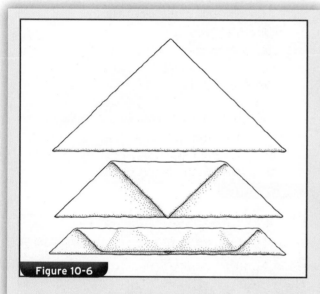

Figure 10-5

Elastic bandages of various sizes.

Figure 10-6

A triangular bandage folded into a cravat.

- **Elastic roller bandages** `Figure 10-5` are used for compression on sprains, strains, and contusions and come in various widths. Elastic bandages are not usually applied over dressings covering a wound.
- **Triangular bandages** `Figure 10-6` are available commercially or can be made from a 36″ to 40″ square of preshrunk cotton muslin. Cut the material diagonally from corner to corner to produce two triangular pieces of cloth. The longest side is called the *base;* the corner directly across from the base is the *point;* and the other two corners are called *ends.* A triangular bandage may be applied two ways:

- Fully opened (not folded). Best used for an arm sling. When used to hold dressings in place, fully opened triangular bandages do not apply sufficient pressure on the wound.
- As a *cravat* (folded triangular bandage). The point is folded to the center of the base and then the fabric is folded in half again from the top to the base to form a cravat. It is used to hold splints in place, to hold dressings in place, to apply pressure evenly over a dressing, or as a swathe (binder) around the victim's body to stabilize an injured arm in an arm sling.
- **Adhesive tape** comes in rolls and in a variety of widths. It is often used to secure roller bandages and small dressings in place. For people allergic to adhesive tape, use paper tape or special dermatologic tape.
- Adhesive strips are used for small cuts and abrasions and are a combination of a dressing and a bandage.

FYI

Removing Adhesive Tape

- When you first apply the tape, fold over one end (sticky sides together) to make a tab. Then when it comes time to remove the tape, you can grasp the starter tab. No need to pick at the tape (and the victim's skin) to get the strip started.
- To remove adhesive tape from the skin, gently lift the tape with one hand as you gently push the skin down and away from the tape with the other hand.
- Lift up a corner of the tape and dab the adhesive with an alcohol wipe. The alcohol dissolves the adhesive as the tape is peeled off.
- When peeling off tape from hairy skin, pull in the direction that the ends of the hair are naturally pointing.
- Firmly hold the skin from which the tape is pulled away.
- Save time and reduce frustration by leaving a tab on the end of the roll of tape for quick access the next time you need it.

Applying a Cravat Bandage

This method employs a cravat bandage (Figure 10-6). The bandage can be applied on the head, forehead, ear, eyes, arm, leg, or hand `Skill Drill 10-1`. For an injured eye, cover both eyes to prevent the injured eye from moving.

4. Place the middle of the bandage over the dressing covering the wound (or eyes) and wrap the bandage around the head (**Step ❶**).

5. Cross the two ends snugly over each other (**Step ❷**).

6. Bring the ends back around to where the dressing is and tie the ends in a knot (**Step ❸**). When wrapping a roller bandage around the head, keep the bandage near the eyebrows and low on the back of the head to prevent the bandage from slipping.

To apply a cravat bandage to the arm or leg using the cravat method, follow the steps in **Skill Drill 10-2**.

1. Wrap the center of the bandage over the dressing (**Step ❶**).

2. With one end, make one turn going up the extremity and another turn going down (**Step ❷**).

3. Tie the bandage off over the dressing (**Step ❸**).

To apply a bandage to the palm of the hand using the cravat method, follow the steps in **Skill Drill 10-3**.

1. Fill the palm with a bulky dressing or pad and close fingers over it (**Step ❶**).

2. Wrap one end of the bandage across the fingers and the other around the wrist (**Step ❷**).

3. Wrap the bandage crossing over the fingers and around the wrist (**Step ❸**).

4. Tie the bandage off at the wrist (**Step ❹**).

Applying a Roller Bandage

With a little ingenuity, you can apply a roller bandage to almost any body part. Self-adhering, conforming roller bandages eliminate the need for many of the complicated bandaging techniques that standard gauze roller, cravat, and triangular bandages require.

The Spiral Method

This method employs a 2″ or 3″ bandage roller for the arm or a 4″ bandage for the leg. To apply a bandage to the arm or leg using the spiral method, follow the steps here:

1. Start at the narrow part of an arm or leg and wrap upward toward the wider part to make the bandage more secure. Start below and at the edge of the dressing **Figure 10-7**.

2. Make two straight anchoring turns with the bandage.

3. Make a series of turns, progressing up the arm or leg. Each turn should overlap the previous wrap. Wrap with criss-cross (figure-eight) turns.

4. Finish with two straight turns and secure the bandage.

Figure 10-7A

Figure 10-7B

Figure 10-7C

Spiral method. **A.** Make two straight anchoring turns with the bandage. **B.** Wrap with criss-cross (figure-eight) turns. **C.** Finish with two straight turns and secure the bandage.

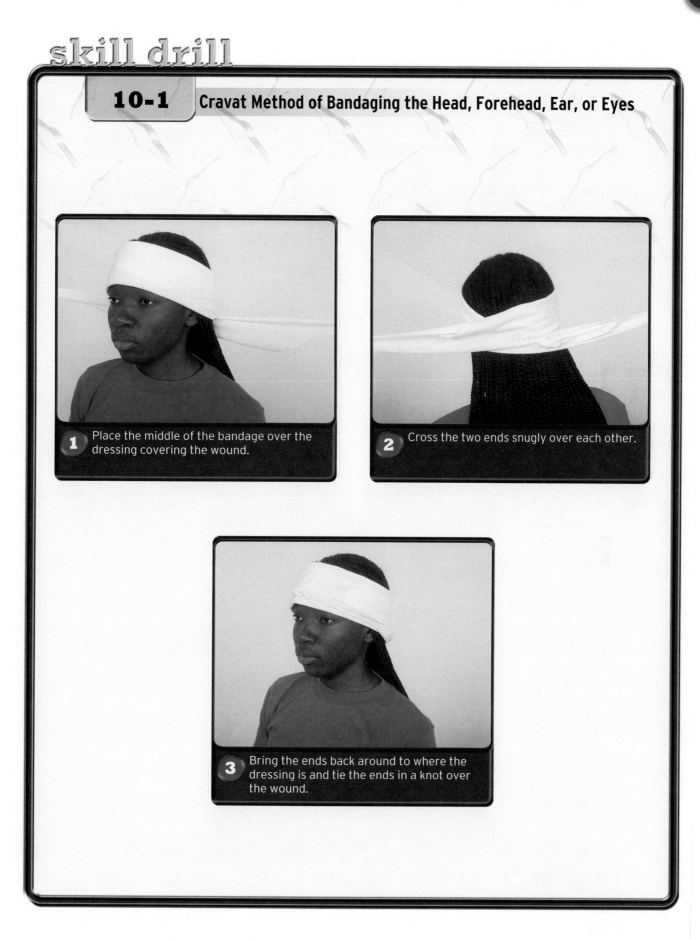

skill drill

10-1   Cravat Method of Bandaging the Head, Forehead, Ear, or Eyes

1 Place the middle of the bandage over the dressing covering the wound.

2 Cross the two ends snugly over each other.

3 Bring the ends back around to where the dressing is and tie the ends in a knot over the wound.

skill drill

10-2   Cravat Method of Bandaging the Arm or Leg

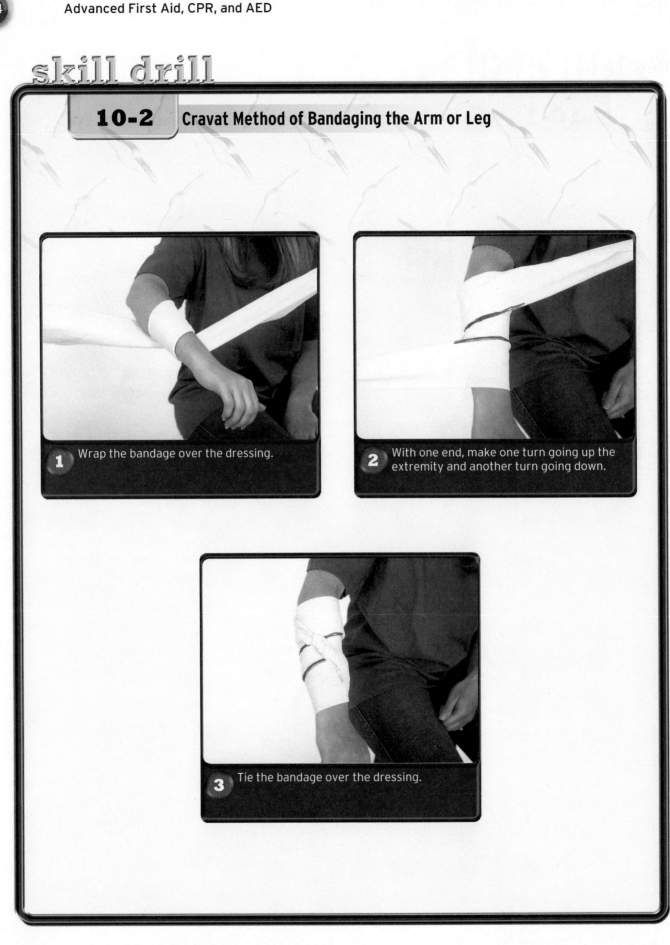

1 Wrap the bandage over the dressing.

2 With one end, make one turn going up the extremity and another turn going down.

3 Tie the bandage over the dressing.

skill drill

10-3   **Cravat Method for Applying a Bandage to the Palm of the Hand**

1 Fill the palm with a bulky dressing or pad.

2 Wrap one end of the bandage around the fingers and the other around the wrist.

3 Wrap the bandage crossing over the fingers and around the wrist.

4 Tie the bandage at the wrist.

The Figure-Eight Method

Use this method of applying a roller bandage to hold dressings or to provide compression at or near a joint such as the ankle. The figure-eight method involves continuous spiral loops of bandage, one up and one down, crossing each other to form an "8." To apply a 4″ or 6″ roller bandage to the elbow or knee using the figure-eight method, follow the steps in **Skill Drill 10-4**:

1. Bend the elbow or knee slightly and make two straight anchoring turns with the bandage over the elbow point or kneecap (**Step ❶**).
2. Bring the bandage above the joint to the upper arm or leg, and make one turn, covering half to three fourths of the bandage from the first turn (**Step ❷**).
3. Bring the bandage just under the joint and make one turn around the lower arm or leg, covering half to three fourths of the first straight turn (**Step ❸**).
4. Continue alternating the turns in a figure-eight maneuver by covering the previous layers (**Steps ❹ and ❺**).
5. Finish by making two straight turns, and secure the end.

To apply a roller bandage to the hand using the figure-eight method, follow the steps in **Skill Drill 10-5**. This method uses a 2″ or 3″ roller bandage.

1. Make two straight anchoring turns with the bandage around the palm of the hand (**Step ❶**).
2. Carry the bandage diagonally across the back of the hand and then around the wrist and back across the palm (**Step ❷**).
3. Complete several figure-eight turns, overlapping each by about three fourths of the previous bandage width. Repeat this figure-eight maneuver as many times as necessary to cover the dressing, overlapping wraps to "stair-step" up the hand (**Step ❸**).
4. Make two straight turns around the wrist, and secure the bandage.

To wrap an ankle or foot using the figure-eight method, follow the steps in **Skill Drill 10-6**. This wrapping will hold a dressing or apply pressure to treat a sprained ankle. It should not be used to support the ankle and foot during sports activity; that type of bandaging involves additional maneuvers. Either 2″ or 3″ roller bandages can be used.

1. Make two straight anchoring turns with the bandage around the foot's instep (**Step ❶**).

2. Make a figure-eight turn by taking the bandage diagonally across the front of the foot, around the ankle, and again diagonally across the foot and under the arch (**Step ❷**).
3. Make several of these figure-eight turns, each time overlapping the previous one by about three fourths the width of the bandage. The bandage advances up the leg (**Step ❸**).
4. Finish with two straight turns around the leg, and secure the bandage.

To securely fasten a roller bandage, you can:

- Apply adhesive tape to secure the bandage **Figure 10-8**.
- Use safety pins to secure the bandage **Figure 10-9**. Be very careful with victims who may have decreased sensation.

Figure 10-8

Apply adhesive tape.

Figure 10-9

Use safety pins.

10-4   **Figure-Eight Method of Bandaging a Knee or Elbow**

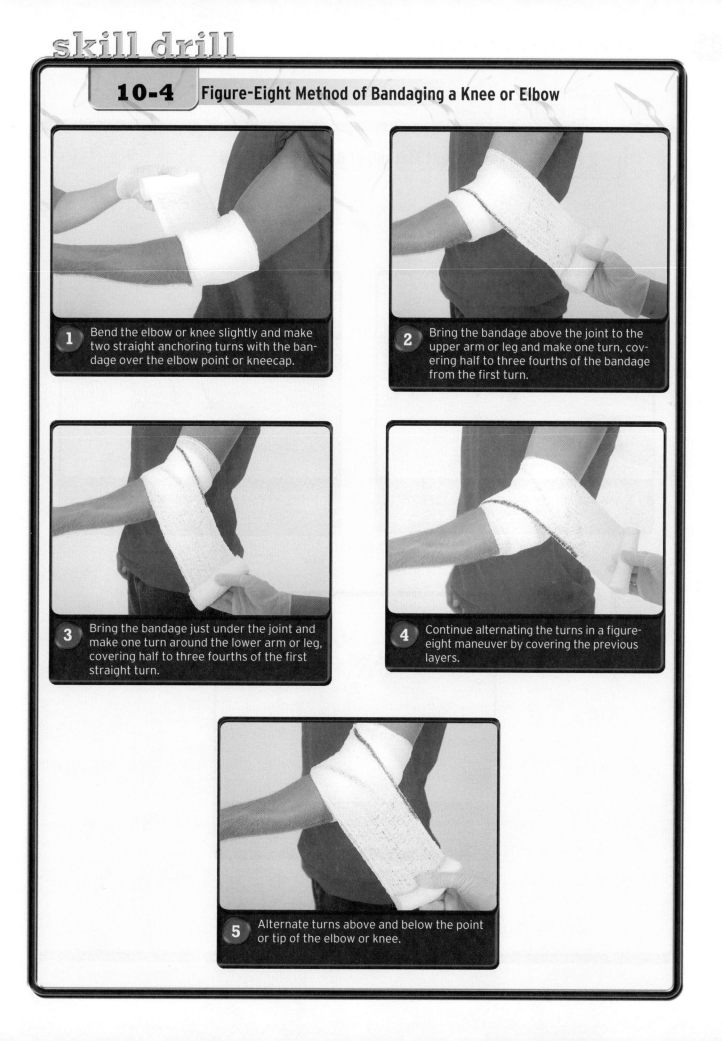

1 Bend the elbow or knee slightly and make two straight anchoring turns with the bandage over the elbow point or kneecap.

2 Bring the bandage above the joint to the upper arm or leg and make one turn, covering half to three fourths of the bandage from the first turn.

3 Bring the bandage just under the joint and make one turn around the lower arm or leg, covering half to three fourths of the first straight turn.

4 Continue alternating the turns in a figure-eight maneuver by covering the previous layers.

5 Alternate turns above and below the point or tip of the elbow or knee.

skill drill

10-5   **Figure-Eight Method of Bandaging a Hand**

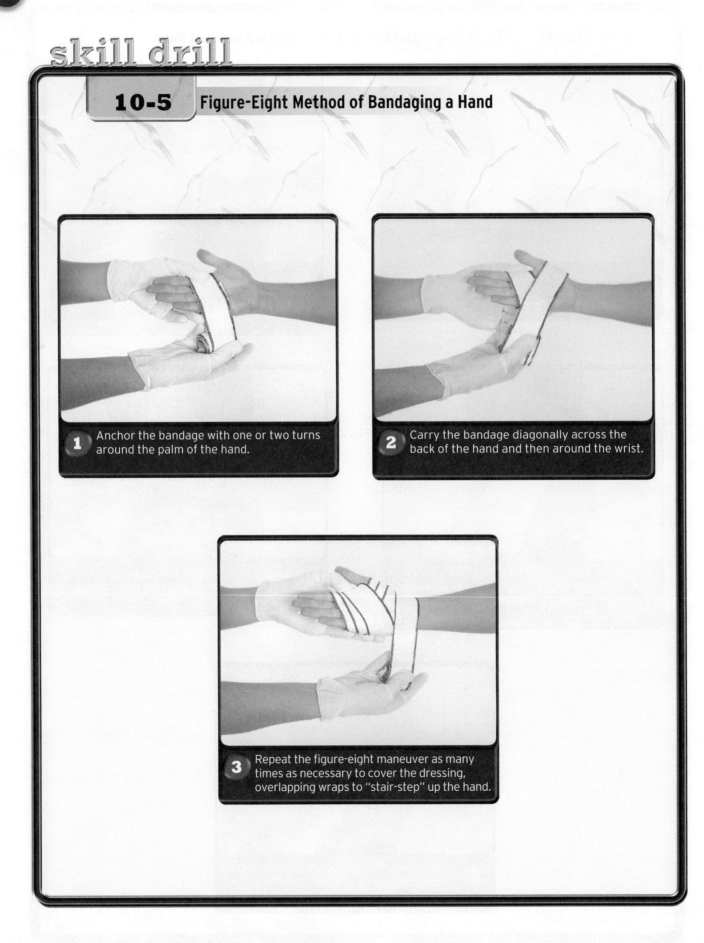

1 Anchor the bandage with one or two turns around the palm of the hand.

2 Carry the bandage diagonally across the back of the hand and then around the wrist.

3 Repeat the figure-eight maneuver as many times as necessary to cover the dressing, overlapping wraps to "stair-step" up the hand.

skill drill

10-6 Figure-Eight Method of Bandaging an Ankle or Foot

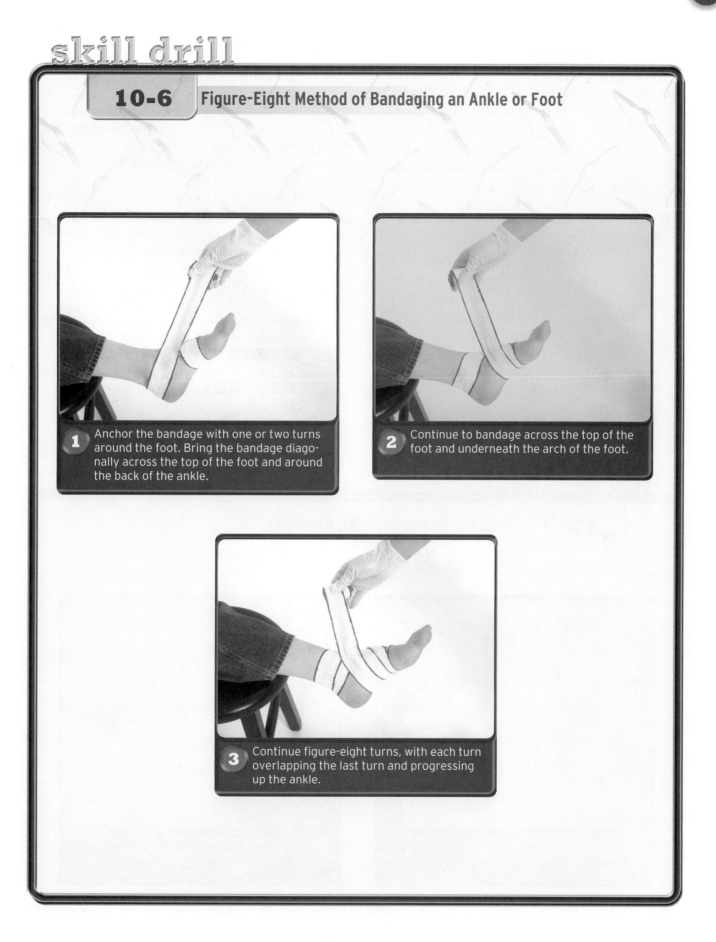

1 Anchor the bandage with one or two turns around the foot. Bring the bandage diagonally across the top of the foot and around the back of the ankle.

2 Continue to bandage across the top of the foot and underneath the arch of the foot.

3 Continue figure-eight turns, with each turn overlapping the last turn and progressing up the ankle.

- Use the special clips provided with elastic bandages **Figure 10-10**.

You can also use either the loop or split-tail methods, described in Skill Drills 10-7 and 10-8. To perform the loop method, follow the steps in **Skill Drill 10-7**:

Figure 10-10

Use special clips.

1. Reverse the direction of the bandage by looping it around a thumb or finger and continue back to the opposite side of the body part (**Step ①**).
2. Encircle the part with the looped end and the free end and tie them together (**Step ②**).

To perform the split-tail method of securing a bandage, follow the steps in **Skill Drill 10-8**:

1. Split the end of the bandage lengthwise for about 12″, then tie a knot to prevent further splitting (**Step ①**).
2. Pass the ends in opposite directions around the body part and tie (**Step ②**).

Applying an Adhesive Strip

1. Remove the wrapping and hold the dressing, pad-side down, by the protective strips **Figure 10-11**.
2. Peel back, but do not remove, the protective strips. Without touching the dressing pad, place it directly onto the wound.
3. Carefully pull away the protective strips. Press the ends and edges down.

skill drill

10-7   Loop Method of Securing Bandages

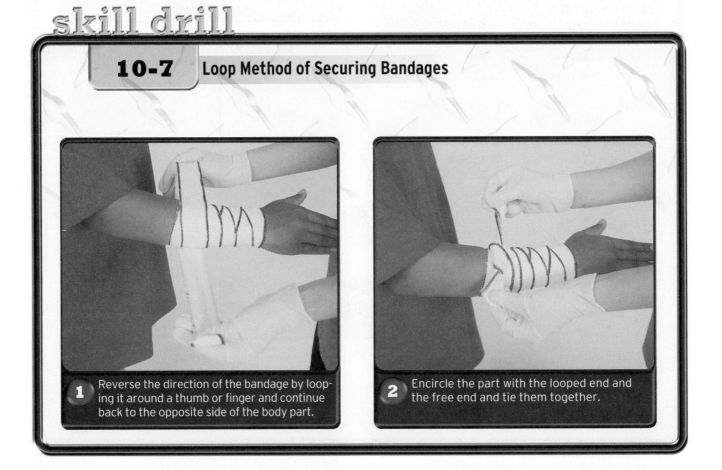

1 Reverse the direction of the bandage by looping it around a thumb or finger and continue back to the opposite side of the body part.

2 Encircle the part with the looped end and the free end and tie them together.

skill drill

10-8   Split-Tail Method of Securing Bandages

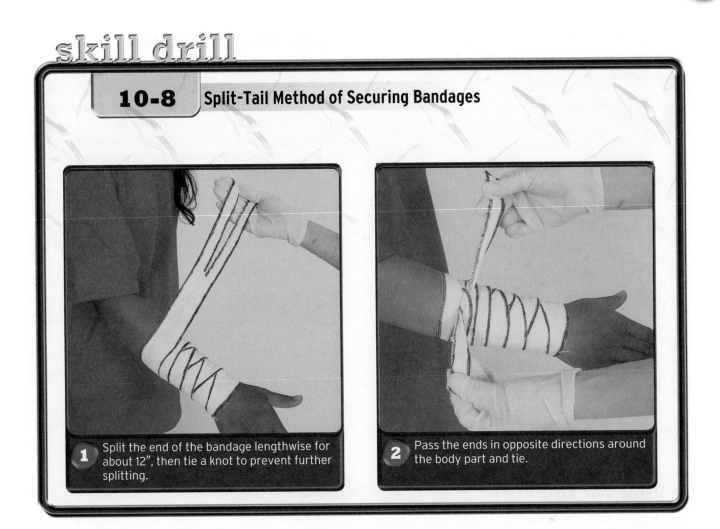

1 Split the end of the bandage lengthwise for about 12", then tie a knot to prevent further splitting.

2 Pass the ends in opposite directions around the body part and tie.

Figure 10-11

Applying an adhesive strip.

FYI

Adhesive Strip Bandage

To make an adhesive strip bandage snug on a chin, knee, or elbow, first cut the adhesive parts of the bandage lengthwise, but do not cut into the pad. Place the pad horizontally over the cut or wound. Then bring the bottom strips of the adhesive strip up and smooth them on the skin. Bring the top parts of the adhesive strips down and smooth them on the skin. Result: An adhesive bandage that contours to the wound.

prep kit

▶ Ready for Review

- A dressing covers an open wound; it touches the wound.
- Dressings used in most first aid situations are commercially prepared, but dressings may need to be improvised.
- A bandage should be clean but need not be sterile.
- The basic types of bandages are roller bandages; self-adhering, conforming bandages; gauze rollers; elastic roller bandages; triangular bandages; adhesive tape; and adhesive strips.
- With a little ingenuity, you can apply a roller bandage to almost any body part.

▶ Vital Vocabulary

adhesive strips A combination of both a sterile dressing and a bandage.

adhesive tape Come in rolls and in a variety of widths.

elastic roller bandages Used for compression on sprains, strains, and contusions and come in various widths.

gauze pads Used for small wounds, sterile, and available in separately wrapped packages of various sizes. Some have a special coating to keep them from sticking to the wound.

gauze rollers Cotton and nonelastic that come in various widths.

roller bandages Come in various widths, lengths, and types of material.

self-adhering, conforming bandages Come as rolls of slightly elastic, gauzelike material in various widths.

trauma dressings Made of large, thick, absorbent, sterile materials.

triangular bandages Available commercially or can be made from a 36″ to 40″ square of preshrunk cotton muslin material.

▶ Assessment in Action

You are enjoying a fly-fishing trip along a popular trout fishing river. It is a Saturday and there are several others fishing the same area. You and your friend decide to descend a steep riverbank to access a less crowded spot. Your friend slips down the river bank. You hurry down the bank and find her clutching her arm, which is bleeding. Another bystander arrives with a first aid kit.

Directions: Circle Yes if you agree with the statement; circle No if you disagree.

Yes No **1.** You should wash your hands with sanitizer and apply exam gloves from the first aid kit.

Yes No **2.** A dressing goes directly on the wound.

Yes No **3.** You can apply a roller bandage on the arm using spiral turns.

Yes No **4.** You should start bandaging from the upper part of the arm and progress down to the wrist.

Yes No **5.** After applying the bandage, you see that your friend's fingers are blue. This is a sign that the bandage is too tight.

▶ Check Your Knowledge

Directions: Circle Yes if you agree with the statement; circle No if you disagree.

Yes No **1.** A dressing does not touch an open wound.

Yes No **2.** Adhesive strips are used for small cuts and abrasions.

Yes No **3.** A bandage should be clean but need not be sterile.

Yes No **4.** Roller bandages come in only one size.

Yes No **5.** Roller bandages can be used only on the arm.

Yes No **6.** A square knot is the preferred knot for bandages.

Yes No **7.** Check the victim's lips for signs of a too-tight bandage.

Yes No **8.** If the victim can wiggle his or her fingers, the bandage is not on correctly.

Yes No **9.** Elastic roller bandages are used for compression on sprains, strains, and contusions.

Yes No **10.** The figure-eight method is used to apply a roller bandage to hold dressings or to provide compression at or near a joint.

11

Burns

Burns

Nearly 2 million burn injuries occur each year in the United States, resulting in 75,000 hospitalizations and more than 3,000 deaths. <u>Burns</u> occur in every age group, across all socioeconomic levels, at home and in the workplace, and in urban, suburban, and rural settings. It has been estimated that about 80% of all burn injuries occur in the home, with house fires responsible for the majority of fire deaths. Most burn victims are injured as a result of their own actions.

The highest-risk age groups for burn injuries are children younger than 5 years and adults older than 55 years. Both groups may have limited ability to recognize and escape from a fire or burn incident. In addition, their relatively thinner skin predisposes them to more serious injuries. Death and complications increase dramatically for burn victims older than 55 years owing to the likelihood of preexisting health problems and their immune systems' decreased ability to fight infection.

Skin death and injury occur as the applied heat exceeds the body's ability to disperse the heat; that point starts at about 113° F. The amount and depth of skin damage depend on the heat's intensity, the duration of contact, and the skin's thickness.

▶ Types of Burns

Burn injuries can be classified as thermal (heat), chemical, or electrical.

- Not all <u>thermal (heat) burns</u> are caused by flames. Contact with hot objects, flammable vapor that ignites and causes a flash or an explosion, and steam and hot liquid are other common causes of burns. Just 3 seconds of exposure to water at 140° F can cause a full-thickness (third-degree) burn in an adult. At 156° F, the same burn occurs in 1 second.

- **Chemical burns.** A wide range of chemical agents can cause tissue damage and death on contact with the skin. As with thermal burns, the amount of tissue damage depends on the duration of contact, the skin thickness in the area of exposure, and the strength of the chemical agent. Chemicals will continue to cause tissue destruction until the chemical agent is removed. Three types of chemicals—acids, alkalis, and organic compounds—are responsible for most chemical burns. Alkalis produce deeper, more extensive burns than acids.

- **Electrical burns.** The injury severity from contact with electric current depends on the type of current (direct or alternating), the voltage, the area of the body exposed, and the duration of contact. Electricity can induce ventricular fibrillation (a type of cardiac arrest), cause respiratory arrest, or "freeze" the victim to the electrical contact point with powerful muscle spasms that increase the length of exposure. Victims of low-voltage electrical injuries may have no skin burns at all but might still have cardiac or respiratory arrest.

Thermal Burns

Evaluate a thermal burn using the following steps. These steps form the basis for treatment of thermal burns.

1. **Determine the depth (degree) of the burn.** Historically, burns have been described as first-degree, second-degree, and third-degree injuries. The terms *superficial, partial thickness,* and *full thickness* are often used by burn-care professionals because they are more descriptive of the tissue damage.

   - **First-degree (superficial) burns** affect the skin's outer layer (epidermis) **Figure 11-1**. Signs and symptoms include: redness, mild swelling, tenderness, and pain. Healing occurs without scarring, usually within a week. The outer edges of deeper burns often are first-degree burns.

Figure 11-1

First-degree burn.

Figure 11-2

Second-degree burn blisters.

- **Second-degree (partial-thickness) burns** extend through the entire outer layer and into the inner skin layer **Figure 11-2**. Signs and symptoms include: blisters, swelling, weeping of fluids, and severe pain. The

Figure 11-3

Third-degree burn.

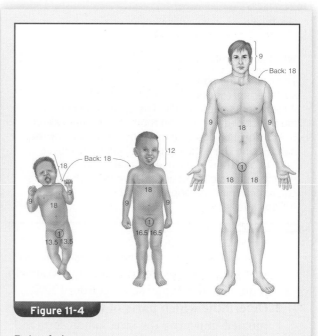

Figure 11-4

Rule of nines.

signs occur because the capillary blood vessels in the dermis are damaged and give up fluid into surrounding tissues. Intact blisters provide a sterile, waterproof covering. Once a blister breaks, a weeping wound results, and the risk of infection increases.

- <u>**Third-degree (full-thickness) burns**</u> are severe burns that penetrate all the skin layers into the underlying fat and muscle **Figure 11-3**. Signs and symptoms include: leathery, waxy, or pearly gray skin that is sometimes charred. It has a dry appearance because capillary blood vessels have been destroyed and no more fluid is brought to the area. The skin does not blanch after being pressed because the area is dead. The victim feels no pain from a third-degree burn because the nerve endings have been damaged or destroyed. Any pain felt is from surrounding burns of lesser degrees. A third-degree burn requires medical care and the removal of dead tissue and often a skin graft to heal properly.

2. **Determine the extent of the burn.** Skin will not ignite unless heated to thousands of degrees. However, if clothing ignites or skin is kept in contact with a heat source, such as scalding water, large areas of the skin will be injured. Determining the extent of a burn means estimating how much body surface area the burn covers. A rough guide known as the *rule of nines* assigns a percentage value of total body surface area (BSA) to each part of an adult's body **Figure 11-4**. The entire head is

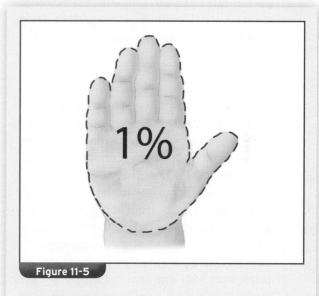

Figure 11-5

Rule of the hand.

9%, one complete arm is 9%, the front torso is 18%, the complete back is 18%, and each leg is 18%. The rule of nines must be modified to take into account the different proportions of a small child. In small children and infants, the head accounts for 18% and each leg is 14%. For small or scattered burns, use the *rule of the hand* **Figure 11-5**. The victim's hand, including the fingers and the thumb held together, represents

Q&A

What is the rule of the palm?

The rule of the palm says that a person's palm surface represents 1% of the BSA, but in actuality, it represents about 0.4%. The entire hand including the closed fingers and thumb represents about 0.8%. This textbook suggests using the rule of the hand–using the entire hand, including the closed fingers and thumb–as an easy method to estimate the extent of a burned area. The extent of a burn is calculated only on people with partial-thickness or full-thickness burns.

about 1% of his or her total body surface. For a very large burn, estimate the unburned area in number of hands and subtract from 100%.

3. **Determine which parts of the body are burned.** Burns on the face, hands, feet, and genitals are more severe than those on other body parts. A circumferential burn (one that goes around a finger, toe, arm, leg, neck, or chest) is considered more severe than a non-circumferential one because of the possible constriction and tourniquet effect on circulation and, in some cases, breathing. All of these burns require medical care.

4. **Determine respiratory involvement.** Respiratory tract damage caused by heat associated with a burn can cause death after a victim is hospitalized. Respiratory damage may result from breathing heat or the products of combustion, from being burned by a flame while in a closed space, or from being in an explosion. In these cases, even with no skin burn injury, there may be respiratory damage. Superheated air is absorbed by the upper respiratory tract (the area from the nose to the trachea), resulting in inflammation. Swelling occurs in 2 to 24 hours, restricting or completely shutting off the airway so that air cannot reach the lungs. All respiratory injuries must receive medical care.

5. **Determine whether other injuries or preexisting medical problems exist or if the victim is elderly** (older than 55 years) **or very young** (younger than 5 years). A medical problem or being in one of the sensitive age groups increases a burn's severity. Burns can aggravate existing medical conditions such as diabetes, heart disease, and lung disease, as well as other medical problems. Concurrent injuries such as fractures, internal injuries, and open wounds increase the severity of a burn.

6. **Determine the burn's severity** `Table 11-1`. This forms the basis for how to treat the burned victim. Most burns are minor, occur at home, and can be managed outside a medical setting. Seek medical care for all moderate and severe burns, as classified by the American Burn Association, or if any of the following conditions applies:
   - The victim has difficulty breathing.
   - Other injuries exist.

Table 11-1 Burn Severity

Minor Burns
- First-degree burn covering less than 50% BSA in adults (face, hands, feet, and genitals not burned)*
- Second-degree burn covering less than 10% BSA in adults
- Second-degree burn covering less than 10% BSA in children and elderly persons

Moderate Burns
- First-degree burn covering more than 50% BSA in adults
- Second-degree burn covering 15% to 30% BSA in adults*
- Second-degree burn covering 10% to 20% BSA in children and elderly persons
- Third-degree burn covering up to 10% BSA in adults (face, hands, and feet not burned)

Critical Burns
- Second-degree burn covering more than 30% BSA in adults
- Second-degree burn covering more than 20% BSA in children and elderly persons
- Third-degree burn covering more than 10% BSA in adults
- Third-degree burn covering more than 2% BSA in children and elderly persons
- Third-degree burn of hands, face, eyes, feet, or genitalia; also most inhalation injuries, electrical injuries, and burns accompanied by major trauma or significant preexisting conditions

Source: Adapted from the American Burn Association.
*Criteria for children have not been established. If in doubt, consult a medical professional.

Table 11-2 First Aid for Burns

Type of Burn	Do ...	Don't ...
First-degree burn (redness, mild swelling, and pain)	Apply cold water and, after cooled, apply aloe vera gel or a body lotion.	Apply butter, oleomargarine, or similar substances.
Second-degree burn (deeper injury; blisters develop)	Apply cold water. After cooled, apply antibiotic ointment. Treat for shock.	Break blisters. Remove shreds of tissue. Use a home remedy.
Third-degree burn (deeper destruction; skin layers destroyed)	Cover the burn with a sterile cloth to protect it. Treat the victim for shock. Watch for breathing difficulty. Obtain medical attention quickly.	Remove charred clothing that is stuck to the burn. Apply ice. Use a home medication.
Chemical burn	Remove chemical by flushing with large quantities of water for at least 20 minutes. Remove surrounding clothing. Quickly obtain medical care.	Apply water under high pressure. Try to neutralize with other chemicals.

- An electrical injury exists.
- The face, hands, feet, or genitals are burned.
- Child abuse is suspected.
- The surface area of a second-degree burn is greater than 10% of the body surface area.
- The burn is third degree.

Care for Thermal Burns

Burn care aims to reduce pain, to provide physical protection, and to provide a favorable environment for healing that minimizes the chances of scarring and infection Table 11-2. Because burns can continue to injure tissue for a surprisingly long time, it is critical to stop the burning. If clothing is burning, have the victim roll on the ground using the "stop, drop, and roll" method. Smother the flames with a blanket or douse the victim with water. Stop a person whose clothes are on fire from running, which only fans the flames. The victim should not remain standing, because he or she is more apt to inhale flames. Once the fire is extinguished, remove all hot or smoldering clothing because the burning may continue if the clothing is left on. If possible, remove jewelry because heat may be held near the skin and cause more damage. Swelling could make jewelry difficult to remove later. Monitor the victim's breathing.

CAUTION

DO NOT remove clothing stuck to the skin. Cut around the areas where clothing sticks to the skin. DO NOT pull on stuck clothing; pulling will further damage the skin.

Care for First-Degree Burns

1. Run cold tap water (60° to 77°F [15° to 25°C]) over the area as soon as possible Figure 11-6 or apply a wet, cold cloth to reduce pain. Apply cold until the part is pain free while in and out of the water (usually in 10 minutes, but it may take up to 45 minutes). Cold stops the progression of the burn into deeper tissue. If cold water is unavailable, use any cold, drinkable liquid to reduce the temperature of the burned skin.

2. Give ibuprofen to relieve pain and inflammation.

3. Have the victim drink as much water as possible without becoming nauseous.

4. After the burn has been cooled, apply an aloe vera gel or an inexpensive skin moisturizer lotion to keep the skin moistened and to reduce itching and peeling. Use a lotion that does not have alcohols or strong fragrances. Lotions with

Cool burn with cold water until pain is relieved.

Cooling usually takes 10–45 minutes.

Figure 11-6

Immerse the burn. Cool burn with cold water until pain is relieved. Cooling usually takes 10-45 minutes.

glycerin and mineral oil are best. Aloe vera has antimicrobial and anti-inflammatory properties and is a mild analgesic.

5. Keep a burned arm or leg raised to reduce swelling and pain.

CAUTION

DO NOT apply cold over a large burn for a prolonged time because it can produce hypothermia.

DO NOT use an ice pack or ice water unless it is the only source of cold available. If you must use it, apply it for only 10 to 15 minutes.

DO NOT apply grease, butter, cream, or a home remedy. Such coatings are unsterile and can lead to infection. They also can seal in heat, causing further damage.

DO NOT cover a first-degree burn.

Care for Small Second-Degree Burns (<10% BSA)

1. Run cold tap water (60° to 77°F [15° to 25°C]) over the area as soon as possible or apply a wet, cold cloth to reduce pain. Apply cold until the part is pain free while in and out of the water (usually in 10 minutes, but it may take up to 45 minutes). Cold stops the progression of the burn into deeper tissue. If cold water is unavailable, use any cold, drinkable liquid to reduce the temperature of the burned skin.

2. Give ibuprofen to relieve pain and inflammation.

3. Have the victim drink as much water as possible without becoming nauseated.

4. After a burn has been cooled, apply a thin layer of an antibiotic ointment. Topical antibiotic therapy does not sterilize a wound, but it decreases the number of bacteria to a level that can be controlled by the body's defense mechanisms and prevents the entrance of bacteria. Physicians may prescribe a silver-based antibiotic, which is the agent of choice for burn wounds.

5. Cover the burn with a dry, nonsticking, sterile dressing or a clean cloth. Covering the burn reduces the amount of pain by keeping air from the exposed nerve endings. The main purpose of a dressing over a burn is to keep the burn clean, prevent evaporative moisture loss, and reduce pain. If fingers or toes have been burned, place dry dressings between them and seek medical care.

6. Seek medical care for second-degree burns covering more than 10% of the BSA.

Care for Large Second-Degree Burns (>10% BSA)

1. Cold can be applied if you monitor the victim for hypothermia (eg, shivering, cold skin on unburned areas).
2. Follow steps 2 and 3 for first-degree and small second-degree burn care.
3. Cover the burn with a dry, nonstick, sterile, or clean dressing.
4. Treat for shock.
5. Seek medical care.

Care for Third-Degree Burns

1. Cover the burn with a dry, nonsticking, sterile dressing or a clean cloth.
2. Treat the victim for shock and keep the victim warm with a clean sheet or blanket.
3. Seek medical care.

Later Thermal Burn Care

For after-thermal burn care, follow a physician's recommendations, if a physician has been consulted (many burns are never seen by a doctor). The following suggestions may apply:

- Wash hands thoroughly before changing any dressing.
- Leave unbroken blisters intact.
- Change dressings once or twice a day unless a physician instructs otherwise.

To change a dressing:

1. Remove the old dressing. If a dressing sticks, soak it off with cool, clean water.
2. Cleanse the area gently with mild soap and water.
3. Pat the area dry with a clean cloth.
4. Apply a thin layer of antibiotic ointment to the burn.
5. Apply a nonsticking sterile dressing.

Watch for signs of infection. Call a physician if any of these appear:

- Increased redness, pain, tenderness, swelling, or red streaks near the burn
- Pus
- Elevated temperature (fever)

Keep the area and dressing as clean and dry as possible. Elevate the burned area, if possible, for the first 24 hours. Give pain medication, if necessary.

Scald Burns

Scald burns are the result of contact with hot liquids. Scald burns can be divided into two types: immersion burns and spill burns. An *immersion burn* results when an area of the body is fully immersed in a hot liquid. It generally has definite demarcations between healthy and injured tissue. This type of burn tends to be deep and is often full thickness. This type of injury is generally caused by abuse and is seen most often in children.

A *spill burn* occurs when a liquid spills, drops, or is thrown on a person. The pattern of this type of burn generally is irregular and may be scattered across large body areas. A spill burn usually is not as deep as an immersion burn.

Neglect and lack of supervision of children in the kitchen and the bathtub are frequent causes of spill burns. Scalds in adults occur more often in the elderly population, who generally have decreased sensation. As a result, many elderly victims are scalded in the bath.

Sunburn

In the United States, about one third of adults and about two thirds of children have a sunburn each summer. Sunburn is the skin's response to the trauma of ultraviolet (UV) radiation that results mainly from exposure to UVB radiation or, rarely, to UVA radiation. Sunburn may be the most common burn sustained by humans, and probably all persons have had one at some time **Figure 11-7**. True sunburn reaction begins 2 to 8 hours after UV radiation exposure. The amount of UV light the skin has received is difficult to gauge accurately. Not until after exposure (4 to 12 hours later) does the redness, tenderness, and discomfort of sunburned skin confirm the overexposure. Painful blistering and swelling peak about 24 hours later.

Sunburn results in first- or second-degree burns. A third-degree burn can occur from a sunburn, but it is rare. The redness of a sunburn is caused by the dilation of the small blood vessels. Blister formation comes from plasma leakage.

Human skin displays marked differences in its response to UV radiation exposure. Some people always burn and never tan, while others rarely experience a painful sunburn. The variability is largely attributed to the degree of pigmentation (melanin) that the skin contains. Darker-hued people generally are more resistant to the sun's rays than are those with light complexions, but all human beings eventually will burn if exposed to enough UVB. Other variables that contribute to individual sensitivity include the area of the body exposed, the underlying condition of the skin, the degree of tanning, and the role of various photosensitizing medicines.

Various skin types respond differently to UV light:

- Type I skin always burns easily and never tans. A type I person normally has blue eyes, red hair, and freckles.
- Type II skin burns easily, tans slightly.
- Type III skin sometimes burns, but always tans gradually and moderately.
- Type IV skin minimally burns and always tans well. Examples of people with type IV skin are people of Hispanic or Asian descent.
- Type V skin rarely burns and tans deeply. Examples of people with type V skin are Middle Easterners and Indians (heavily pigmented).
- Type VI skin does not burn (although it can burn or peel with significant exposure). An example of people with type VI skin is people of African descent (deeply pigmented).

Care for Sunburns

1. Cool compresses for up to 45 minutes are quite soothing to sunburned skin. Frequent cool showers or soaking in a tub may provide remarkable relief. Some experts advise against the use of topical analgesics, sprays, or lotions, especially those containing benzocaine. Benzocaine may sensitize the skin, resulting in contact dermatitis that compounds the original problem. Topical anesthetic sprays or lotions may provide temporary relief, but they are expensive and generally ineffective. Over-the-counter (OTC) analgesics such as ibuprofen should suffice in most cases because they reduce pain and inflammation. Drinking lots of water is also suggested.
2. First- and second-degree sunburns can be quite painful. When a large area of skin is involved,

Figure 11-7

Sunburn.

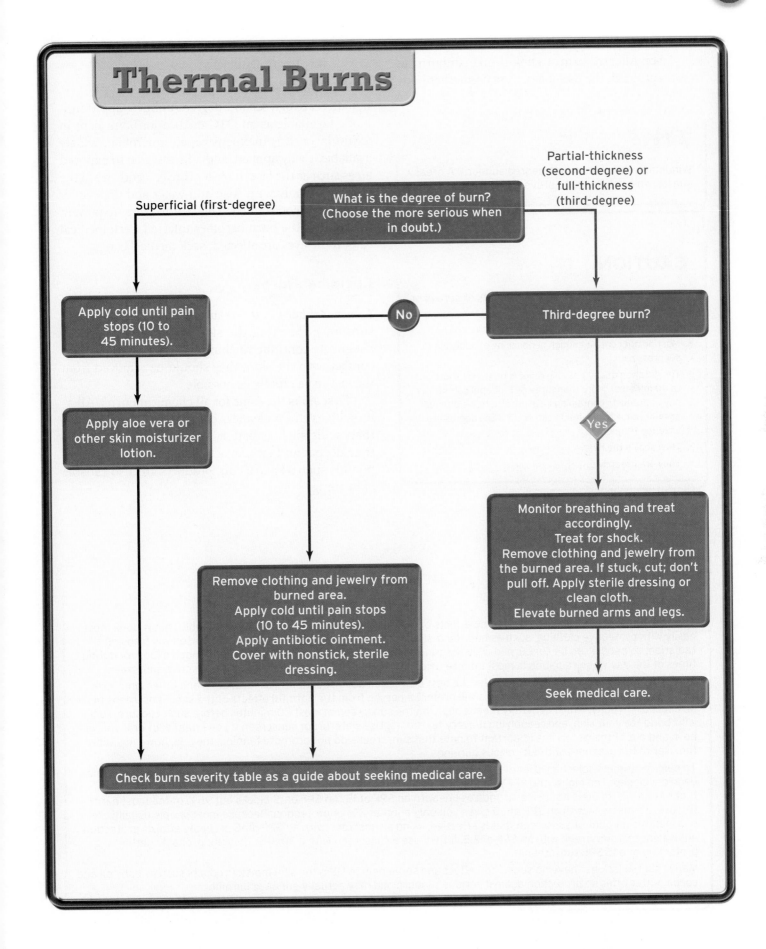

Thermal Burns

What is the degree of burn? (Choose the more serious when in doubt.)

Superficial (first-degree)

Partial-thickness (second-degree) or full-thickness (third-degree)

Apply cold until pain stops (10 to 45 minutes).

Apply aloe vera or other skin moisturizer lotion.

No

Third-degree burn?

Yes

**Remove clothing and jewelry from burned area.
Apply cold until pain stops (10 to 45 minutes).
Apply antibiotic ointment.
Cover with nonstick, sterile dressing.**

**Monitor breathing and treat accordingly.
Treat for shock.
Remove clothing and jewelry from the burned area. If stuck, cut; don't pull off. Apply sterile dressing or clean cloth.
Elevate burned arms and legs.**

Seek medical care.

Check burn severity table as a guide about seeking medical care.

the person may feel ill and have chills and fever. After the pain of a first-degree sunburn has subsided, the use of aloe vera or another body

FYI

Windburn resembles a first-degree sunburn. A greasy sunscreen can be used to prevent and treat it.

CAUTION

DO NOT use topical OTC burn ointments or sprays or anesthetic sprays because:

- Some products may cause allergic reactions.
- Most do not contain enough benzocaine or lidocaine to suppress pain.
- The duration of any possible relief is relatively short (30 to 40 minutes). More than three or four applications per day of products containing local anesthetics is discouraged because toxic effects can occur if the agents are used too frequently.
- They seal in the heat.
- They are expensive.

lotion can keep the skin moist. Do not use butter or petroleum jelly.

Sunburn Aftercare

For aftercare of a second-degree sunburn, apply antibiotic (available as an OTC medication) ointment in a thin layer. It is inexpensive, antimicrobial, widely available, easily applied, and adheres even to exposed areas such as the face. If blisters break, gently wash the area twice daily with soap and water and then cover with an antibiotic ointment and sterile gauze to prevent infection. If the burn becomes infected, seek medical care. If the eyes are affected, seek medical care.

Chemical Burns

A *chemical burn* is the result of an acid or an alkali substance touching the skin . Because chemicals continue to "burn" as long as they are in contact with the skin, they should be removed from the victim as rapidly as possible.

First aid is the same for all chemical burns. Alkalis such as drain cleaners cause more serious burns than acids such as battery acid because they penetrate deeper and remain active longer. Organic compounds such as petroleum products are also capable of burning.

FYI

Sunburn Prevention

The best protection against the damaging effects of UV radiation is to limit exposure to sunlight. That is done most easily with protective clothing, such as hats, long-sleeved shirts, and long pants. Wet, white cotton will transmit UV radiation, so people can be sunburned while wearing such clothing. People should avoid prolonged exposure during times of the day when radiation is most intense (usually between 10 AM and 2 PM) and apply effective sunscreens.

Sunscreens are readily available and offer the best protection against sunburn, skin cancers, and other long-term skin injury. The proper use of sunscreens will protect a person from the harmful effects of the sun. Sunscreens must be applied correctly, which generally means applying the sunscreen at least 20 minutes before sun exposure, so it will "bond" to your skin, and reapplying it every few hours. Use waterproof sunscreen if you sweat a lot or if you will be in and out of the water. It is important to note that sunscreens do not promote tanning; they do, however, allow the user to tan gradually without serious burning.

To help consumers select an effective sunscreen, the system of rating products by the *skin protection factor (SPF)* has been developed. The higher the SPF number, the greater the protection against sunburn. However, a sunscreen that has an SPF of 30 is not twice as good as one with an SPF of 15. An SPF of 15 blocks out 95% of the most harmful rays; a sunscreen with an SPF of 30 gives you only another 3% of protection. Because most people usually use only half the amount of sunscreen that is effective, using a sunscreen with an SPF of 15 probably affords protection equivalent to a sunscreen with an SPF of 7.5. If they use a sunscreen with a 30 SPF, they are probably getting the protection of a 15 SPF sunscreen.

Many "suntan lotions" have no sunscreen effect and serve only to keep the skin moist. Products such as baby oil and cocoa butter offer no protection against serious sunburn and may actually enhance burning.

Figure 11-8

Chemical burn from sulfuric acid.

Figure 11-9

Flushing a chemical burn.

Q&A

How can you determine how deep a burn is?

There are two layers of skin: the epidermis and the dermis. The epidermis, the outer layer of skin, serves primarily as a barrier between the body and the environment. The dermis has blood vessels and contains nerves, sweat glands, sebaceous glands, and hair roots.

The individual layers of skin are not visible to the naked eye, so when determining depth of a burn, it is helpful to remember that the dermis is the layer that will bleed. Full-thickness burns do not bleed because the blood vessels have been destroyed.

Care for Chemical Burns

1. Immediately remove the chemical by flushing the body portion with water . If available, use a hose or a shower. Brush dry powder chemicals from the skin before flushing. Water may activate a dry chemical and cause more damage to the skin. Take standard precautions to protect yourself from exposure to the chemical.
2. Remove the victim's contaminated clothing and jewelry while flushing with water. Clothing can hold chemicals, allowing them to continue to burn as long as they are in contact with the skin.
3. Flush for 20 minutes or longer. Let the victim wash with a mild soap before a final rinse. Washing with large amounts of water dilutes the chemical concentration and washes it away.
4. Cover the burned area with a dry, sterile dressing or, for large areas, a clean lint-free cloth, such as a pillowcase.
5. If the chemical is in an eye, flood it for at least 20 minutes, using a gentle stream of water.
6. Seek medical care immediately for all chemical burns.

Chemical Burns

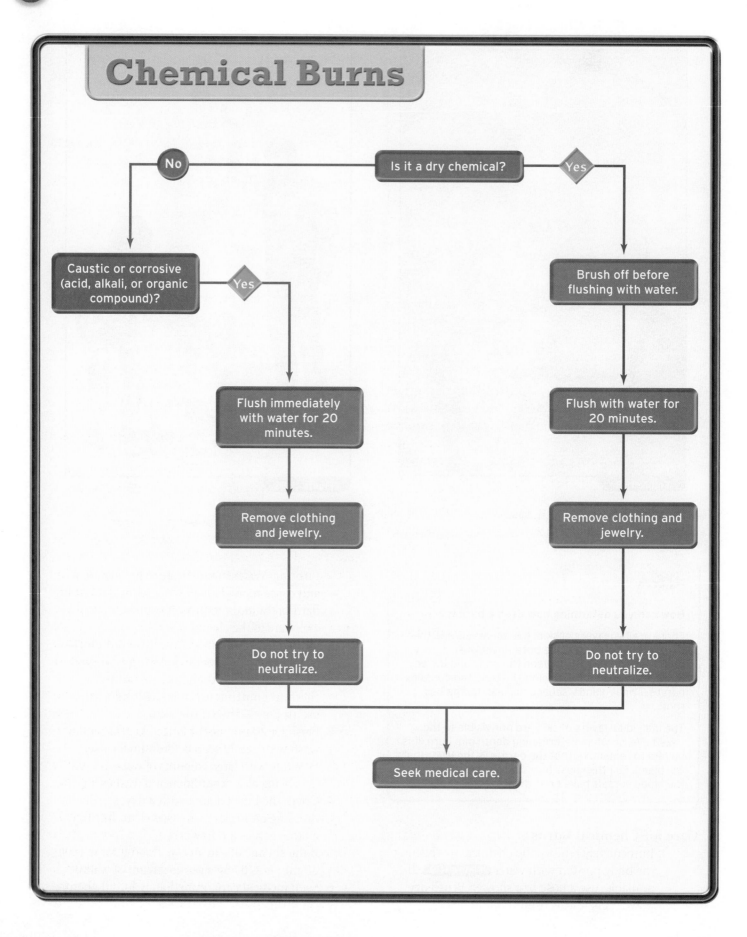

> **CAUTION**
>
> DO NOT waste time! A chemical burn is an emergency!
>
> DO NOT apply water under high pressure; it will drive the chemical deeper into the tissue.
>
> DO NOT try to neutralize a chemical even if you know which chemical is involved; heat may be produced, resulting in more damage. Some product labels for neutralizing may be wrong. Save the container or the label for the chemical's name.

Electrical Burns

Even a mild electrical shock can cause serious internal injuries **Figure 11-10**. A current of 1,000 volts or more is considered high voltage, but even the 110 volts found in ordinary household current can be deadly. There are three types of electrical injuries: thermal burn (flame), arc burn (flash), and true electrical injury (contact). A *thermal burn* (flame) results when clothing or objects in direct contact with the skin are ignited by an electric current. These injuries are caused by the flames produced by the electric current and not by the passage of the electric current or arc.

An *arc burn* (flash) occurs when electricity jumps, or arcs, from one spot to another and not from the passage of an electric current through the body. Although the duration of the flash may be brief, it usually causes extensive superficial injuries.

A true *electrical injury* (contact) happens when an electric current passes directly through the body. This type of injury is characterized by an entrance wound and an exit wound. The important factor with this type of injury is that the surface injury may be just the tip of the iceberg. High-voltage electric currents passing through the body may disrupt the normal heart rhythm and cause cardiac arrest, internal burns, and other injuries.

During an electrical shock, electricity enters the body at the point of contact and travels along the path of least resistance (nerves and blood vessels). The major damage occurs inside the body—the entrance burn may appear small. Usually, the electricity exits where the body is touching a surface or is in contact with a ground (for example, a metal object). The exit wound can be extensive. Sometimes, a victim has more than one exit site.

Care for Electrical Burns

1. Make sure the area is safe. Unplug, disconnect, or turn off the power. If that is impossible, call 9-1-1 for help. Never touch an energized wire, object, or victim yourself.
2. Check breathing and, if absent, begin CPR.
3. If the victim fell, check for a spinal injury.
4. Treat the victim for shock.
5. Place dry, sterile dressings on all burn wounds.
6. Place blankets under and over the victim.
7. Seek medical care immediately. Electrical injuries may require treatment in a burn center.

Contact With an Outdoor Power Line

If the electrical shock is from contact with a downed power line, the power must be turned off before a rescuer approaches anyone who may be in contact with the wire. If a power line falls across a car containing a person, tell the person to stay in the car until the power can be shut off. The only exception is if fire threatens the car. In that case, tell the victim to jump out of the car without making contact with the car or the wire.

If you feel a tingling sensation in your legs and lower body as you approach a victim, stop. The sensation signals that you are on energized ground and that an electric current is entering through one foot, passing through your lower body, and leaving through the other foot. Raise one foot off the ground, turn around, and hop to a safe place.

If you can safely reach the victim, do not attempt to move any wires, even with wooden poles, tools with wood handles, or tree branches. Wood can conduct electricity and the rescuer will be electrocuted. Do *not* attempt to move downed wires unless you are trained and equipped with tools able to handle the

Figure 11-10

Electrical burns. **A.** Exit wound on a foot. **B.** Electrical burn caused by chewing through an electrical cord.

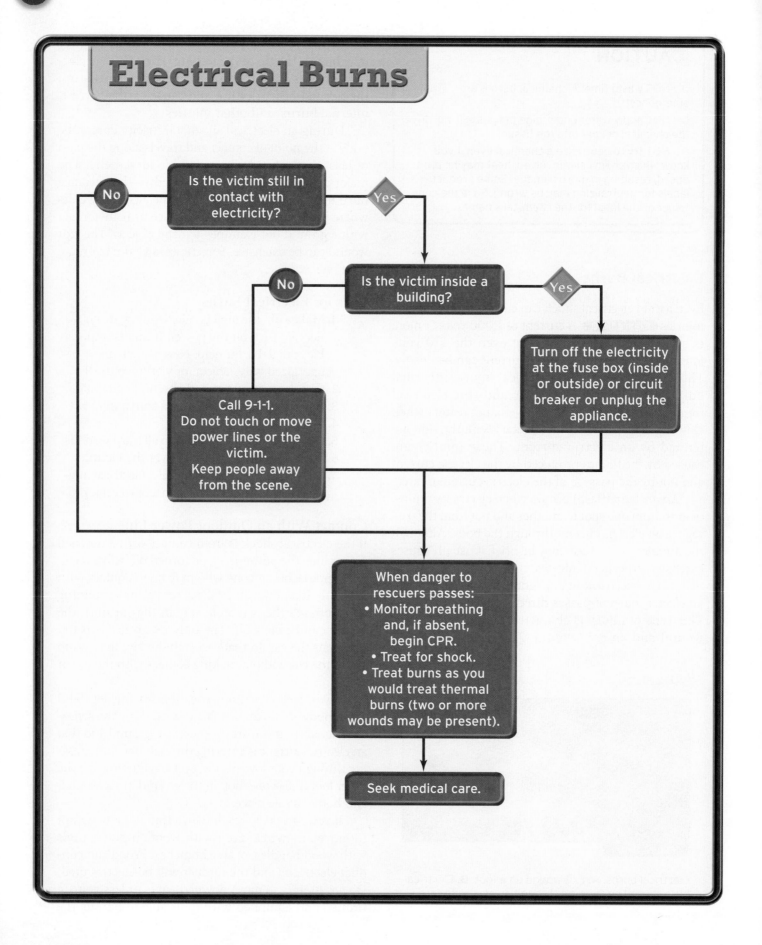

Electrical Burns

Is the victim still in contact with electricity? — No → / Yes →

Is the victim inside a building? — No → / Yes →

Yes → **Turn off the electricity at the fuse box (inside or outside) or circuit breaker or unplug the appliance.**

No → **Call 9-1-1. Do not touch or move power lines or the victim. Keep people away from the scene.**

When danger to rescuers passes:
- Monitor breathing and, if absent, begin CPR.
- Treat for shock.
- Treat burns as you would treat thermal burns (two or more wounds may be present).

Seek medical care.

Skin

Muscle

Tissue
damage

Skin

Entrance wound

Exit wound

Figure 11-11

The external signs of an electrical burn may be deceiving. The entrance wound may be a small burn, while the damage to deeper tissue may be massive.

high voltage. Wait until trained personnel with the proper equipment can cut the wires or disconnect them. Prevent bystanders from entering the danger area.

Contact Inside Buildings

Most electrical burns that occur indoors are caused by faulty electrical equipment or careless use of electrical appliances. Turn off the electricity at the circuit breaker, fuse box, or outside switch box, or unplug the appliance if the plug is undamaged. Do not touch the appliance or the victim until the current is off.

Once there is no danger to rescuers, first aid can begin. Electric current flows quickly into the body's tissues and then exits. The surface injuries of the skin involve small surface areas (entrance and exit points); the major damage occurs deep under the skin **Figure 11-11** . See Chapter 24, *Wilderness First Aid,* for lightning burns and their care.

▶ Emergency Care Wrap-up

Condition	What to Look For	What to Do
Thermal (Heat) Burns	**First-degree burn (superficial)** • Redness • Mild swelling • Pain	1. Cool the burn with cold water. 2. Apply aloe vera gel or a skin moisturizer. 3. If available, give an OTC medication to reduce pain and swelling.
	Second-degree burn (partial thickness) • Blisters • Swelling • Pain • Weeping of fluid	1. Cool burn with cold water and monitor victims with large, second-degree burns for hypothermia. 2. Apply antibiotic ointment. 3. Cover with a dry, nonstick sterile dressing. 4. If available, give an OTC medication to reduce pain and swelling. 5. Seek medical care.
	Third-degree burn (full thickness) • Dry, leathery skin • Gray or charred skin	1. Monitor breathing and provide care as needed. 2. Cover burn with a dry, nonstick sterile, or clean dressing. 3. Treat for shock. 4. Seek medical care.
Chemical Burns	• Stinging pain	1. Brush dry chemicals off skin. 2. Flush with a large amount of water for 20 minutes (gentle water flow). 3. Remove the victim's contaminated clothing and jewelry while flushing. 4. Cover the area with a dry, sterile, or clean dressing. 5. Seek medical care.
Electrical Burns	• Possible third-degree burn with entrance and exit wounds	1. Safety first! Unplug, disconnect, or turn off the electricity. 2. Open the airway, check breathing, and provide care as needed. 3. Care for burns as you would a third-degree burn. 4. Seek medical care.

▶ Ready for Review

- Burns occur in every age group; across all socioeconomic levels; at home and in the workplace; and in urban, suburban, and rural settings.
- Burn injuries can be classified as thermal, chemical, or electrical.
- Treatment depends on the depth of burns.
- A chemical burn is the result of a caustic or corrosive substance touching the skin.
- There are three types of electrical injuries: thermal burn (flame), arc burn (flash), and true electrical injury (contact).

▶ Vital Vocabulary

<u>burns</u> Injuries in which soft tissue receives more energy than it can absorb from thermal heat, chemicals, or electricity.

<u>chemical burns</u> Damage caused to the skin by chemicals.

<u>electrical burns</u> Injury caused from contact with electric current.

<u>first-degree (superficial) burns</u> Burns affecting only the epidermis. Characterized by skin that is red but not blistered or burned through.

<u>second-degree (partial-thickness) burns</u> Burns affecting the epidermis and some portion of the dermis but not the subcutaneous tissue. Characterized by blisters and skin that is white to red and moist.

<u>thermal (heat) burns</u> Damage to the skin caused by contact with hot objects, flammable vapor, steam, hot liquid, or flames.

<u>third-degree (full-thickness) burns</u> Burns that affect all skin layers and may affect the subcutaneous layers, muscle, bone, and internal organs, leaving the area dry, leathery, and white, dark brown, or charred.

prep kit

▶ Assessment in Action

After a long, hot day at the water park, your friend complains of severe sunburn on his back and shoulders. He failed to apply sunscreen while at the water park. Blisters have formed, and your friend refuses to sit up in a chair and complains of severe pain.

Directions: Circle Yes if you agree with the statement; circle No if you disagree.

Yes   No   **1.** The blisters and pain are signs that this is a first-degree burn.

Yes   No   **2.** You should break the blisters to relieve pressure and clean the burn.

Yes   No   **3.** Cool compresses can be used to relieve pain.

Yes   No   **4.** You can apply antibiotic ointment and aloe vera to keep the skin moist.

Yes   No   **5.** This person does not need medical care.

▶ Check Your Knowledge

Directions: Circle Yes if you agree with the statement; circle No if you disagree.

Yes   No   **1.** Victims of a burn should immediately drink water.

Yes   No   **2.** Petroleum jelly can be applied over a burn.

Yes   No   **3.** The rule of the hand can help determine the size of a burned area.

Yes   No   **4.** Neutralize an acid on the skin by using baking soda.

Yes   No   **5.** Use a large amount of water to flush chemicals off the body.

Yes   No   **6.** Brush a dry chemical off the skin before flushing with water.

Yes   No   **7.** When someone gets electrocuted, there can be two burn wounds: entrance and exit.

Yes   No   **8.** When a victim is in contact with a power line, use a tree branch to remove the wires.

Yes   No   **9.** Ibuprofen helps relieve pain and swelling.

Yes   No   **10.** Cold water can be used, in moderation, on any burn of any size.

Head and Spinal Injuries

Head Injuries

Any head injury is potentially serious. If not properly treated, injuries that seem minor could become life threatening. Head injuries include scalp wounds, skull fractures, and brain injuries. Spinal injuries (that is, neck and back injuries) can also be present in head-injured victims.

▶ Scalp Wounds

Scalp wounds bleed profusely because the scalp has many blood vessels. A bleeding scalp wound does not affect the blood supply to the brain. The brain obtains its blood supply from arteries in the neck, not the scalp. A severe scalp wound may have an accompanying concussion, skull fracture, an impaled object, a brain injury or a spinal injury.

Care for Scalp Wounds

1. Control the bleeding by applying direct pressure with a dry, sterile or clean dressing. If the dressing becomes blood filled, do not remove it. Add another dressing on top of the first one **Figure 12-1**.

2. If you suspect a skull fracture, apply pressure around the edges of the wound and over a broad area rather than on the center of the wound **Figure 12-2**.

Figure 12-1

Apply direct pressure with a dry, sterile dressing to control the bleeding.

Figure 12-2

Apply pressure around the edges of the wound to control bleeding from a suspected skull fracture.

3. Keep the head and shoulders slightly elevated to help control the bleeding if no spinal injury is suspected.
4. Seek medical care.

Figure 12-3

Raccoon eyes.

▶ Skull Fracture

A **skull fracture** is a break or a crack in the cranium (bony case surrounding the brain). Skull fractures may be open (with an accompanying scalp laceration) or closed (without an accompanying scalp laceration).

Recognizing Skull Fracture

It is difficult to determine a skull fracture except by X-ray or a CT scan unless the skull deformity is severe. Signs and symptoms of a skull fracture include the following:

- Pain at the point of injury
- Deformity of the skull
- Bleeding from the ears or nose
- Clear, pink, watery cerebrospinal fluid (CSF) leaking from an ear or the nose. A drop of CSF on a handkerchief, pillowcase, or other white or light-colored cloth will form a pink ring around a slightly blood-tinged center, resembling a target; this is called the *halo sign (ring sign)*.
- Discoloration around the eyes ("raccoon eyes") appearing several hours after the injury **Figure 12-3**.
- Discoloration behind an ear (known as **Battle's sign**), appearing several hours after the injury **Figure 12-4**.
- Heavy scalp bleeding if the skin is broken. A scalp wound may expose the skull or brain tissue.
- Penetrating wound such as from a bullet or an impaled object.

Figure 12-4

Battle's sign.

Care for Skull Fracture

1. Monitor the victim's breathing and, if absent, begin CPR.
2. Stabilize the victim's neck to prevent movement.
3. Keep the head and shoulders slightly elevated if no spinal injury is suspected.
4. Cover the wounds with a sterile dressing.
5. To control bleeding, apply pressure around the edges of the wound, not directly on it.

CAUTION

DO NOT stop the flow of blood or CSF from an ear or nose. Blocking the flow could increase pressure within the skull.

DO NOT remove an impaled object from the head. Stabilize it in place with bulky dressings.

DO NOT clean an open skull fracture; infection of the brain could result.

DO NOT press on the fractured area.

▶ Brain Injuries

It is not injury specifically to the head that causes most short- and long-term problems, but injuries to the brain itself. Most head injuries are a result of motor vehicle crashes and falls. Many of these injuries are minor—shallow lacerations or localized bruising and swelling. However, about 50,000 people die each year in the United States of head trauma, and twice that many have brain injuries that leave them with permanent damage.

The brain is a delicate organ. When the head is struck with sufficient force, the brain bounces against the inside of the skull. Brain injuries can be serious and difficult first aid emergencies to handle. The victim is often confused or unresponsive, making assessment difficult. Many brain injuries are life threatening. Mishandling a victim with a brain injury could result in permanent damage or death.

The brain, like other body tissues, will swell from bleeding when it is injured. Unlike other tissues, however, the brain is confined in the skull where there is little room for swelling. Any swelling of brain tissue or accumulation of blood inside the skull compresses the brain and increases the pressure inside the skull, which interferes with brain functioning. Furthermore, because the skull is hard, the brain and its surface blood vessels may be damaged if they strike the inside of the skull, which can occur when the head is struck directly or is rapidly accelerated or decelerated (such as in a vehicle accident). The phenomenon of a person "seeing stars" when struck on the back of the head results because the occipital lobe of the brain (the part that controls vision) strikes the back of the skull.

The nerve cells of the brain and the spinal cord, unlike most other cells in the body, are unable to regenerate. When those cells die, they are lost forever and cannot be replaced. Injuries to the brain can be caused by a penetrating foreign object, by bony fragments from a skull fracture, or by the brain striking the inside of the skull after a person's head has hit a stationary object (such as the ground)—a *deceleration injury*—or has been hit by something like a baseball bat or a teammate's knee—an *acceleration injury*. Sometimes there will be two points of injury: one at the point of impact and one where the brain rebounds off the skull on the opposite side.

▶ Types of Brain Injury

All brain injuries are unique. The brain can receive several types of injuries depending on the type and amount of force that impacts the head. The type of injury the brain receives may affect just one functional area of the brain, various areas, or even the entire brain. Two types of brain injury are traumatic brain injury and acquired brain injury.

Traumatic Brain Injury

The following sections on traumatic brain injury are adapted from Centers for Disease Control and Prevention, National Injury and Violence Prevention.

Concussion

A **concussion** is considered a mild traumatic brain injury (MTBI) and occurs when a blow to the head alters the function of the brain (Table 12-1).

FYI

Suspect a Concussion (MTBI)

- High-speed activities (motor vehicle crashes, bicycle riding, skateboarding)
- Sports and recreation activities
- Falls (including those among older adults), especially from a significant distance (eg, off a ladder, from a tree)
- Suspected child maltreatment (eg, shaking, hitting, throwing)
- Exposure to blasts (including military personnel returning from war zones)
- Injuries to the external parts of the head and/or scalp (eg, lacerations) and orthopaedic injuries (eg, fractures, dislocations)

Source: Centers for Disease Control and Prevention, U.S. Department of Health and Human Services. *Heads Up: Facts for Physicians about Mild Traumatic Brain Injury (MTBI).* (5) (Accessed January 14, 2011: http://www.cdc.gov/concussion/headsup/pdf/Facts_for_Physicians_booklet-a.pdf)

Recovery from a concussion can last anywhere from several minutes to days, weeks, months, or even longer. Children, adolescents, and older adults tend to take longer to recover than adults. Concussion victims who have already experienced previous concussions may need increased recovery time as well. Although most concussion victims make a full recovery, it is possible for victims to experience post-concussion syndrome, in which concussion symptoms last longer than 3 months.

Sometimes additional problems can occur in a concussion victim. A concussion victim experiencing any of the following signs and symptoms may have a blood clot that is pushing the brain against the skull:

- Loss of consciousness, even if brief
- Persistent, worsening headache
- Weakness, numbness, or decreased coordination
- Vomiting or nausea
- Slurred speech
- Very drowsy or cannot be awakened
- Increasingly confused, restless, or agitated
- Unusual behavior
- One pupil larger than the other
- Convulsions or seizures
- Inability to recognize people or places
- Will not stop crying and cannot be consoled (child)
- Will not nurse or eat (child)

Victims experiencing any of these signs and symptoms should seek immediate medical care.

Table 12-1 Symptoms of MTBI

Thinking/Remembering	Physical	Emotional/Mood	Sleep Disturbance
• Difficulty thinking clearly • Feeling slowed down • Difficulty concentrating • Difficulty remembering new information	• Headache • Nausea or vomiting (early on) • Balance problems • Dizziness • Fuzzy or blurry vision • Feeling tired, having no energy • Sensitivity to noise or light	• Irritability • Sadness • More emotional • Nervousness or anxiety	• Sleeping more than usual • Sleeping less than usual • Trouble falling asleep

Source: Centers for Disease Control and Prevention, National Center for Injury Prevention and Control

If the victim is wearing a helmet, such as a motorcycle or football helmet, it should not be removed by a first aider unless:

- You suspect an obstructed airway.
- The helmet is so loose that you cannot stabilize the spine.

If the helmet must be removed to provide lifesaving care of an airway problem, make sure to stabilize the head and neck as the helmet is carefully removed.

Other Traumatic Brain Injuries

Other types of traumatic brain injuries include the following:

- <u>Contusion</u>: A direct blow to the head can cause a bruise to the brain.
- Coup-contrecoup: A blow to the head is strong enough to cause a contusion at the site of impact, as well as move the brain, causing it to hit the opposite side of the skull. This second hit causes a second contusion.
- Diffuse axonal: Shaking or strong rotation of the head causes this tearing injury. One example of diffuse axonal injury is Shaken Baby Syndrome.
- Penetration: Objects such as a bullet, knife, or other sharp object enters the brain. The wound is then contaminated by hair, skin, bone, and pieces of the penetrating object. These contaminants may not be retrievable.

Q&A

How does blunt head trauma cause death?

Blunt trauma can cause bleeding into or around the brain, or can lead to swelling of the brain (called edema). The skull is a rigid capsule that protects the brain. Bleeding in or around the brain causes a rapid rise of pressure within the rigid skull. The only escape route for this excess pressure is through the foramen magnum, an opening at the base of the skull through which the brainstem and spinal cord exit. The pushing of brain material through this opening compresses the brainstem, resulting in the cessation of breathing, followed by death.

Acquired Brain Injuries

Acquired brain injuries are injuries that develop during or after birth and are not due to injuries. This is in contrast to congenital problems, which are due to abnormal brain development before birth. Acquired injuries include infection, stroke, tumors, and anoxia (lack of oxygen). Anoxia can be due to conditions such as respiratory arrest, problems during birth, or drowning. Acquired brain injuries can cause signs and symptoms that are similar to traumatic brain injuries. Care is mainly supportive and requires immediate medical attention.

Further Care

Several signs appearing within 48 hours of a head injury indicate a need to seek medical care.

- **Headache:** Expect a headache. If it lasts more than 1 or 2 days or increases in severity, seek medical advice.
- **Nausea, vomiting:** If nausea lasts more than 2 hours, seek medical advice. Vomiting once or twice, especially in children, may be expected after a head injury. Vomiting does not indicate the severity of the injury. However, if vomiting begins again hours after the initial episodes have ceased, seek medical care.
- **Drowsiness:** Allow a victim to sleep, but wake the victim at least every 2 hours to check the state of consciousness and sense of orientation by asking his or her name and to use information-processing skills (for example, "Recite the months of the year backward"). If the victim cannot respond or appears confused or disoriented, seek medical advice.
- **Vision problems:** If the victim "sees double," if the eyes do not move together, or if one pupil appears to be larger than the other, seek medical advice.
- **Mobility:** If the victim cannot use his or her arms or legs as well as previously or is unsteady when walking, seek medical care.
- **Speech:** If the victim has slurred speech or is unable to talk, seek medical care.
- **Seizures (convulsions):** If the victim has a violent involuntary contraction (spasm) or series of contractions of the skeletal muscles, seek medical care.

Eye Injuries

Of all the parts of the human body, an injured eye probably causes the most anxiety and concern in a victim. The eyes—arguably the most important human

Head Injuries

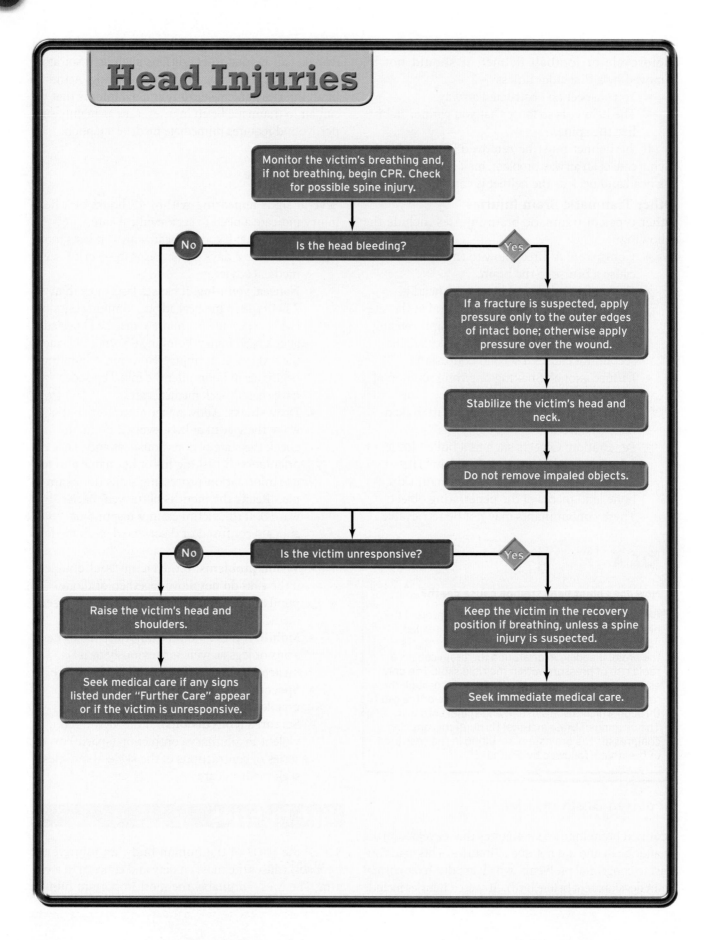

Monitor the victim's breathing and, if not breathing, begin CPR. Check for possible spine injury.

Is the head bleeding?

No

Yes

If a fracture is suspected, apply pressure only to the outer edges of intact bone; otherwise apply pressure over the wound.

Stabilize the victim's head and neck.

Do not remove impaled objects.

Is the victim unresponsive?

No

Yes

Raise the victim's head and shoulders.

Keep the victim in the recovery position if breathing, unless a spine injury is suspected.

Seek medical care if any signs listed under "Further Care" appear or if the victim is unresponsive.

Seek immediate medical care.

Figure 12-5

Stabilizing a long, penetrating object against movement (using a paper cup to protect the object from being hit).

CAUTION

DO NOT assume that any eye injury is innocent. When in doubt, seek medical care immediately.

DO NOT remove an object stuck in the eye or try to wash out an object with water.

DO NOT exert pressure on an injured eyeball or a penetrating object.

sense organs—are easily damaged by trauma. A very slight penetration by a metal fragment, for example, means hospitalization. Medical care may include surgery; despite technical advances, blindness or the loss of an eye remains a possibility whenever there is an eye injury. Have an opthamologist or other physician examine the eye as soon as possible, even if an injury seems minor at first.

▶ Penetrating Eye Injuries

Penetrating eye injuries are severe injuries that result when a sharp object, such as a knife or a needle, penetrates the eye. Most penetrating injuries, although not all, are obvious. Suspect penetration any time you see a lid laceration or cut.

Care for Penetrating Eye Injuries

1. Seek immediate medical care. Any penetrating eye injury should be managed in the hospital.
2. Stabilize the object. Stabilize a long, protruding object with bulky dressings or clean

cloths. You can place a protective paper cup or cardboard folded into a cone over the affected eye to prevent bumping of the object **Figure 12-5**. For short objects, surround the eye without touching the object with roller gauze bandage or cloths held in place with a roller bandage.

▶ Blows to the Eye

Blows to the eye can range in severity from minor to sight threatening. One such injury is the common *shiner* or *black eye,* which occurs when some of the many delicate blood vessels around the eye rupture. The bleeding itself is insignificant and will disappear, but it may hide damage to the eyeball **Figure 12-6**. A fist, ball, or other blunt object can break the bone

Figure 12-6

Blow to the eye.

Figure 12-7

Lacerated eyelid.

around the eyeball. Symptoms that indicate such a break are double vision and the inability to look upward.

Care for Blows to the Eye

1. Apply an ice or cold pack for about 15 minutes to reduce the pain and swelling. Do not apply any pressure on the eye.
2. Seek medical care immediately if there is double vision, pain, or reduced vision.

▶ Cuts of the Eye or Lid

The signs of a cut eyeball or lid include the following **Figure 12-7** :

- "Cut" appearance of the cornea (clear part of the eye) or sclera (white part of eye).
- Inner liquid filling of the eye may come out through the wound.
- Lid is cut.

Care for Cuts of the Eye or Lid

1. If the eyeball is cut, do not apply pressure. If only the eyelid is cut, apply a sterile or clean dressing with gentle pressure.
2. Bandage both eyes lightly.
3. Seek medical care immediately.

▶ Chemical in the Eyes

Chemicals in the eyes can threaten sight. First aid may determine the fate of the eye and vision. Alkalis cause greater damage than acids because they penetrate deeper and continue to burn longer. Common alkalis include drain cleaners, cleaning agents, ammonia,

Eye Injuries

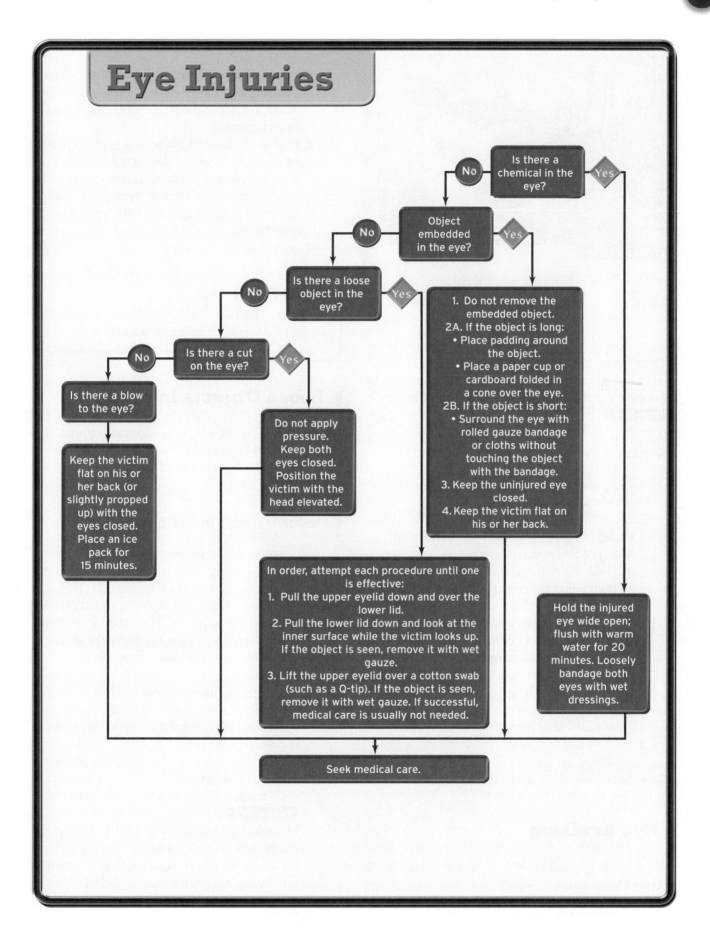

Is there a chemical in the eye? — No / Yes

Object embedded in the eye? — No / Yes

Is there a loose object in the eye? — No / Yes

Is there a cut on the eye? — No / Yes

Is there a blow to the eye? — No

Keep the victim flat on his or her back (or slightly propped up) with the eyes closed. Place an ice pack for 15 minutes.

Do not apply pressure. Keep both eyes closed. Position the victim with the head elevated.

1. Do not remove the embedded object.
2A. If the object is long:
 • Place padding around the object.
 • Place a paper cup or cardboard folded in a cone over the eye.
2B. If the object is short:
 • Surround the eye with rolled gauze bandage or cloths without touching the object with the bandage.
3. Keep the uninjured eye closed.
4. Keep the victim flat on his or her back.

In order, attempt each procedure until one is effective:
1. Pull the upper eyelid down and over the lower lid.
2. Pull the lower lid down and look at the inner surface while the victim looks up. If the object is seen, remove it with wet gauze.
3. Lift the upper eyelid over a cotton swab (such as a Q-tip). If the object is seen, remove it with wet gauze. If successful, medical care is usually not needed.

Hold the injured eye wide open; flush with warm water for 20 minutes. Loosely bandage both eyes with wet dressings.

Seek medical care.

Figure 12-8

Flushing the eye to treat a chemical burn.

cement, plaster, and caustic soda. Common acids include hydrochloric acid, nitric acid, sulfuric (battery) acid, and acetic acid. Because damage can occur in 1 to 5 minutes, the chemical must be removed immediately Figure 12-8 .

Care for Chemical in the Eye

1. Use your fingers to keep the eye open as widely as possible.
2. Flush the eye with water immediately. If possible, use warm water. If water is not available, use any nonirritating liquid.
   - Hold the victim's head under a faucet or pour water into the eye from any clean container for at least 20 minutes, continuously and gently. It is impossible to use too much water on these injuries.
   - Irrigate from the nose side of the eye toward the outside to avoid flushing the material into the other eye.
   - Tell the victim to roll the eyeball as much as possible to help wash out the eye.
3. Loosely bandage both eyes with cold, wet dressings.
4. Seek immediate medical care.

▶ Eye Avulsion

A blow to the eye can *avulse* it (knock it out) from its socket. This is a serious injury.

Care for Eye Avulsion

1. Cover the eye loosely with a sterile or clean dressing that has been moistened with clean water. Do not try to push the eyeball back into the socket.
2. Protect the injured eye with a paper cup, a piece of cardboard folded into a cone, or a doughnut-shaped pad made from a roller gauze bandage or a cravat bandage.
3. Cover the undamaged eye with a patch to stop movement of the damaged eye.
4. Seek medical care immediately.

CAUTION

DO NOT try to remove an object stuck in the eye.

▶ Loose Objects in the Eye

Loose objects in the eye are the most frequent eye injury and can be very painful. Tearing is common because it is the body's way of trying to remove the object.

Care for Objects in the Eye

Try one or more of the following methods to remove the object:

1. Lift the upper lid over the lower lid so that the lower lashes can brush the object off the inside of the upper lid. Have the victim blink a few times and let the eye move the object out. If the object remains, keep the eye closed.
2. Try flushing the object out by rinsing the eye gently with warm water. Hold the eyelid open and tell the victim to move the eye as it is rinsed.
3. Examine the lower lid by pulling it down gently. If you can see the object, remove it with moistened sterile gauze or a clean cloth Figure 12-9 .
4. Many foreign bodies lodge under the upper eyelid; however, expertise is required to invert the lid and remove the object. Examine the underside of the upper lid by

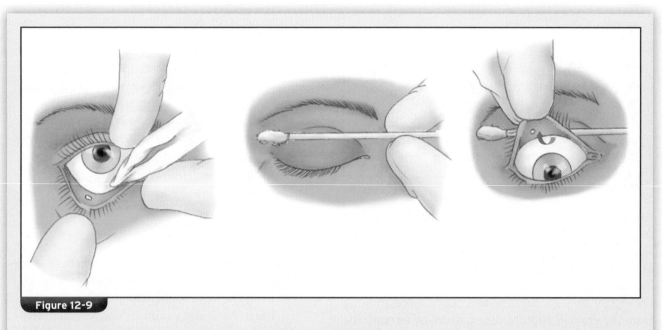

Figure 12-9

Removing loose objects from the eye. Lower lid: If tears or gentle flushing do not remove the object, gently pull down the lower lid. Remove an object by gently flushing with lukewarm water or by using wet, sterile gauze. Upper lid 1: Tell the person to look down. Pull gently downward on the upper eyelashes. Lay a swab or matchstick across the top of the lid. Upper lid 2: Fold the lid over the swab or matchstick. Remove an object by gently flushing with lukewarm water or by using wet, sterile gauze.

CAUTION

DO NOT allow the victim to rub the eye.

DO NOT try to remove an embedded foreign object.

DO NOT use dry cotton (cotton balls or cotton-tipped swabs) or instruments such as tweezers to remove an object from an eye.

FYI

An Unresponsive Victim's Eyes

An unconscious victim may lose the reflexes such as blinking that protect the eye. If the eyes do not stay closed, keep them closed by covering them with moist dressings.

grasping the lashes of the upper lid, placing a matchstick or cotton-tipped swab across the upper lid, and rolling the lid upward over the stick or swab. If you can see the object, remove it with moistened sterile gauze or a clean cloth.

▶ Light Burns to the Eye

Burns can result if a person looks at a source of ultraviolet light such as sunlight, arc welding, bright snow, or tanning lamps. Severe pain occurs 1 to 6 hours after exposure.

Care for Light Burns

1. Cover both eyes with cold, wet packs. Tell the victim not to rub the eyes.
2. Have the victim rest in a darkened room. Do not allow light to reach the victim's eyes.
3. Give pain medication, if needed.
4. Seek medical care.

Ear Injuries

Most ear problems are not life threatening. Fast action may be needed, however, to relieve pain and to prevent or reverse hearing loss. Head trauma may involve the ear. Foreign bodies in the ear canal usually produce overzealous removal attempts. Except for disk batteries (which damage moist tissue by creating a current) and live insects, few foreign bodies must be extracted immediately. First aiders should seek medical care for the victim because attempts to remove a foreign body from the ear can rupture the eardrum or lacerate the ear canal.

A live insect crawling around in the ear canal can be very uncomfortable for the victim. Shine a small light into the ear. Sometimes the insect will crawl out toward the light. If it will not leave the ear, drown the insect by placing several drops of light mineral oil or vegetable oil (not motor oil) into the ear. Often the insect will crawl out before it dies. When it stops moving and the insect is near the opening, carefully irrigate the ear with warm water. The insect should wash out. If that is unsuccessful, use a bulb syringe to suck the insect out. If the insect cannot be removed, seek medical care.

Children insert all sorts of things into their ears that may be impossible for you to remove safely. If the object is visible near the ear canal opening and you feel it is safe, cautiously try to remove the object with tweezers. Small objects can sometimes be removed by irrigating the ear with warm water. Do not try irrigation if the object blocks the entire ear canal or if the object is vegetable matter such as a kernel of corn or a bean, which will swell when wet.

Nose Injuries

▶ Nosebleeds

A severe nosebleed frightens the victim and often challenges the first aider's skill. Most nosebleeds are self-limiting and seldom require medical attention. In cases of accompanying head or neck injuries, stabilize the head and neck for protection. In some cases, loss of blood could cause shock.

There are two types of nosebleeds:
- **Anterior nosebleed** (front of nose) is the most common type (90%). Blood flows from the nose through one nostril.
- The **posterior nosebleed** (back of nose) involves massive bleeding, usually backward into the mouth or down the back of the throat. A posterior nosebleed is serious and requires medical care.

Care for Nosebleeds

To care for an anterior nosebleed, follow these guidelines from the American Academy of Otolaryngology:
1. Keep the head higher than the level of the heart. Have the victim sit and lean slightly forward to prevent blood draining into the throat.
2. Pinch the soft parts of the nose together between your thumb and two fingers **Figure 12-10** .
3. Continue compressing the pinched parts for 5 to 10 minutes.
4. Apply ice (crushed in a plastic bag or washcloth) to the nose and cheeks.

If bleeding continues:
1. Clear the nose of all blood clots by gently blowing the nose.
2. If available, spray a decongestant spray (such as Afrin or Neo-Synephrin) into the nostril.
3. Pinch the nose again for 10 minutes.
4. If the nosebleed continues, seek medical care.

Figure 12-10

Control bleeding from the nose by pinching the nostrils together.

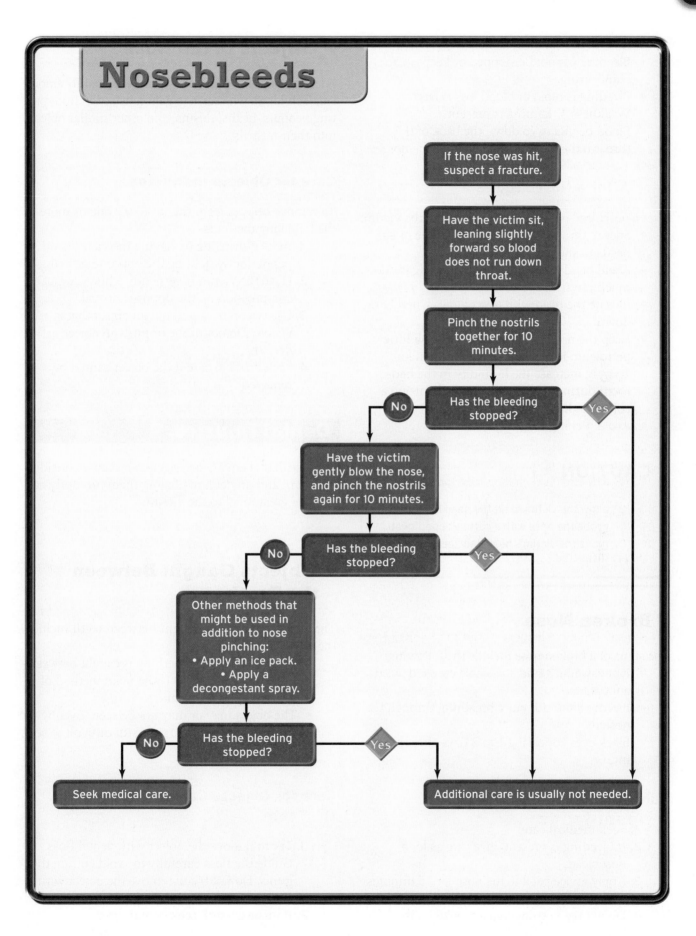

Nosebleeds

If the nose was hit, suspect a fracture.

Have the victim sit, leaning slightly forward so blood does not run down throat.

Pinch the nostrils together for 10 minutes.

No ← Has the bleeding stopped? → **Yes**

Have the victim gently blow the nose, and pinch the nostrils again for 10 minutes.

No ← Has the bleeding stopped? → **Yes**

Other methods that might be used in addition to nose pinching:
• Apply an ice pack.
• Apply a decongestant spray.

No ← Has the bleeding stopped? → **Yes**

Seek medical care.

Additional care is usually not needed.

Seek professional medical help if:
- Bleeding cannot be stopped or keeps reappearing.
- Bleeding is rapid or blood loss is large.
- Weakness or fainting is present.
- Blood begins to go down the back of the throat rather than out the front of the nose.

Care After a Nosebleed

After a nosebleed has stopped, suggest that the victim:
- Sneeze through an open mouth, if he or she needs to sneeze.
- Avoid bending over and participating in too much physical exertion.
- Elevate the head with two pillows when lying down.
- Keep the nostrils moist by applying a little petroleum jelly just inside the nostril for 1 week; increase the humidity in the bedroom during the winter months by using a cold-mist humidifier.
- Avoid picking or rubbing the nose.

CAUTION

DO NOT allow the victim to tilt the head backward.
DO NOT probe the nose with a cotton-tipped swab.
DO NOT move the victim's head and neck if a spinal injury is suspected.

▶ Broken Nose

The signs of a broken nose include the following:
- Pain, swelling, and a possible crooked appearance
- Bleeding and difficulty breathing through the nostrils
- Black eyes appearing 1 to 2 days after the injury

Care for a Broken Nose

1. Seek medical care.
2. If bleeding is present, give care as for a nosebleed.
3. Apply an ice pack to the nose for 15 minutes at a time throughout the day.
4. Do not try to straighten a crooked nose.

▶ Objects in the Nose

A foreign object in the nose is a problem mainly among small children, who seem to gain satisfaction from putting peanuts, beans, raisins, and other similar objects into their nostrils.

Care for Objects in the Nose

To remove objects from the nose, try one or more of the following methods:
1. Induce sneezing by having the victim sniff pepper or by tickling the opposite nostril.
2. Have the victim blow gently while you put compression on the opposite nostril.
3. Use tweezers to pull out an object that is visible. Do not probe or push an object deeper.
4. Seek medical care if the object cannot be removed.

Dental Injuries

Because dental emergencies generally cause considerable pain and anxiety, managing them promptly can provide great relief to the victim.

▶ Objects Caught Between the Teeth

The signs of an object caught between teeth include the following:
- Victim says that something is caught between his or her teeth. This is the main method of detecting the problem.
- The object may or may not be seen. Even with the use of a flashlight, it is still difficult to see a small object.

Care for Objects Caught Between the Teeth

1. Try to remove the object with dental floss. Guide the floss carefully to avoid cutting the gums. Do not try to remove the object with a sharp or pointed instrument.
2. If unsuccessful, seek dental care.

▶ Bitten Lip or Tongue

The signs of a bitten lip or tongue include the following:

- Immediate pain when it happens.
- Blood may be seen.

Care for a Bitten Lip or Tongue

1. Apply direct pressure to the bleeding area with sterile gauze or a clean cloth.
2. Clean the area with a cloth.
3. If swelling is present, apply an ice pack or have the victim suck on a popsicle or ice chips.
4. If the bleeding does not stop, seek medical care.

▶ Loosened Tooth

Trauma can cause teeth to become loosened in their sockets. Applying pressure on either side of each tooth with the fingers can determine looseness. Any tooth movement, even if it is barely felt, indicates a possibly loose tooth.

Care for a Loosened Tooth

1. Have the victim bite down on a piece of gauze to keep the tooth in place.
2. Consult a dentist or an oral surgeon.

▶ Knocked-Out Tooth

A knocked-out tooth is a dental emergency but it is also a common one. A majority of the teeth knocked out each year in the United States could be saved with proper treatment **Figure 12-11**. Emergency care for knocked-out teeth has changed dramatically in recent years. The first question you want to ask when a tooth has been knocked out is, "Where is the tooth?" Time is crucial for successful reimplantation. After a tooth is knocked out, ligament fiber fragments remain attached to the tooth and to the bone in the socket. These ligament fibers begin to die soon after the injury. Therefore, it is important to prevent the tooth from drying and to protect the ligament fibers from damage. Moisture alone is not sufficient to preserve the tooth's ligament fibers. Steps must be taken to prevent the

Figure 12-11

Knocked-out tooth.

tooth from becoming dehydrated and to protect the ligament fibers from damage.

Care for a Knocked-Out Tooth

1. Have the victim rinse his or her mouth, and, if bleeding, put a rolled gauze pad in the socket to control the bleeding.
2. Find the tooth and handle it by the crown, not the root, to minimize damage to the ligament fibers.
3. A tooth often can be successfully reimplanted if it is replaced in its socket within 30 minutes after the injury; the odds of successful reimplantation decrease about 1% for every minute the tooth is absent from the socket.
   - One of the worst things you can do to a knocked-out tooth is to transport it dry. Consider using the victim's own saliva for the short term (less than 1 hour). Whole milk is much better because it maintains the vitality of the ligaments for 3 hours. Ideally, the milk should be kept cold to minimize bacterial growth. Do not use reconstituted powdered milk or milk by-products such as yogurt; they can damage the ligaments.
   - The best transport medium is Hank's solution, a balanced-pH cell-culture medium that helps restore the ligament fibers. The use of Hank's solution extends the viability of the ligament fibers for 6 to 12 hours. The solution, which is available commercially as the Save-a-Tooth kit, has been approved by the US Food and Drug

Administration for use up to 24 hours after an injury, and there is some evidence that using it enables successful reimplantation, even after 96 hours. A tooth-saving kit is available in drugstores or online and deserves consideration as a standard item at schools, sporting events, and summer camps.

- Some experts recommend that the tooth be placed in the victim's mouth to keep it moist until dental treatment is available. Do not use this method for children or others who may swallow the tooth.

4. Take the victim and the tooth immediately to a dentist.

5. If you are in a remote location, try to replace the tooth into the socket, using adjacent teeth as a guide. Apply pressure on the tooth so the top is even with the adjacent teeth. Asking the victim to bite down gently on gauze is helpful. Immediate reinsertion is not always possible, however. The victim may be reluctant to put the knocked-out tooth back into its socket, especially if it has fallen on the ground and is covered with debris—or the tooth may repeatedly fall out, putting the victim at risk of inhaling or swallowing it. Do not use this method for children or others who may swallow the tooth. In victims with multiple trauma, the presence of more serious injuries may prevent reinsertion.

Figure 12-12

Broken teeth.

▶ Broken Tooth

The front teeth are frequently broken by falls or direct blows **Figure 12-12** . Such damage is not unusual in the victims of violent acts or motor vehicle crashes. It is also common in children, especially those with an overbite.

Care for a Broken Tooth

1. Rinse the mouth with warm water to clean the area.
2. Apply an ice pack on the face in the area of the injured tooth to decrease swelling.
3. If you suspect a jaw fracture, stabilize the jaw by wrapping a bandage under the chin and over the top of the head.
4. Seek immediate dental care.

CAUTION

DO NOT handle a knocked-out tooth roughly.

DO NOT put a knocked-out tooth in water, mouthwash, alcohol, or povidone iodine (Betadine).

DO NOT put a knocked-out tooth in skim milk, reconstituted powdered milk, or milk by-products such as yogurt.

DO NOT rinse a knocked-out tooth unless you are reinserting it in the socket.

DO NOT place a knocked-out tooth in anything that can dry or crush the outside of the tooth.

DO NOT scrub a knocked-out tooth or remove any attached tissue fragments.

DO NOT remove a partially extracted tooth. Push it back into place and seek a dentist so the loose tooth can be stabilized.

FYI

First Aid

If you are in a remote area with no dentist nearby, you can make a temporary cap from melted candle wax or paraffin and a few strands of cotton. When the wax begins to harden but can still be molded, press a wad of it onto the tooth. Other improvisations include using ski wax or chewing gum (preferably sugarless).

Dental Injuries

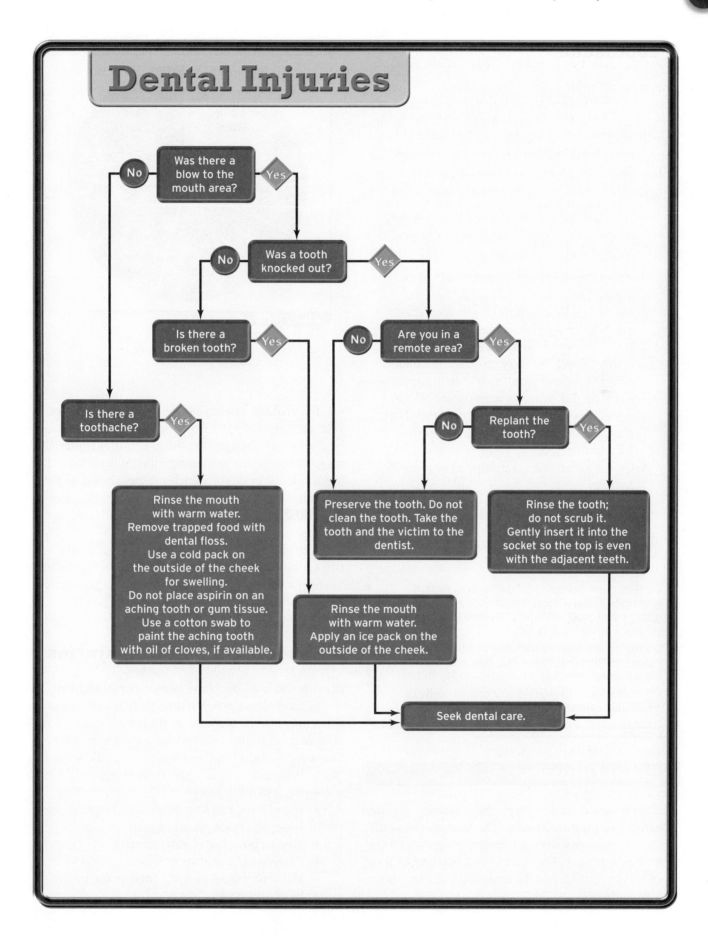

▶ Toothache

The most common reason for toothaches is dental decay. Victims frequently report pain limited to one area of the mouth, although it can be more widespread; pain can also affect the ear, eye, neck, or even the opposite side of the jaw. The tooth will be sensitive to heat and cold. Identify the diseased tooth by tapping the area with a spoon handle or similar object. A diseased tooth will hurt.

Care for a Toothache

1. Rinse the mouth with warm water to clean it out.
2. Use dental floss to remove any food that might be trapped between the teeth.
3. If you suspect a cavity, paint the tooth by using a small cotton swab soaked in oil of cloves (eugenol) (or Orajel) to help suppress the pain. Take care to keep the oil off the gums, lips, and inside surfaces of the cheeks. If applicable, follow the same procedures as for a broken tooth.
4. Give the victim acetaminophen or ibuprofen for pain.
5. Seek dental care.

CAUTION

DO NOT place pain medication (such as aspirin, acetaminophen, or ibuprofen) on the aching tooth or gum tissues or allow them to dissolve in the mouth. A serious acid burn can result.

DO NOT cover a cavity with cotton if there is any pus discharge or facial swelling. See a dentist immediately.

DO NOT stick anything into an exposed cavity or into a softened exposed root.

Spinal Injuries

The *spine* is a column of vertebrae stacked on one another from the tailbone to the base of the skull. Each vertebra has a hollow center through which the spinal cord passes. The spinal cord consists of long tracts of nerves that join the brain with all other body organs and parts.

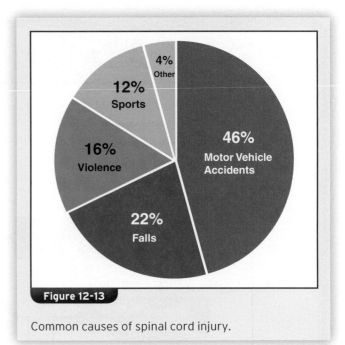

Figure 12-13

Common causes of spinal cord injury.

If a broken vertebra pinches spinal nerves, paralysis can result. All unresponsive victims should be treated as though they have a spinal injury. All responsive victims sustaining injuries from falls, diving accidents, or motor vehicle crashes should be carefully checked for a spinal injury before being moved **Figure 12-13**. Suspect a spinal injury in all head-injury victims.

A mistake in the handling of a spinal injury victim could mean a lifetime of paralysis for the victim. Suspect a spinal injury whenever a significant cause of injury occurs.

▶ Recognizing Spinal Injuries

Because the head may have been snapped suddenly in one or more directions, anytime there is a head injury, there may also be a spinal cord injury. About 15% to 20% of head-injury victims also have a spinal injury. Other signs and symptoms include the following:

- Pain radiating into the arms or legs
- Neck or back pain
- Numbness, tingling, weakness, burning, or lessened sensation in the arms or legs
- Loss of bowel or bladder control
- Paralysis of the arms or legs
- Deformity (odd-looking angle of the victim's head and neck)

Ask a responsive victim these questions and follow these steps **Skill Drill 12-1**:

- Is there pain? Neck (cervical spine) injuries radiate pain to the arms; upper-back (thoracic spine) injuries radiate pain around the ribs; lower-back injuries usually radiate pain down the legs. Often, the victim will describe the pain as "electric."
- Can you wiggle your fingers? Moving the fingers is a sign that nerve pathways are intact **(Step ❶)**.
- Can you feel this pressure on your finger? Pinch the tip of the victim's finger to check for spinal injury **(Step ❷)**.
- Can you squeeze my hand? Ask the victim to grip your hand. A strong grip indicates that an upper spinal injury is unlikely **(Step ❸)**.
- Can you wiggle your toes? Moving the toes is a sign that nerve pathways are intact **(Step ❹)**.
- Squeeze the victim's toes **(Step ❺)**.
- Can you push your foot against my hand? Ask the victim to press a foot against your hand **(Step ❻)**. If the victim cannot perform this movement or if the movement is extremely weak against your hand, the victim may have a spinal injury.

If the victim is unresponsive, do the following:

- Look for cuts, bruises, and deformities.
- Test responses by pinching the victim's hand (the palm or back of the hand) and bare foot (the sole or the top of the foot). No reaction could mean spinal cord damage **Skill Drill 12-2**:

1. Pinch the victim's hand for a response **(Step ❶)**.
2. Pinch the victim's foot for a response **(Step ❷)**.
3. Test the spinal cord by using the *Babinski test* **(Step ❸)**: Stroke the bottom of the foot firmly toward the big toe with a key or similar blunt object. The body's normal response is to move the big toe down (except in infants). If the spinal cord or brain is injured, the big toe in an adult and a child will flex upward.
4. Ask bystanders what happened. If you still are not sure about a possible spinal injury, assume the victim has one until it is proved otherwise.

▶ Care for a Spinal Injury

1. Monitor breathing. For an unresponsive victim, open the airway and check for breathing.
2. Stabilize the victim to prevent movement by using one of the following methods. Whichever method you use, tell the victim not to move.
   - Grasp the victim's head over the ears and hold the head and neck still until the EMS arrives **Figure 12-14**.
   - If you anticipate a long wait for EMS or you are tired from holding the victim's head in place, kneel with the victim's head between your knees or place objects on each side of the victim's head to prevent it from rolling from side to side.

CAUTION

DO NOT move the victim, even if the victim is in water. (For a water-related rescue, manually stabilize the victim while floating on the water's surface.)Wait for EMS personnel to arrive; they have the proper training and equipment. Victims with suspected spinal injury require cervical collars and stabilization on a spine board. It is better to do nothing than to mishandle a victim with a spinal injury, unless the victim's location puts him or her in additional danger.

Figure 12-14

Steady and support the victim's head and neck as soon as possible. Have a bystander steady and support the feet. The head and feet should be continuously supported until medical help takes over. Stabilize by holding the head. Keep your arms steady by placing them on your thighs. To free yourself to help others, place heavy objects on each side of the head.

skill drill

12-1 Checking for Spinal Injuries in a Responsive Victim

1 Victim wiggles fingers.

2 Rescuer squeezes fingers.

3 Victim squeezes rescuer's hand.

4 Victim wiggles toes.

5 Rescuer squeezes toes.

6 Victim pushes foot against rescuer's hand.

skill drill

12-2 Checking for Spinal Injuries in an Unresponsive Victim

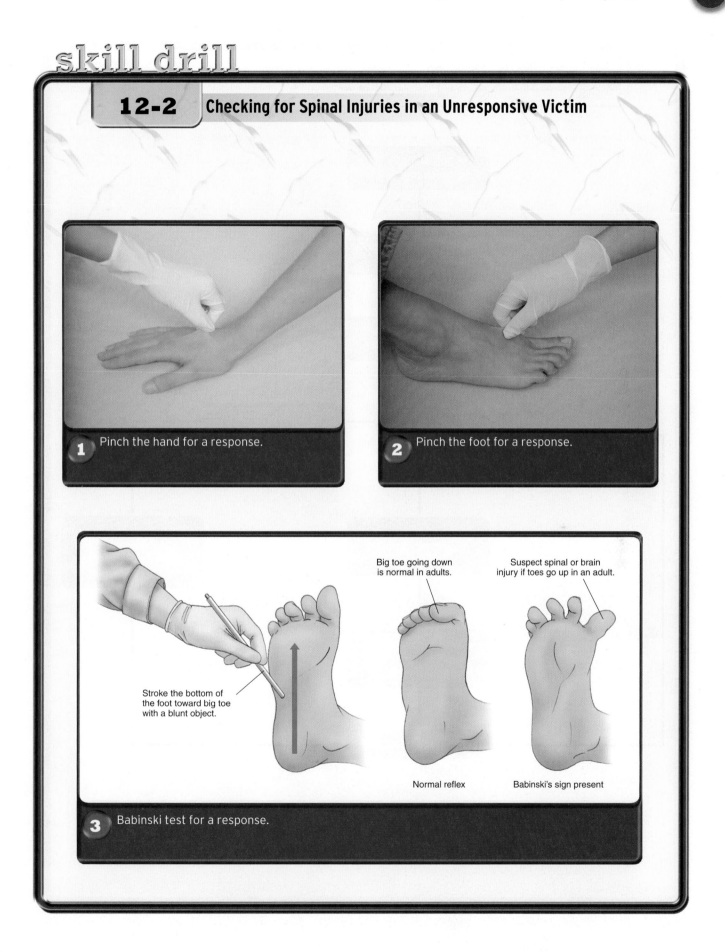

1 Pinch the hand for a response.

2 Pinch the foot for a response.

Stroke the bottom of the foot toward big toe with a blunt object.

Big toe going down is normal in adults.

Suspect spinal or brain injury if toes go up in an adult.

Normal reflex

Babinski's sign present

3 Babinski test for a response.

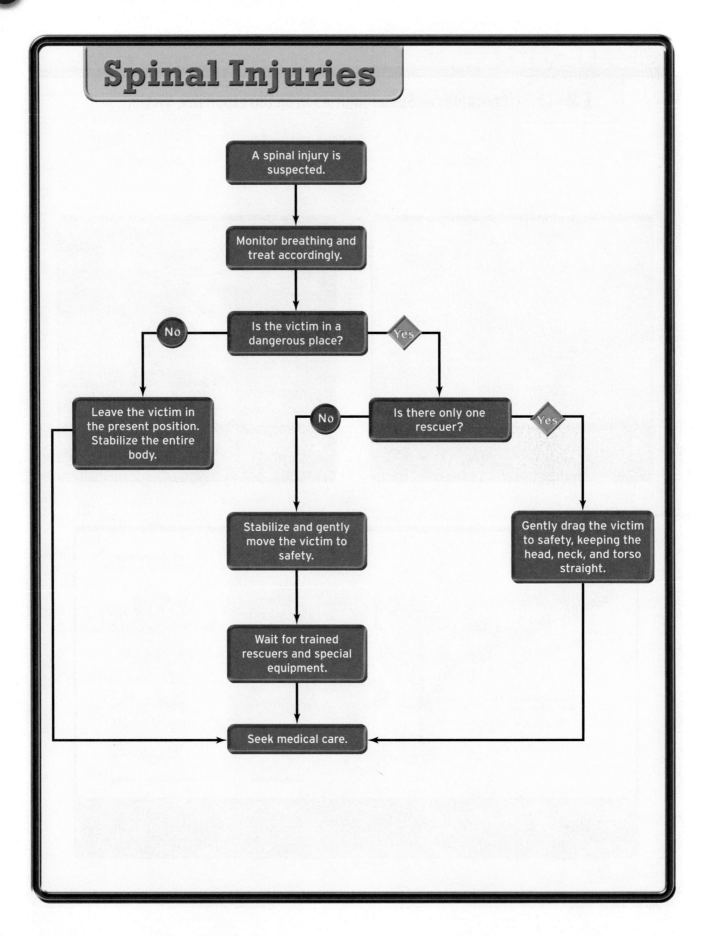

Spinal Injuries

A spinal injury is suspected.

↓

Monitor breathing and treat accordingly.

↓

No ← Is the victim in a dangerous place? → Yes

Leave the victim in the present position. Stabilize the entire body.

No ← Is there only one rescuer? → Yes

Stabilize and gently move the victim to safety.

Gently drag the victim to safety, keeping the head, neck, and torso straight.

Wait for trained rescuers and special equipment.

Seek medical care.

▶ Emergency Care Wrap-up

Condition	What to Look For	What to Do
Head Injuries	Scalp wound	1. Apply a sterile or clean dressing and direct pressure to control bleeding. 2. Keep the head and shoulders raised. 3. Seek medical care.
	Skull fracture	1. Monitor breathing and provide care if needed. 2. Control bleeding by applying pressure around the edges of the wound. 3. Stabilize the victim's head and neck against movement. 4. Seek medical care.
	Brain injury (concussion)	1. Monitor breathing and provide care if needed. 2. Stabilize the victim's head and neck against movement. 3. Control any scalp bleeding. 4. Seek medical care.
Eye Injuries	Loose object in eye	1. Look for object underneath both lids. 2. If seen, remove with wet gauze.
	Penetrating eye injury	1. If object is still in eye, protect eye and stabilize long objects. 2. Call 9-1-1.
	Blow to the eye area	1. Apply an ice or cold pack. DO NOT place ice or cold pack on eyeball. 2. Seek medical care if vision is affected.
	Eye avulsion	1. Cover eye loosely with wet dressing. 2. DO NOT try to put eye back into socket. 3. Call 9-1-1.
	Cuts of eye or lid	1. If eyeball is cut, DO NOT apply pressure. 2. If only eyelid is cut, apply dressings with gentle pressure. 3. Call 9-1-1.
	Chemical in eye	1. Flush with warm water for 20 minutes. 2. Seek medical care.
	Eye burns from light	1. Cover eyes with cold, wet dressings. 2. Seek medical care.

▶ Emergency Care Wrap-up

Condition	What to Look For	What to Do
Nose Injuries	**Nosebleeds**	1. Keep the victim sitting up with the head level or tilted forward slightly. 2. Pinch the soft parts of the nose for 5 to 10 minutes. 3. Seek medical care if: • Bleeding does not stop • Blood is going down throat • Bleeding is associated with a broken nose
	Broken nose	1. Care as for a nosebleed. 2. Apply an ice or cold pack for 15 minutes at a time. 3. Seek medical care.
Dental Injuries	**Bitten lip or tongue**	1. Apply direct pressure. 2. Apply an ice or cold pack.
	Knocked-out tooth	1. Control bleeding (place rolled gauze in socket). 2. Find tooth and preserve it in milk or the victim's saliva. Handle the tooth by the crown, not the root. 3. Take the tooth with the victim to a dentist.
	Toothache	1. Rinse the mouth and use dental floss to remove trapped food. 2. Give pain medication. 3. Seek dental care.
Spinal Injuries	**Spinal injury** • Inability to move arms and/or legs or painful to move them • Numbness, tingling, weakness, or burning feeling in arms and/or legs • Deformity (head and neck at an odd angle)	1. Stabilize the head and neck against movement. 2. If unresponsive, open the victim's airway and check breathing. 3. Call 9-1-1.

▶ Ready for Review

- Any head injury is potentially serious. If not properly treated, injuries that seem minor could become life threatening.
- Scalp wounds bleed profusely because the scalp has a rich supply of blood.
- A skull fracture is a break or crack in the cranium. Skull fractures may be open or closed.
- Injuries to the brain cause short- and long-term problems.
- An injured eye probably causes the most anxiety and concern in a victim.
- Penetrating eye injuries are severe injuries that result when a sharp object penetrates the eye.
- Blows to the eye can range in severity from minor to sight threatening.
- Cuts of the eye or lid require medical care.
- Chemicals in the eyes can threaten sight.
- A blow to the eye can knock it from its socket.
- Loose objects in the eye are the most frequent eye injury and can be very painful.
- Burns to the eye can result if a person looks at a source of ultraviolet light.
- Most ear injuries are not life threatening but fast action may be needed to relieve pain or to prevent or reverse hearing loss.
- Most nosebleeds are self-limiting and seldom require medical attention.
- A foreign object in the nose is a problem mainly among small children who put small objects up their nostrils.
- Because dental emergencies generally cause considerable pain and anxiety, managing them promptly can provide great relief to the victim.
- Trauma can cause teeth to become loosened in their sockets.
- A knocked-out tooth is a dental emergency.
- The front teeth are frequently broken by falls or direct blows.
- The most common reason for toothaches is dental decay.
- A mistake in the handling of a spinal injury victim could mean a lifetime of paralysis for the victim.

▶ Vital Vocabulary

anterior nosebleed Bleeding from the front of the nose.

Battle's sign A contusion on the mastoid area of either ear; sign of a basilar skull fracture.

concussion A temporary disturbance of brain activity caused by a blow to the head.

contusion A bruise; an injury that causes a hemorrhage in or beneath the skin but does not break the skin.

posterior nosebleed Bleeding from the back of the nose, which may flow out of the nostrils and into the mouth or throat.

skull fracture A break of part of the skull (head bones).

▶ Assessment in Action

While working at a construction site, you witness a fellow worker fall to the ground after being struck by a piece of wood thrown by a table saw. He was not wearing his safety glasses and you see a cut to his eyeball and eyelid.

Directions: Circle Yes if you agree with the statement; circle No if you disagree.

Yes	No	1. Apply pressure immediately to the injured eyeball.
Yes	No	2. Tell the victim to keep both eyes closed. Both eyes can be covered with a cravat or roller bandage.
Yes	No	3. Position the victim with his head elevated.
Yes	No	4. Medical care is not necessary in this case.

▶ Check Your Knowledge

Directions: Circle Yes if you agree with the statement; circle No if you disagree.

Yes   No   **1.** Remove objects embedded in an eyeball.

Yes   No   **2.** Scalp wounds have very little bleeding.

Yes   No   **3.** Scrub and rinse the roots of a knocked-out tooth.

Yes   No   **4.** After a blow to the area around an eye, apply a cold pack.

Yes   No   **5.** Tears are sufficient to flush a chemical from the eye.

Yes   No   **6.** Use clean, damp gauze to remove an object from the eyelid's surface.

Yes   No   **7.** Preserve a knocked-out tooth in mouthwash.

Yes   No   **8.** Do not move a victim with a suspected spinal injury.

Yes   No   **9.** Inability to move the hands or feet, or both, may indicate a spinal injury.

Yes   No   **10.** To care for a nosebleed, have the injured person sit down and tilt his or her head back.

Chest, Abdominal, and Pelvic Injuries

Chest Injuries

Chest injuries fall into two categories: open or closed. In open chest injuries, the chest wall is penetrated by some object (eg, knife, bullet). A closed chest injury is one in which the skin is not broken. The injury is caused by blunt trauma (eg, falling object, struck during a fight or assault).

All victims with chest injuries should have their airway, breathing, and circulation (ABCs) checked and rechecked. A responsive victim with a chest injury should usually sit up or, if the injury is on a side, be placed with the injured side down. This position prevents blood inside the chest cavity from seeping into the uninjured side and allows the uninjured side to expand.

► Closed Chest Injuries

In a **closed chest injury,** the skin is not broken. Closed chest injuries include rib fractures and flail chest.

Rib Fractures

The upper four ribs are rarely fractured because they are protected by the collarbone and the shoulder blades. The upper four ribs are so enmeshed with the muscles that they rarely need to be splinted or

Figure 13-1

Stabilize the ribs with a soft object such as a pillow, coat, or blanket (hold or tie). Tell the victim to occasionally take a deep breath and to cough.

Q&A

How could broken ribs become life threatening?

A rib fracture is extremely painful, especially because it cannot be stabilized while it heals. Inhaling air causes the muscles between the ribs to expand the chest and a fractured rib, making it a very painful process. In an attempt to avoid the pain, a victim may develop shallow breathing, which does not fully inflate the small air sacs (alveoli) in the lungs. This can result in an accumulation of fluid, leading to pneumonia.

The pain is usually localized to the area of the fracture. If the sharp end of the broken rib protrudes into the chest cavity, it may puncture the lung, causing it to collapse and allow air between the lung and the chest wall (known as a pneumothorax). A minor collapsing of a lung is painful but not severely disabling. A complete collapse of the lung is painful and exhibits very noticeable shortness of breath. A life-threatening condition known as tension pneumothorax occurs when air or blood progressively accumulates between the chest cavity and the lung (pleural cavity) during inhalation and cannot escape during exhalation. This compresses the heart, uninjured lung, aorta, and vena cava, causing a decrease in blood return to the heart and thereby decreasing cardiac output.

realigned like other broken bones. The lower two ribs are difficult to fracture because they are attached on only one end and have the freedom to move, which is why they are called *floating ribs*. Broken ribs usually occur along the side of the chest. The main symptom of a rib fracture is pain at the injured rib site; when the victim breathes, coughs, or moves; or when the area is touched.

Recognizing Rib Fractures

The signs of rib fracture include:
- Sharp pain, especially when the victim takes a deep breath, coughs, or moves
- Victim holds the injured area, trying to reduce the pain
- Victim reports being hit where the pain is
- Area tender when pressed
- Shallow breathing

To assess for a rib fracture, gently press inward on both sides of the chest at the same time.

Care for Rib Fractures

1. Help the victim find a comfortable position. Stabilize the ribs by having the victim hold a pillow or other similar soft object against the injured area or use bandages to hold the pillow in place. You can also tie an arm over the injured area. Do not apply tight bandages around the chest because they will restrict breathing **Figure 13-1**.
2. Give pain medication.
3. Seek medical care.

Flail Chest

A **flail chest** is a serious injury that involves several ribs in the same area broken in more than one place. The area over the injury may move in a direction opposite to that of the rest of the chest wall during breathing (known as *paradoxical movement*). This injury is very painful and makes breathing difficult.

Rib Fractures

Fractured ribs are a common injury and most frequently occur between ribs 3 and 10. The location for most fractures is on the sides of the body. The first two pairs of ribs are protected by the clavicles, whereas the last two pairs move freely and give with impact. Little can be done to assist the healing of broken ribs other than binding them to restrict movement. Tightly binding the chest limits breathing and, because exhalation is inadequate, fluid accumulates in the air sacs (alveoli) and can result in pneumonia. This often explains pneumonia deaths in elderly persons.

Recognizing Flail Chest

The signs and symptoms of a flail chest include:
- Paradoxical chest motion takes place. The area over the injury may move in a direction opposite to that of the rest of the chest wall during breathing.
- Breathing is very painful and difficult.
- Bruising of the skin over the injury may occur.

Care for Flail Chest

1. Support the chest by one of several methods:
   - Apply hand pressure. This is useful for a short time.
   - Place the victim on the injured side with a blanket or clothing underneath.
2. Monitor breathing.
3. Seek medical care.

▶ Open Chest Injuries

In an **open chest injury**, the skin has been broken and the chest wall is penetrated by an object such as a knife or bullet.

Impaled Object in the Chest

If an object penetrates the chest wall, air and blood escape into the space between the lungs and the chest wall. The air and blood cause the lung to collapse. Lung collapse can lead to shock and death.

Recognizing an Impaled Object in the Chest

An impaled object is usually easily recognized. However, in some cases the object may be below the skin surface and is difficult to see. Carefully look at wounds that could be hiding the object that caused the damage.

Care for an Impaled Object in the Chest

1. Stabilize the object in place with bulky dressings or clothes **Figure 13-2** . *Do not try to remove an impaled object.* Doing so can result in bleeding and air in the chest cavity.
2. Call 9-1-1.

Sucking Chest Wound

A **sucking chest wound** results when a chest wound allows air to pass into and out of the chest with each breath **Figure 13-3** . Bubbles may be seen at the wound during exhalations and a sucking sound heard during inhalations.

Recognizing a Sucking Chest Wound

The signs of a sucking chest wound include:
- Blood bubbling out of a chest wound during exhalation
- Sucking sound heard during inhalations

Figure 13-2

Stabilize a penetrating object with bulky padding. Secure the padding and object.

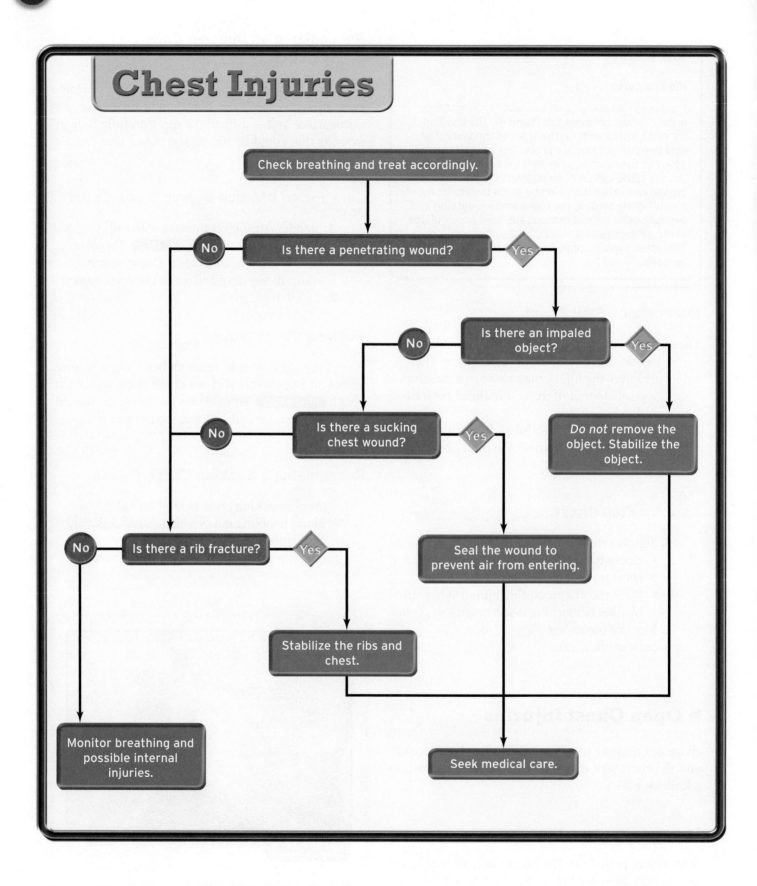

Chest Injuries

Check breathing and treat accordingly.

Is there a penetrating wound?

No

Yes

Is there an impaled object?

No

Yes

Is there a sucking chest wound?

No

Yes

Do not remove the object. Stabilize the object.

Is there a rib fracture?

No

Yes

Seal the wound to prevent air from entering.

Stabilize the ribs and chest.

Monitor breathing and possible internal injuries.

Seek medical care.

Figure 13-3

A sucking chest wound.

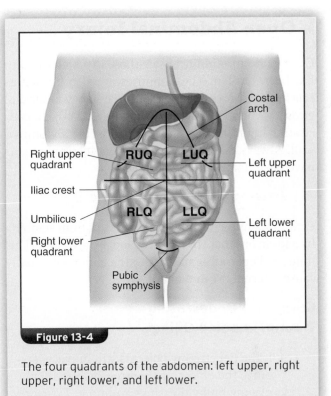

Figure 13-4

The four quadrants of the abdomen: left upper, right upper, right lower, and left lower.

Care for a Sucking Chest Wound

1. Seal the wound with anything available to stop air from entering the chest cavity. Plastic wrap or a plastic bag works well. Tape it in place, but leave one side untaped to create a flutter valve to prevent air from being trapped in the chest cavity. The open side of the dressing should be allowed to drain to gravity. If plastic wrap is not available, you can use your gloved hand.
2. Lean or lay the victim on the injured side.
3. If the victim has trouble breathing or seems to be getting worse, remove the plastic cover (or your hand) to let air escape, and then reapply.
4. Call 9-1-1.

Abdominal Injuries

Injuries to the abdomen are either open or closed and can involve hollow and/or solid organs. An internal abdominal injury is one of the most frequently unrecognized injuries; when missed, it becomes one of the main causes of death. A hollow organ rupture (for example, of the stomach or intestines) spills the contents of the organ into the abdominal cavity, causing inflammation. Solid organ rupture (such as of the liver or spleen) results in severe internal bleeding.

▶ Closed Abdominal Injury

Closed abdominal injuries occur when the internal abdominal tissues are damaged but the skin is unbroken. These are also known as *blunt injuries*. Such an injury might come from striking the handlebar of a bicycle or the steering wheel of a car, or when the victim is struck by a board or baseball bat.

A Blow to the Abdomen

Bruising and damage to internal organs can result from a severe blow to the abdomen.

Recognizing a Closed Abdominal Injury

Examine the abdomen by gently pressing all four quadrants of the abdomen with your fingertips Figure 13-4 . A normal abdomen is soft and not tender when pressed. Signs of a closed abdominal injury include:

- Bruises or other marks
- Pain, tenderness, muscle tightness, or rigidity
- Distention (swelling)

Care for a Closed Abdominal Injury

1. If unresponsive, place the victim on the left side in a comfortable position with the legs bent and in a "fetal position."
2. If responsive, place the victim on one side in a comfortable position with the legs slightly bent. Roll onto side in case of vomiting.
3. Call 9-1-1.

▶ Open Abdominal Injury

<u>Open abdominal injuries</u> are those in which the skin has been broken. These injuries are also known as *penetrating injuries*. Examples include stab wounds and gunshot wounds. It is difficult to know whether a penetrating injury involves more than just the abdominal wall. Always assume the worst—that internal organs have been damaged.

A Penetrating Wound/Impaled Object

Open abdominal wounds usually result from stabbing by a knife or other sharp object and are always serious injuries. Penetrating injuries to the abdomen usually cause internal organ damage.

Care for a Penetrating Wound/Impaled Object

1. If the penetrating object is still in place, stabilize the object and control the bleeding by placing bulky dressings around it. *Do not try to remove the object.*
2. Call 9-1-1.

Protruding Organs

A <u>protruding organ injury</u> (evisceration) refers to a severe injury to the abdomen in which internal organs escape or protrude from the wound.

Care for Protruding Organs

1. Call 9-1-1.
2. Allow the victim to stay in a comfortable position with the legs pulled up toward the abdomen.

Figure 13-5

Do not reinsert protruding organs. Cover them with a moist, sterile dressing.

3. Cover the protruding organs with a moist, sterile dressing or clean cloth, or a piece of plastic **Figure 13-5**.
4. Treat for shock.

Pelvic Injuries

Pelvic fractures are usually caused by falling or a motor vehicle crash.

Recognizing Pelvic Injuries

The signs of a pelvic injury include:
- Pain in the hip, groin, or back that increases with movement
- Inability to stand or walk
- Signs of shock

Check the pelvis by gently pressing inward and downward on the tops of the hips. See Skill Drill 4-2, Steps 5a and 5b.

CAUTION

DO NOT try to reinsert protruding organs into the abdomen—you could introduce infection or damage the intestines.

DO NOT cover the organs tightly.

DO NOT cover the organs with any material that clings or disintegrates when wet.

DO NOT give anything by mouth.

CAUTION

DO NOT roll the victim—additional internal damage could result.

DO NOT move the victim. Whenever possible, wait for trained EMS personnel with their ambulance, backboard, and other specialized equipment.

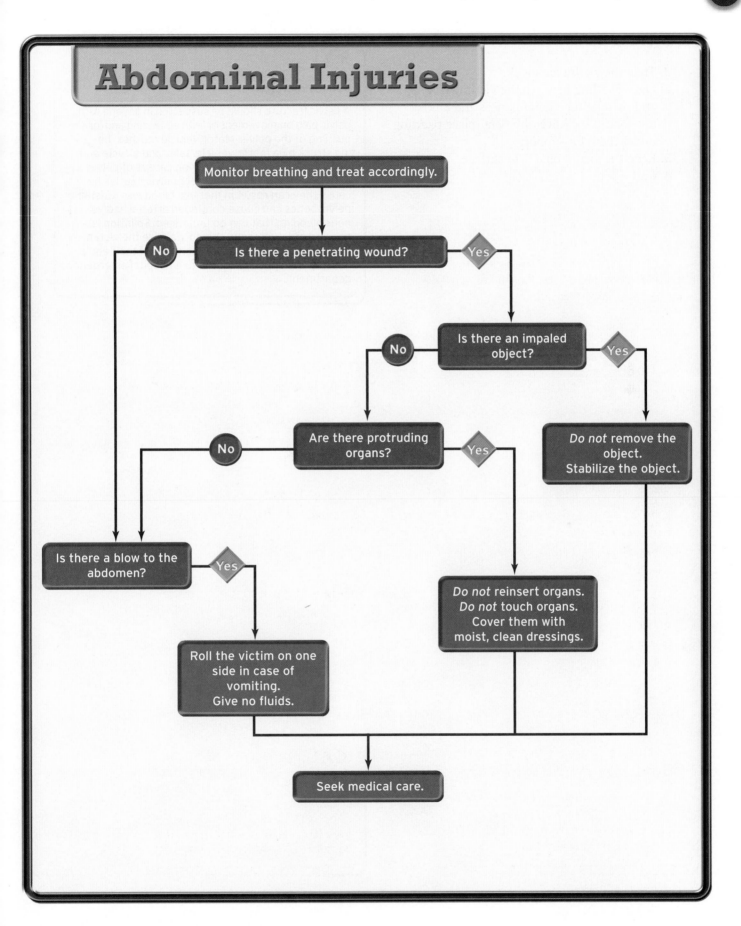

Abdominal Injuries

Monitor breathing and treat accordingly.

No — Is there a penetrating wound? — Yes

No — Is there an impaled object? — Yes

No — Are there protruding organs? — Yes

Do *not* remove the object.
Stabilize the object.

Is there a blow to the abdomen? — Yes

Do not reinsert organs.
Do not touch organs.
Cover them with moist, clean dressings.

Roll the victim on one side in case of vomiting.
Give no fluids.

Seek medical care.

Care for Pelvic Injuries

1. Treat the victim for shock.
2. Place padding between the victim's thighs, and then tie the victim's knees and ankles together. If the knees are bent, place padding under them for support.
3. Keep the victim on a firm surface.
4. Call 9-1-1.

FYI

Pelvic Fractures

A pelvic fracture should be suspected in anyone with pelvic pain on movement or with squeezing and/or pushing of the pelvis. Motor vehicle crashes, being struck by a motor vehicle, falls, and bicycle and motorcycle crashes are common causes of pelvic injury. It is important to suspect pelvic injuries because they can result in massive blood loss. Unstable pelvic bones can cause continued arterial and venous bleeding that can go unnoticed. Splinting is necessary. Laypersons should stabilize the victim and wait for trained EMS personnel and their equipment to transport the victim to a hospital emergency department.

▶ Emergency Care Wrap-up

Condition	What to Look For	What to Do
Chest Injuries	**Rib fractures** • Sharp pain with deep breaths, coughing, or moving • Shallow breathing • Holding of injured area to reduce pain	1. Place victim in comfortable position. 2. Support ribs with a pillow, blanket, or coat (either holding or tying with bandages). 3. Seek medical care.
	Embedded (impaled) object • Object remains in wound	1. DO NOT remove object from wound. 2. Use bulky dressings or cloths to stabilize the object. 3. Call 9-1-1.
	Sucking chest wound • Blood bubbling out of wound • Sound of air being sucked in and out of wound	1. Seal wound to stop air from entering chest; tape three sides of plastic or use gloved hand. 2. Remove cover to let air escape if victim worsens or has trouble breathing. 3. Call 9-1-1.
Abdominal Injuries	**Blow to abdomen (closed)** • Bruise or other marks • Muscle tightness and rigidity felt while gently pushing on abdomen	1. Place victim in comfortable position with legs pulled up toward the abdomen. 2. Treat for shock. 3. Seek medical care.
	Protruding organs (open) • Internal organs escaping from abdominal wound	1. Place victim in a comfortable position with the legs pulled up toward the abdomen. 2. DO NOT reinsert organs into the abdomen. 3. Cover organs with a moist, sterile or clean dressing. 4. Treat for shock. 5. Call 9-1-1.
Pelvic Injuries	**Pelvic fractures** • Pain in hip, groin, or back that increases with movement • Inability to walk or stand • Signs of shock	1. Keep victim still. 2. Treat for shock. 3. Call 9-1-1.

prep kit

▶ Ready for Review

- Chest injuries fall into two categories: open or closed.
- Closed chest injuries include rib fractures and flail chest.
- In an open chest injury, the skin has been broken and the chest wall is penetrated by an object such as a knife or bullet.
- Injuries to the abdomen are either open or closed and can involve hollow and/or solid organs.
- Closed abdominal injuries occur when the internal abdominal tissues are damaged but the skin is unbroken.
- Open abdominal injuries are those in which the skin has been broken and the abdominal wall penetrated.
- Pelvic fractures are usually caused by falling or a motor vehicle crash.

▶ Vital Vocabulary

<u>closed abdominal injuries</u> Injuries to the abdomen that occur as a result of a direct blow from a blunt object. There is no break in the skin.

<u>closed chest injury</u> An injury to the chest in which the skin is not broken; usually due to blunt trauma.

<u>flail chest</u> A condition that occurs when several ribs in the same area are broken in more than one place.

<u>open abdominal injuries</u> Injuries to the abdomen that include penetrating wounds and protruding organs.

<u>open chest injury</u> An injury to the chest in which the chest wall itself is penetrated by an external object such as a bullet or knife.

<u>protruding organ injury</u> A severe injury to the abdomen in which the internal organs escape or protrude from the wound; evisceration.

<u>sucking chest wound</u> A chest wound that allows air to pass into the chest cavity with each breath.

▶ Assessment in Action

You are on the first aid team at a local scout camp. The scout leaders are conducting a funny skit on a stage at the main lodge. One of the scouts in the skit jumps in the air and lands on his side. As he runs off the stage toward you, he is in obvious pain and is clutching his side. He lies down and a knife falls to the ground. You hear a sucking sound coming from the wound on his side whenever the victim inhales.

Directions: Circle Yes if you agree with the statement; circle No if you disagree.

Yes No **1.** You should check the victim's breathing and treat accordingly.

Yes No **2.** Blood bubbling out of the wound during breathing is a sign of a sucking chest wound.

Yes No **3.** This wound should be sealed on three sides to prevent air from being trapped in the chest cavity.

Yes No **4.** If the victim begins to have trouble breathing, do not remove the seal to reapply.

Yes No **5.** This is a medical emergency and 9-1-1 should be called immediately.

▶ Check Your Knowledge

Directions: Circle Yes if you agree with the statement; circle No if you disagree.

Yes No **1.** Stabilize a broken rib with a soft object, such as a pillow or blanket, tied to the chest.

Yes No **2.** Cover a sucking chest wound with a piece of plastic taped down on three sides.

Yes No **3.** Remove a penetrating or impaled object from the chest or the abdomen.

Yes No **4.** A flail chest refers to a single broken rib.

Yes No **5.** Keep the victim with a broken pelvis still.

Yes No **6.** Sharp pain while breathing can be a sign of a rib fracture.

Yes No **7.** Rib fractures should be treated by tightly taping the chest.

Yes No **8.** Most victims with abdominal injuries are more comfortable with their knees bent.

Yes No **9.** Leave a chest wound alone if you hear air being sucked in and out.

Yes No **10.** A broken pelvis can threaten life because of the large amount of blood lost.

Bone, Joint, and Muscle Injuries

Bone Injuries

Bone, joint, and muscle injuries are among the most common reasons for seeking medical care. Although rarely fatal, they often result in short- or long-term disability.

► Fractures

The real problems are not the broken bones themselves but rather the potential injury to the vital organs next to them. People usually do not die of broken bones. They die of airway obstruction, blood loss, and brain injury. However, broken bones can be painful and debilitating and can cause lifelong aggravation, disability, and deformity.

The terms <u>fracture</u> and *broken bone* have the same meaning: a break or crack in a bone. There are two categories of fractures:

- <u>Closed fracture</u>. The skin is intact, and no wound exists anywhere near the fracture site **Figure 14-1A**.
- <u>Open fracture</u>. The skin over the fracture has been broken. The wound may result from the bone protruding through the skin or from a direct blow that cut the skin at the time of the fracture. The bone may not always be visible in the wound **Figure 14-1B**.

It is not possible to determine the exact nature of a broken bone outside a medical facility. It may be helpful, however, for first aiders to be familiar with the terminology that physicians use to describe fractures **Figure 14-2**.

A *transverse fracture* cuts across the bone at right angles to its long axis and is often caused by direct injury. *Greenstick fractures* are incomplete fractures that commonly occur in children, whose bones (like green sticks) are pliable. A *spiral fracture* usually results from a twisting injury, and the fracture line has the appearance of a spring. The fracture line of an *oblique fracture* crosses the bone in a slanting direction (or at an oblique angle, thus the name). A *comminuted*

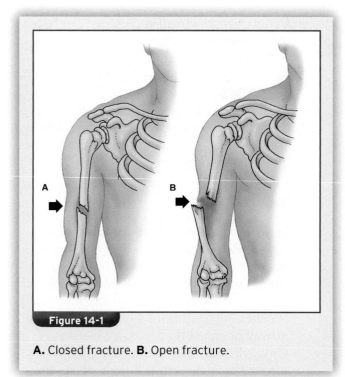

Figure 14-1

A. Closed fracture. **B.** Open fracture.

Q&A

Which is the most frequently fractured bone in the body?

Due to its vulnerable position and its relative thinness, the clavicle is the most frequently fractured bone in the body. Fractured clavicles are caused by either a direct blow or a transmitted force resulting from a fall on the outstretched arm.

Greenstick   Transverse   Oblique   Comminuted   Impacted

Figure 14-2

Types of fractures.

fracture is one in which the bone is fragmented into more than two pieces (that is, splintered or crushed). In an *impacted fracture,* the broken ends of the bone are jammed together and the bone may function as if no fracture were present.

Recognizing Fractures

It may be difficult to tell if a bone is broken **Figure 14-3**. When in doubt, treat the injury as a fracture. Use the mnemonic DOTS to assess for an injury—Deformity, Open wound, Tenderness, Swelling.

- *Deformity* might not be obvious. Compare the injured part with the uninjured part on the other side.
- *Open wound* may indicate an underlying fracture.
- *Tenderness* and pain are commonly found only at the injury site. The victim usually will be able to point to the site of the pain. A useful procedure for detecting a fracture is to feel along the bone gently; a victim's complaint about pain or tenderness serves as a reliable sign of a fracture.
- *Swelling* caused by bleeding happens rapidly after a fracture.

Additional signs and symptoms include the following:

- *Loss of use* may or may not occur.
- *Guarding* occurs when motion produces pain; the victim refuses to use the injured part. Sometimes, however, the victim is able to move a fractured limb with little or no pain.

- A *grating sensation,* called **crepitus,** can be felt and sometimes even heard when the ends of the broken bone rub together. Do not move the injured limb in an attempt to detect it **Figure 14-4**.
- The *history* of the injury can lead you to suspect a fracture whenever a serious accident has happened. The victim may have heard or felt the bone snap.

Care for Fractures

1. Perform a primary check for life-threatening conditions. A fracture, even an open fracture, seldom presents an immediate threat to life. Treatment should be deferred until after you have handled any life-threatening conditions such as opening an airway or controlling massive bleeding. Only when all life-threatening conditions have been dealt with is it appropriate to identify and stabilize fractures. Determine what happened and the location of the injury.
2. Gently remove clothing covering the injured area. Cut clothing at the seams if necessary.
3. Examine the area by looking and feeling for DOTS.
   - Look at the injury site. Swelling and black-and-blue marks, which indicate escape of blood into the tissues, may come from the

Figure 14-3

X-rays of a victim's forearm showing the fracture before and after setting.

Figure 14-4

Forearm fracture.

bone end or associated muscular and blood vessel damage. Shortening or severe deformity (*angulation*) between the joints or deformity around the joints, shortening of the extremity, and rotation of the extremity when compared with the opposite extremity indicate a bone injury. Lacerations or even small puncture wounds near the site of a bone fracture are considered open fractures.

- Feel the injured area. If a fracture is not obvious, gently press, touch, or feel along the length of the bone for deformities, tenderness, and swelling.

4. Check blood flow and nerves. Use the mnemonic CSM (circulation, sensation, movement) as a way of remembering what to do **Skill Drill 14-1**:

- *Circulation.* For an arm injury, feel for the radial pulse (located on the thumb side of the wrist); use the posterior tibial pulse (located between the inside ankle bone and the Achilles tendon) for a leg injury. A pulseless arm or leg is a significant emergency that requires immediate surgical care. If there is no pulse, gently realign the extremity to try to restore the blood flow. Some experts recommend the capillary refill test. (Press on a fingernail or toenail, then release it. If circulation is normal, the nail bed should return to its normal color within 2 seconds.) Performing the capillary refill test in the dark or the cold may limit its accuracy (**Step ❶**).

- *Sensation.* This is the most useful early sign. Lightly touch or squeeze one of the victim's toes or fingers and ask the victim what he or she feels (**Step ❷**). Loss of sensation is an early sign of nerve damage.

- *Movement.* Inability to move develops later. Check for nerve damage by asking the victim to wiggle his or her toes or fingers (**Step ❸**). If the toes or fingers are injured, do not have the victim attempt to move them. A quick nerve and circulatory check is extremely important. The most serious complication of a fracture is inadequate blood flow in an extremity. The major blood vessels of an extremity tend to run close to the bones, which means that any

time a bone is broken, the adjacent blood vessels are at risk of being torn by bone fragments or pinched off between the ends of the broken bone. The tissues of the arms and legs cannot survive for more than 3 hours without a continuing blood supply. If you note any disruption in the nerve or circulatory supply, seek immediate medical attention. Major nerve pathways also travel close to bone and may be torn or pinched off between the ends of the broken bone.

5. Stabilize the injured part to prevent movement.

- If emergency medical services (EMS) will arrive soon, stabilize the injured part with your hands until they arrive.

- If EMS will be delayed or if you are taking the victim to medical care, stabilize the injured part with a splint.

6. If the injury is an open fracture, do not push on any protruding bones **Figure 14-5**. Cover the wound and exposed bones with a dressing. Place rolls of gauze around the bone and bandage the injury without applying pressure on the bone.

7. Apply an ice pack, if possible, to help reduce swelling and pain.

8. Seek medical care. Call 9-1-1 for any open fractures or large bone fractures (such as the femur) or when transporting the victim would be difficult or would aggravate the injury.

Figure 14-5

Open tibia, fibula fracture of the leg.

14-1 Checking CSM in an Extremity

1 Check an upper extremity for:
Circulation—radial pulse.

1 Check a lower extremity for:
Circulation—posterior tibial pulse.

2 Sensation—squeeze fingers.

2 Sensation—squeeze toes.

3 Movement—wiggle fingers.

3 Movement—wiggle toes.

Joint Injuries

A joint is where two or more bones come together.

▶ Dislocations

A *dislocation* occurs when a joint comes apart and stays apart with the bone ends no longer in contact. The shoulders, elbows, fingers, hips, kneecaps (patellas), and ankles are the joints most frequently affected.

Recognizing Dislocations

Dislocations cause signs and symptoms similar to those of fractures: deformity, severe pain, swelling, and inability of the victim to move the injured joint. The main sign of a dislocation is deformity. Its appearance will be different from that of an uninjured joint **Figure 14-6**.

Care for Dislocations

1. Check the CSM. If the end of the dislocated bone is pressing on nerves or blood vessels, numbness or paralysis may exist below the dislocation. Always check the pulses. If there is no pulse in the injured extremity, transport the victim to a medical facility immediately.
2. Use the RICE (rest, ice, compression, elevation) procedures.
3. Use a splint to stabilize the joint in the position in which it was found.

Figure 14-6

Dislocation.

4. Do not try to reduce the joint (put the displaced parts back into their normal positions) because nerve and blood vessel damage could result. For instance, when medical help is more than 1 hour away, experts in wilderness medicine have identified easy and safe ways to treat the following dislocations: kneecap, fingers and toes, and anterior shoulder (see Chapter 24, *Wilderness First Aid*).
5. Seek medical care to reduce the dislocation. Call 9-1-1 for dislocations when transporting the victim would be difficult or would aggravate the injury.

▶ Sprains

A **sprain** occurs when a joint is twisted or stretched beyond its normal range of motion. Bones are held together at joints by tough bands of tissue called ligaments. When a joint is sprained, the ligaments are either partially or completely torn. There are different degrees of sprains, but it is difficult for a first aider to classify the degree of a sprain. Sprains most often occur in the knee and the ankle, but can occur in any joint.

Ankle sprains most often occur when the foot turns inward and stress is placed on the outside (lateral side) of the ankle. A severe lateral ankle sprain, if not correctly treated, can result in a chronically unstable ankle that is prone to sprains. Any ligament or bone injury on the inner side of the ankle usually represents a serious problem and requires medical care.

Recognizing Sprains

It is often difficult to distinguish between a severe sprain and a fracture because their signs and symptoms are similar.

- Severe pain
- Pain prevents the victim from moving or using the joint.
- Swelling
- Skin around the joint may be discolored because of bleeding from torn blood vessels.

Care for Sprains

1. Follow the RICE procedures. Apply an ice pack for 20 minutes; apply compression with an elastic bandage for 3 to 4 hours; repeat the cycles of an ice pack for 20 minutes and 3 hours of compression. Raise the injured part to reduce the flow of blood to the injury. For more information on the RICE procedure, see page 210.
2. Swelling in a joint can lead to stiffness in a matter of hours. It is important to keep a joint from swelling by using cold promptly; it is equally important to help the swelling recede as quickly as possible with compression and elevation.

Muscle Injuries

Although muscle injuries pose no real emergency, first aiders have ample opportunities to care for them.

▶ Strains

A *muscle strain,* also known as a *muscle pull,* occurs when a muscle is stretched beyond its normal range of motion and tears the muscle. There are different degrees of strains, but it is difficult for a first aider to classify the degree of a strain. When muscle fibers tear, fluid from nearby tissues leaks out and starts to build up near the injury. The area becomes inflamed, swollen, and tender. Inflammation begins immediately after an injury, but it can take 24 to 72 hours for enough tissue fluid to build up to cause pain and stiffness.

Recognizing Strains

Any of the following signs and symptoms may indicate a muscle strain:

- Sudden, sharp pain in the affected muscle
- Extreme tenderness when the area is touched
- Swelling
- Weakness and inability to use the injured part
- Stiffness and pain when the victim moves the muscle
- After a few days, the skin around the injury may be discolored because of bleeding from torn blood vessels.

Care for Strains

To care for strains, simply follow the RICE procedures.

▶ Cramps

A cramp occurs when a muscle goes into an uncontrolled spasm and contraction. Although scientific literature has yet to confirm the causes of muscle cramps, several factors are associated with them. For example, muscle cramping is associated with certain diseases such as diabetes and atherosclerosis. Muscle cramps are often associated with physical activity. Roughly, muscle cramps can be divided into two categories: *night cramps,* which include any cramp occurring at night or while an individual is at rest, and *heat cramps,* which are related to dehydration and electrolyte imbalance. (The electrolytes potassium and sodium carry an electric charge that helps trigger muscles to contract and relax.)

Recognizing Cramps

- Sudden, severe pain, usually in the legs.
- A knotting of the muscle may be felt and sometimes seen.
- Restricted movement

Care for Cramps

Many treatments for cramps are available. Try one or more of the following:

1. Have the victim gently stretch the affected muscle. Because a muscle cramp is an

uncontrolled muscle contraction or spasm, a gradual extension of the muscle may help lengthen the muscle fibers and relieve the cramp.

2. Relax the muscle by pressing and massaging it.
3. Apply an ice pack to help relieve the cramping pain (unless you are in a cold environment).
4. Pinch the upper lip hard (an acupressure technique) to reduce calf-muscle cramping.
5. Drink lightly salted cool water (dissolve ¼ teaspoon salt in a quart of water) or a commercial sports drink.

▶ Contusions

A muscle contusion or bruise results from a blow to the muscle.

Recognizing Contusions

- Swelling
- Pain and tenderness
- After a few days, the skin in the area may become discolored due to bleeding from torn blood vessels.

Care for Contusions

To care for muscle contusions, follow the RICE procedures.

CAUTION

DO NOT give salt tablets to a person with muscle cramps. They can cause stomach irritation, nausea, and vomiting.

▶ Emergency Care Wrap-up

Condition	What to Look For	What to Do
Bone Injuries	**Fractures (broken bones)** • DOTS (deformity, open wound, tenderness, swelling) • Inability to use injured part normally • Grating or grinding sensation felt or heard • Victim heard or felt bone snap	1. Expose and examine the injury site. 2. Bandage any open wound. 3. Splint the injured area. 4. Apply ice or cold pack. 5. Seek medical care: Depending on the severity, call 9-1-1 or transport to medical care.
Joint Injuries	**Dislocation or sprain** • Deformity • Pain • Swelling • Inability to use injured part normally	**Dislocation** 1. Expose and examine the injury site. 2. Splint the injured area. 3. Apply ice or cold pack. 4. Seek medical care. **Sprain** 1. Use RICE procedures.
Muscle Injuries	**Strain** • Sharp pain • Extreme tenderness when area is touched • Indentation or bump • Weakness and loss of function of injured area • Stiffness and pain when victim moves the muscle	1. Use RICE procedures.
	Contusion • Pain and tenderness • Swelling • Bruise on injured area	1. Use RICE procedures.
	Cramp • Uncontrolled spasm • Pain • Restriction or loss of movement	1. Stretch and/or apply direct pressure to the affected muscle.

▶ Ready for Review

- Broken bones can be painful and debilitating and can cause lifelong aggravation, disability, and deformity.
- A joint is where two or more bones come together. Joints can be dislocated or sprained.
- Muscles can be strained, bruised, or cramped.

▶ Vital Vocabulary

<u>closed fracture</u> A fracture in which there is no wound in the overlying skin.

<u>cramp</u> A painful spasm of a muscle.

<u>crepitus</u> A grating sound heard and the sensation felt when the fractured ends of a bone rub together.

<u>fracture</u> A break or rupture in a bone.

<u>open fracture</u> A fracture exposed to the exterior; an open wound lies over the fracture.

<u>sprain</u> A trauma to a joint that injures the ligaments.

▶ Assessment in Action

While walking through your neighborhood, you see two boys yelling for help on the sidewalk. One is on the ground in pain and clutching his arm. The other boy explains that the injured boy lost control while skateboarding and crashed. The victim said he heard a snap when he crashed and landed on his arm.

Directions: Circle Yes if you agree with the statement; circle No if you disagree.

Yes No **1.** You should look and feel for DOTS.

Yes No **2.** You notice a severe deformity on the victim's forearm but the skin is not broken. This is a closed fracture.

Yes No **3.** You should check the injured arm for circulation, sensation, and movement.

Yes No **4.** You should not splint the arm because of the deformity.

Yes No **5.** Applying ice helps reduce swelling.

prep kit

▶ Check Your Knowledge

Directions: Circle Yes if you agree with the statement; circle No if you disagree.

Yes   No   **1.** Apply cold on a suspected sprain.

Yes   No   **2.** The letters RICE stand for rest, ice, compression, and elevation.

Yes   No   **3.** DOTS stands for deformity, open wound, tenderness, and swelling.

Yes   No   **4.** Guarding occurs when motion produces pain.

Yes   No   **5.** Crepitus cannot be heard, but it can be felt by the victim.

Yes   No   **6.** A dislocation is cared for much differently than a fracture.

Yes   No   **7.** Check a suspected fracture by having the victim move the extremity.

Yes   No   **8.** Treat a muscle cramp by stretching the affected muscle.

Yes   No   **9.** CSM stands for cold, swelling, and motion.

Yes   No   **10.** Do not push on a protruding bone.

15

Extremity Injuries

Extremity Injuries

Injuries to the extremities are common because people are involved in active lifestyles that include sports and wilderness activities. This chapter focuses on bone, joint, and muscle injuries of the extremities; bleeding, wounds, and other soft-tissue injuries are covered elsewhere. Most of the conditions discussed result from sudden trauma, although some chronic injuries incurred over time, such as tennis elbow, are included.

▶ Assessment

Use these guidelines to assess injuries to the extremities:
- Look for signs and symptoms of fractures and dislocations.
- Examine the extremities, using the mnemonic DOTS (Deformity, Open wound, Tenderness, Swelling). Look at and gently feel the extremity, starting at the distal end (fingers or toes) and working upward.
- Compare one extremity with the other to determine size and shape differences.
- Use the "rule of thirds" for extremity injuries. Imagine each long bone as being divided into thirds. If deformity, tenderness, or swelling is located in the upper or lower third of a long bone, assume that the nearest joint is injured.

- Consider the cause of injury (COI) when evaluating the possibility of a fracture and its location. Forces that cause musculoskeletal injuries are direct forces (for example, a car bumper striking a pedestrian's leg), indirect forces along the long axis of bones (for example, a person falling onto an outstretched hand and fracturing the collarbone), and twisting forces (for example, a person's foot fixed in one spot with the leg suddenly twisting).
- Use the mnemonic CSM as a reminder to check the extremity for circulation, sensation, and movement of fingers or toes.

▶ Types of Injuries

Types of injuries to the extremities range from simple contusions to complex open fractures:

- **Contusions,** or bruising of the tissue
- **Strains,** in which muscles are stretched or torn
- **Sprains,** which involve the tearing or stretching of the joints, causing mild to severe damage to the ligaments and joint capsules
- **Tendinitis,** which is inflammation of a tendon (cord that attaches muscle to bone) caused by overuse
- **Dislocations,** in which bones are displaced from their normal joint alignment, out of their sockets, or out of their normal positions
- **Fractures,** which are breaks in bones that may or may not be accompanied by open wounds

Care for Extremity Injuries

1. Use the RICE procedures for injuries described in this chapter (see Skill Drill 15-1, page 213).
2. Apply a splint to stabilize fractures and dislocations.

RICE Procedure for Bone, Joint, and Muscle Injuries

RICE is the acronym for rest, ice, compression, and elevation—the recommended immediate treatment for bone, joint, and muscle injuries. The steps during the first 48 to 72 hours after an injury can do a lot to relieve—even prevent—aches and pains. Treat all extremity bone, joint, and muscle injuries with the RICE procedure. In addition to RICE, fractures and dislocations should be splinted to stabilize the injured area.

▶ R = Rest

Injuries heal faster if rested. *Rest* means the victim does not use or move the injured part. Using any part of the body increases the blood circulation to that area, which can cause more swelling of an injured part. Crutches may be used to rest leg injuries.

▶ I = Ice

An ice pack should be applied to the injured area as soon as possible after the injury for 20 to 30 minutes as often as possible while awake, removing the ice pack for 5–10 minutes between each 20–30 minute period, during the first 24 to 48 hours. Never apply ice directly to the skin. Skin treated with cold passes through four stages: cold, burning, aching, and numbness. When the skin becomes numb, usually in 20 to 30 minutes, remove the ice pack. After removing the ice pack, compress the injured part with an elastic bandage and keep it elevated (the "C" and "E" of RICE).

Cold constricts the blood vessels to and in the injured area, which helps reduce the swelling and inflammation, and it dulls the pain and relieves muscle spasms. Cold should be applied as soon as possible after the injury; healing time often is directly related to the amount of swelling that occurs. Heat has the opposite effect when applied to fresh injuries: It increases circulation to the area and increases the swelling and the pain.

Use either of the following methods to apply cold to an injury:

- Put crushed ice (or cubes) into a double plastic bag, hot water bottle, or wet towel. A layer of cloth should separate the ice from the skin. Secure it in place with an elastic bandage for 20 to 30 minutes. Ice bags can conform to the body's contours.
- Use a chemical "snap pack," a sealed pouch that contains two chemical envelopes. Squeezing the pack mixes the chemicals, producing a chemical reaction that has a cooling effect. Although they do not cool as well as other methods, they are convenient to use

CAUTION

DO NOT apply an ice pack for more than 20 to 30 minutes at a time. Frostbite or nerve damage can result.

DO NOT apply an ice pack on the back outside part of the knee. Nerve damage can occur.

DO NOT apply cold if the victim has a history of circulatory disease, Raynaud disease (spasms in the arteries of the extremities that reduce circulation), or abnormal sensitivity to cold, or if the injured part has been frostbitten previously.

DO NOT stop using an ice pack too soon. A common mistake is the early use of heat, which may result in swelling and pain. Use an ice pack three to four times a day for the first 24 hours, preferably up to 48 hours, before applying any heat. For severe injuries, using ice for up to 72 hours is recommended.

FYI

Homemade Ice Packs

- Ice bags kept in a freezer freeze solid and cannot be shaped to fit the injured area. One part isopropyl (rubbing) alcohol to three parts water prevents freezing, and the ice bag can be easily molded. Bags can be reused for months.
- An unopened bag of frozen vegetables is inexpensive; keeps its basic shape (unlike ice chips, which melt); molds to the shape of the injured area; is reusable; and is packaged in a fairly puncture-resistant, watertight bag.
- For cold therapy over a fairly large area, soak a face towel in cold water, wring it out, fold it, and place it in a large self-sealing plastic bag. Store the bag in the freezer. To use the cold pack, wrap it in a light cotton towel and apply for 20 minutes, after which it can be refrozen. A washcloth in a smaller bag can be used to treat a smaller area.
- Fill a plastic bag with snow.
- Fill a polystyrene plastic cup with water and freeze it. When you need an ice pack, peel the cup to below ice level; the remaining part of the cup forms a cold-resistant handle. Rub the ice over the injured area (movement is necessary to prevent skin damage). These ice "packs" are inexpensive and convenient and take up little space.
- To make a funnel for filling an ice bag, push out the bottom of a paper cup and fit it into the neck of the ice bag. The ice will slide through the cup and into the bag.

FYI

Heat and Cold: When to Use Which?

Many people use heat devices or ice packs to speed recovery from sports injuries—but when is the right time to use each technique? Cold usually should be applied immediately after an acute injury, such as an ankle sprain. Icing reduces pain, swelling, and muscle spasm immediately after injury, but its use should be discontinued after 2 or 3 days. Heat applications (heat packs, radiant heat, or whirlpool baths) can then be used to reduce muscle spasms and pain. In addition, heat increases blood flow and joint flexibility. Vigorous heat is used to treat chronic injuries, but mild heat can reduce muscle spasm. Heat is also effective for acute back pain, but ice massage is preferred if the back pain persists for 2 weeks or more.

Source: Kaul M P, Herring S A: Superficial heat and cold. *Physician and Sportsmedicine.* 22(12);65.

when ice is not readily available. They lose their cooling power quickly, however, and can be used only once. Also, they may be impractical because they are expensive.

▶ C = Compression

Compressing the injured area squeezes fluid out of the injury site. Compression limits the ability of the skin and other tissues to expand and reduces internal bleeding. Apply an elastic bandage to the injured area, especially the foot, ankle, knee, thigh, hand, or elbow. Fill the hollow areas with padding such as a sock or washcloth before applying the elastic bandage.

Elastic bandages come in various sizes for different body areas:
- 2″ width for the wrist, hand, and foot
- 3″ width for the elbow and arm
- 4″ width for the ankle, knee, and leg

Start the elastic bandage several inches below the injury and wrap in an upward, overlapping (about one half to three fourths of the bandage's width) spiral, starting with even and somewhat tight pressure, then gradually wrapping more loosely above the injury. Stretch the elastic bandage no more than one third its ability to stretch.

Applying compression may be the most important step in preventing swelling. The victim should wear the elastic bandage continuously for the first 18 to 24 hours (except when cold is applied). At night, have the victim loosen but not remove the elastic bandage.

For an ankle injury, place a horseshoe-shaped pad around the ankle knob and secure it with the elastic bandage **Figure 15-1** . The pad can be made from various materials (eg, twisting a wash cloth, socks). The pad will compress the soft tissues and the bones. Wrap the bandage tightest nearest the toes and loosest above the ankle. It should be tight enough to decrease swelling but not tight enough to inhibit blood flow. For a contusion or a strain, place a pad between the injury and the elastic bandage.

CAUTION

DO NOT apply an elastic bandage too tightly. If applied too tightly, elastic bandages will restrict circulation. Stretch a new elastic bandage to about one third its maximum length for adequate compression. Leave fingers and toes exposed so possible color change can be easily observed. Compare the toes or fingers of the injured extremity with those on the uninjured one. Pale skin, pain, numbness, and tingling are signs that the bandage is too tight. If any of these symptoms appears, immediately remove the elastic bandage. Leave the elastic bandage off until all the symptoms disappear, then rewrap the area less tightly. Always wrap from below the injury and move toward the heart.

▶ E = Elevation

Gravity slows the return of blood to the heart from the lower parts of the body. Once fluids get to the hands or feet, they have nowhere else to go, and those parts of the body swell. Elevating the injured area, in combination with ice and compression, limits circulation to that area, which in turn helps limit internal bleeding and minimize swelling.

It is simple to prop up an injured leg or arm to limit bleeding. Whenever possible, elevate the injured part above the level of the heart for the first 24 hours after an injury. If a fracture is suspected, do not elevate an extremity until it has been stabilized with a splint. Along with the use of RICE procedures, fractures and dislocations should be splinted.

To perform the RICE procedure, follow the steps in **Skill Drill 15-1** :
1. R = Rest. Stop using the injured area.
2. I = Ice. Place an ice pack on the injured area. Use an elastic bandage to hold the ice pack in place for 20 to 30 minutes (**Step** ❶).

A.

B.

Figure 15-1

A. Place a horseshoe-shaped pad around the ankle knob. B. Secure the pad with an elastic bandage.

3. C = Compression. Remove the ice, apply a compression bandage, and leave in place for 3 to 4 hours (**Step** ❷).
4. E = Elevation. Raise the injured area higher than the heart, if possible (**Step** ❸).

Shoulder Injuries

▶ Shoulder Dislocation

Three bones come together at the shoulder: the scapula (shoulder blade), the clavicle (collarbone), and the humerus (upper arm bone). The shoulder is the most freely movable joint in the body. The extreme range of its possible movements makes the shoulder joint highly susceptible to dislocation (separation). A *dislocation* of the shoulder occurs when the bones of the

skill drill

15-1 The RICE Procedure

1 Place an ice pack on the injured area. Use an elastic bandage to hold the ice pack in place for 20 to 30 minutes.

2 Remove the ice, apply a compression bandage, and leave in place for 3 to 4 hours.

3 Raise the injured area higher than the heart, if possible.

shoulder come apart as a result of a blow or a particular movement. Shoulder dislocation is second in frequency only to finger dislocations.

Recognizing a Shoulder Dislocation

- In about 95% of shoulder dislocations, the victim holds the upper arm away from the body, supported by the uninjured arm. This position differentiates a dislocation from a fracture of the humerus, in which the victim holds the arm against the chest.
- The dislocated arm cannot be brought across the chest wall to touch the opposite shoulder (that is, the sling position).
- Extreme pain in the shoulder area.
- In a dislocation, the shoulder looks squared off, rather than rounded.
- An injury to the shoulder resulting in complete loss of function is more apt to be a dislocation than a fracture.
- The victim may describe a history of previous dislocations.
- Numbness or paralysis in the arm from pressure, pinching blood vessels or nerves.

Care for a Shoulder Dislocation

1. Do not try to force, twist, or pull the shoulder back in place because it may cause bone, nerve, or blood vessel injury.
2. Place a folded or rolled blanket or a pillow between the upper arm and the chest to support the arm.
3. Apply an arm sling and swathe (binder). See Chapter 16, *Splinting Extremities* for more details. Use the arm sling which has one end tucked between the arm and body and ties in the back. This keeps pressure off the area.
4. Apply an ice pack for 20 minutes.
5. Seek immediate medical care.

▶ Clavicle Fracture

Fractures of the clavicle (collarbone) are common and usually are the result of falling with the arm and hand outstretched. The victim falls onto his or her hand, and the force from the fall is transmitted to the shoulder. Most clavicle fractures (80%) occur in the middle third of the bone.

Recognizing a Clavicle Fracture

Usually the fracture is easy to detect because the clavicle lies immediately under the skin and a deformity can be seen.

The victim:
- Fell on an outstretched arm
- Received a direct blow to the clavicle or shoulder

AND if the victim has:
- Severe pain over the injured area
- Been holding the injured arm against the chest with the uninjured arm to stabilize the injury
- Not moved the arm because of the pain
- Swelling
- Visible deformity
- Tenderness
- "Dropped" or drooped shoulder
- Bruising

Care for a Clavicle Fracture

1. Treat for shock.
2. Apply an arm sling and swathe (binder). This keeps pressure off the area.
3. Apply an ice pack to the area for 20 minutes, three to four times during the next 24 hours.
4. Seek immediate medical care.

▶ Contusions

Direct blows cause contusions, or bruises, about the shoulder. Often called *shoulder pointers*, contusions of this type may cause severe discomfort.

Recognizing Contusions

- Swelling
- Pain at the injury site
- Feeling of firmness when pressure is exerted on the shoulder
- Tenderness
- Discoloration under the skin (black and blue)

Care for Contusions

1. Apply an ice pack to the area for 20 minutes, three to four times during the first 24 hours.
2. Place the arm in a sling and swathe (binder). Use the arm sling which has one end tucked between the arm and body and ties in the back. This keeps pressure off the area.

▶ Tendinitis

The general cause of tendinitis (inflammation) in the shoulder is continuous overuse or unusual use. Repeated arm movement often results in painful shoulders. Examples of these include many of the throwing sports (such as seen with a baseball pitcher or a football quarterback) and in other sports in which the shoulder is used extensively (such as swimming).

Recognizing Tendinitis

- Constant pain or pain with motion of the shoulder
- Limited motion of the shoulder
- "Crackling" sound when the joint is moved
- Tenderness over the area

Care for Tendinitis

1. Use an ice massage for 10 minutes before and after exercise. Fill a Styrofoam cup with water and freeze. Tear a small amount of foam from the top so ice protrudes. Massage firmly over the injured area in a circle about the size of a baseball.
2. Use a sling and swathe (binder) to rest the shoulder.
3. Use pain medication such as ibuprofen.
4. Seek medical advice if needed.

▶ Humerus Fracture

The shaft of the humerus (upper arm) can be felt throughout its entire length along the inner side of the upper arm.

Recognizing a Humerus Fracture

The victim received a:
- Direct blow to the area
- Twist or fall on the outstretched arm

AND any one or combination of these occurred:
- Severe pain
- Swelling
- Visible deformity. The deformity may be hidden by swelling or by the large muscles surrounding the upper part of the arm.
- Tender if touched
- May be unable to move the arm
- Will hold the arm against the chest for comfort

Care for a Humerus Fracture

1. Assess and treat for shock if indicated.
2. Apply an ice pack for 20 minutes.
3. Stabilize the arm by applying one rigid splint on the part of the arm away from the body. Apply an arm sling and swathe (binder).
4. Seek immediate medical care.

Elbow Injuries

▶ Elbow Fractures and Dislocations

All elbow fractures and dislocations should be considered serious and treated with extreme care. Inappropriate care can result in injury to the nearby nerves and blood vessels.

Recognizing Elbow Fractures and Dislocations

- Immediate swelling
- Severe pain
- Possible visible deformity; compare it with the uninjured elbow
- Restricted, painful motion
- Numbness or coldness of the hand and fingers below the elbow

Care for Elbow Fractures and Dislocations

1. Do not move the elbow.
2. Treat for shock.

3. Splint the elbow in the position found to prevent nerve and blood vessel damage:
   - If straight, keep the splinted elbow straight.
   - If bent, keep the elbow bent.
4. Apply an ice pack for 20 minutes.
5. Seek immediate medical care.

▶ Tennis Elbow

Tennis elbow results from sharp, quick twists of the wrist (not just from playing tennis). The muscles that bend the wrist back and straighten the fingers all begin in one spot, no bigger than a dime, on the outside bony prominence (protrusion), of the elbow. Tennis elbow, which is an inflammation of the tendons on this outer side of the elbow, can be very painful whenever the wrist and the elbow are used.

Recognizing Tennis Elbow

- Pain increases while using the arm
- Causes gradual grip weakness
- The injured elbow fatigues quicker than normal
- Very tender on outer protrusion of elbow

Care for Tennis Elbow

1. Apply heat before an activity; the victim might wear a brace or rubber sleeve on the sore elbow.
2. Apply an ice pack for 20 minutes after completion of the activity.
3. Seek medical advice for an appropriate rehabilitation program.

▶ Golfer's Elbow

Repetitive motion produces pain. This injury is the equivalent of the more common tennis elbow but with pain on the inside of the elbow. It is tendinitis affecting the tendons attached to the bony protrusion on the inside of the elbow.

Recognizing Golfer's Elbow

- Pain increases while using the arm
- Causes gradual grip weakness
- The injured elbow fatigues quicker than normal

Care for Golfer's Elbow

1. Apply heat before an activity; the victim might wear a brace or rubber sleeve on the tender elbow.
2. Apply an ice pack for 20 minutes after completion of an activity.
3. Seek medical advice for an appropriate rehabilitation program.

▶ Radius and Ulna Fractures

There are two large bones (radius and ulna) in the forearm, and either or both bones may be broken. When only one bone is broken, the other acts as a splint and there may be little or no deformity. However, a marked deformity may be present in a fracture near the wrist. When both bones are broken, the arm usually appears deformed.

Recognizing Radius and Ulna Fractures

The victim has pain in the forearm or wrist from:
- A direct blow
- Falling on an outstretched hand

AND has
- A visible deformity
- Severe pain radiating up and down from the injury site
- An inability to move the wrist or it is painful while moving the wrist

Care for Radius and Ulna Fractures

1. Assess and treat for shock if indicated.
2. Apply an ice pack to the area for 20 minutes.
3. Apply two rigid splints on both sides of the arm from the tip of the elbow to the fingers. Place the arm in a sling and swathe (binder) with the hand in a thumb-up position.
4. Seek medical care.

▶ Wrist Fracture

The wrist usually is broken when the victim falls with the arm and hand outstretched.

Recognizing a Wrist Fracture

- Injury to the wrist associated with a snapping or popping sensation within the wrist
- Pain in the wrist that is aggravated by movement
- Tenderness
- Swelling
- Unable or unwilling to move the wrist
- Lumplike deformity on the back of the wrist

Care for a Wrist Fracture

1. Use the RICE procedures (with the exception of compression).
2. Stabilize the wrist with a splint.
3. Seek medical care.

Hand Injuries

▶ Crushed Hand

The hand may be fractured by a direct blow or by a crushing injury.

Recognizing a Crushed Hand

- Pain
- Swelling
- Loss of motion
- Open wounds
- Broken bones

Care for a Crushed Hand

1. Control the bleeding.
2. Apply an ice pack for 20 minutes.
3. Seek medical care.

Finger Injuries

The three bones that make up each finger are the most commonly broken bones in the body. Many of the tendons attached to the finger bones can tear with or without a fracture, and the three joints—the *distal interphalangeal,* the *proximal interphalangeal,* and the *metacarpal phalangeal*—can also be injured. A so-called finger sprain may be a complicated fracture or dislocation.

▶ Finger Fracture

Contrary to popular belief, broken bones—especially the fingers—can move when they are broken.

Recognizing Finger Fractures

The finger or thumb has:
- A visible deformity; finger has a twisted look
- Immediate pain and hurts with or without movement
- Numbness
- Swelling
- Pinpointed tenderness that usually indicates a fracture

Test for a finger fracture:
- If possible, straighten the fingers and place them on a hard surface.
- Tap the tip of the injured finger toward the hand. Pain lower down in the finger or into the hand can indicate a fracture.

Care for Finger Fractures

1. Do not try to realign the finger.
2. Gently apply an ice pack.
3. Splint the finger by either:
   - "Buddy" taping the fractured finger to another for support. For a thumb, tape it with three to four figure-eight patterns around the joint. Monitor the finger for swelling and circulation issues.

   OR

   - Keeping the hand and fingers in the position of function (cupping shape as though holding a baseball) with extra padding in the palm. Secure the hand, fingers, and arm to a rigid splint.
4. Seek medical care.

▶ Finger Dislocation

Finger dislocations are common. The same causes of fractured fingers can also cause a dislocated finger.

Recognizing a Finger Dislocation

The finger or thumb has:
- A visible deformity
- Immediate pain
- Swelling

- Shortening of the finger
- May be unable to bend the finger in the injured area; motion is impossible

Care for a Finger Dislocation

1. Do not try to realign the dislocation.
2. Apply an ice pack for 20 minutes.
3. If possible, splint the finger by either:
   - "Buddy" taping the finger for support. For a thumb, tape it with three to four figure-eight patterns around the joint. Monitor the finger for swelling and circulation issues.

   OR

   - Keeping the hand and fingers in the position of function (cupping shape as though holding a baseball) with extra padding in the palm. Secure the hand, fingers, and arm to a rigid splint.
4. Seek medical care.

▶ Sprained Finger

The upper joints of the fingers have a ligament on each side of the joint.

Recognizing a Sprained Finger

The finger or thumb has been:
- "Jammed" or compressed
- Stepped on
- Forced or twisted sideways

AND the victim:
- Has pain and swelling over a joint (especially tenderness on both sides of a joint)
- Is unable to make a fist
- Has a weakness while curling the injured finger alone
- Experiences a weakness or pain when gripping

Care for a Sprained Finger

1. Apply an ice pack for 20 minutes.
2. Reevaluate after the ice pack application and seek medical care if pain and weakness exist.
3. Tape fingers with "buddy" taping for support. Tape thumb with three to four figure-eight patterns around joint.

▶ Nail Avulsion

A victim may have had a blow to the nail, the nail may have been torn away by a piece of machinery, or a long toenail may have caught on a loop of carpet or other fixed object. An injury in which a nail is partly or completely torn loose is known as a *nail avulsion.*

Recognizing a Nail Avulsion

- The nail may be completely detached or partially held in place by the skin.

Care for a Nail Avulsion

1. Secure the damaged nail in place with an adhesive bandage.
2. If part or all of the nail has been completely torn away, apply antibiotic ointment. Secure a partly torn loose nail with an adhesive bandage. Do not trim away the loose nail. Consult a physician for further advice.

▶ Splinters

Sharp splinters (usually wooden) can be impaled into the skin or under a fingernail or toenail.

Recognizing Splinters

- There is a small puncture wound. The sliver may be seen, or in other cases, neither seen nor felt.

Care for Splinters

1. If embedded in the skin, use tweezers to remove it. In some cases, you may need to tease it out with a sterile needle until the end can be grasped with tweezers or fingers. Clean the wound with soap and water.
2. If the splinter is impaled under a fingernail or toenail and breaks off flush, cut a V-shaped notch in the nail to gain access to the splinter. Remove the embedded splinter by grasping its end with tweezers.

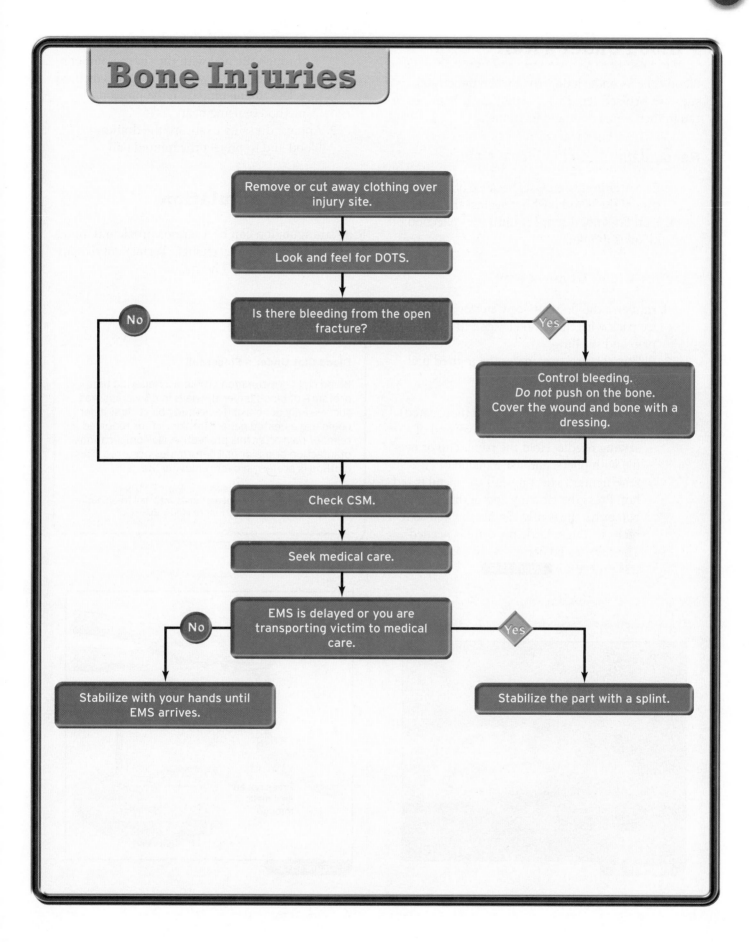

▶ Blood Under a Nail

Blood collects under a fingernail when underlying tissues are bruised (eg, finger struck by a hammer or caught between a door and its frame).

Recognizing Blood Under a Nail

- Excruciating pain exists because of the pressure of the blood pushing against the nail.
- Pain does not disappear until the collection of blood is drained.

Care for Blood Under a Nail

1. Immerse the finger in ice water or apply an ice pack with the hand elevated to reduce pain and swelling.
2. Relieve the pressure under the injured nail by using one of the following methods :
   - Straighten the end of a metal (noncoated) paper clip or use the blunt (eye) end of a sewing needle. Hold the paper clip or needle with pliers, and use a match or cigarette lighter to heat it until the metal is red hot. Press the glowing end of the paper clip or needle gently against the nail so it melts through. Little pressure is needed. The nail has no nerves, so this is a painless procedure **Figure 15-3**.

   - By using a rotary action, carefully drill through the nail with the sharp point of a small knife or sewing needle. This method is less threatening than the previous method of using heat.
3. Apply a dressing to absorb the draining blood and to protect the injured nail.

▶ Ring Strangulation

Ring strangulation can be a serious problem if it cuts off the blood supply long enough. Permanent damage may result within 4 or 5 hours.

FYI

Blood Clot Under a Fingernail

Blood clots are common problems. Relieving the pressure of blood under the nails in 45 victims was successfully done using a heated object (first aiders could use a heated paperclip). All victims reported relief of pain after this procedure. No complications of infection or major nail deformities occurred. This method is preferred over removing the nail.

Source: Seaberg D C, Angelos W J, Paris P M. 1991. Treatment of subungual hematomas with nail trephination: a prospective study. *Am J Emerg Med* 9:209-210.

Figure 15-2

Relieve pain by releasing the blood under a nail.

Figure 15-3

Making a hole in a fingernail.

Red-hot, noncoated metal paper clip

Press hot end so it melts through

Recognizing Ring Strangulation

- The ring has become tight on the finger after an injury or after some other cause of swelling, such as a local reaction to a bee sting.

Care for Ring Strangulation

Try one or more of the following methods to remove a ring:

- Lubricate the finger with soap and water, grease, oil, butter, petroleum jelly, or some other slippery substance, and then try to remove the ring.
- Immerse the finger in cold water or apply an ice pack for several minutes to reduce the swelling.
- Liberally spray window or glass cleaner onto the finger, and then try to slide off the ring.
- Massage the finger from the tip toward the hand to move the swelling; lubricate the finger again and try removing the ring.
- Smoothly wind thread around the finger, starting about an inch from the ring edge and going toward the ring, keeping each round of thread touching the next. Wind smoothly and tightly right up to the edge of the ring. This action will push the swelling toward the hand. Slip the end of the thread under the ring with a matchstick or toothpick, then slowly unwind the thread on the hand side of the ring. You should be able to twist the ring gently over the thread and off the finger.
- Lubricate the finger well, then pass a rubber band under the ring. Hold both ends of the rubber band and, while maintaining tension on the rubber band toward the end of the finger, pull the rubber band around and around the finger.
- If you do not have access to timely medical care, consider cutting the narrowest part of the ring with a ring saw, jeweler's saw, ring cutter, or fine hacksaw blade. Be sure to protect the exposed portions of the finger.
- Inflate an ordinary balloon (preferably a slender, tube-shaped one) about three fourths full. Tie the end. Insert the victim's swollen finger into the end of the balloon until the balloon evenly surrounds the entire finger. In about 15 minutes, the air pressure in the balloon should return the finger to its normal size and the ring can be removed.

FYI

Ring Removal From an Extremely Swollen Finger

Rings on swollen fingers are not uncommon, but they must be removed or serious problems can result. Generally, the removal method is simply to cut the ring off the finger or to use one of several nondestructive removal methods using string or a rubber band. A simple method that eliminates the swelling and permits the removal of a ring involves wrapping the entire finger starting at the nail and wrapping toward the ring with a tight, elastic band, which reduces the swelling and frees the ring.

Source: Cresap CR. 1995. Removal of a hardened steel ring from an extremely swollen finger. *Am J Emerg Med* 13(3):318-320.

Hip Joint Injuries

▶ Hip Dislocation

A hip can be dislocated by a fall, a blow to the thigh, or direct force to the foot or knee. The hip joint is a stable ball-and-socket joint that requires great force to dislocate. Often a hip is dislocated when the knee strikes the dashboard during a motor vehicle crash. It is difficult to differentiate a hip dislocation from a hip fracture.

Recognizing a Hip Dislocation

- Severe pain at the injury site
- Swelling at the injury site
- Hip is flexed and the knee bent and rotated inward toward the opposite hip
- Injury usually quite visible

Care for a Hip Dislocation

1. Assess and treat for shock if indicated.
2. Stabilize the injury.
3. Check for an ankle pulse (posterior tibial).
4. Seek medical care. This injury is best transported by EMS personnel.

▶ Hip Fracture

A *hip fracture* is a fracture of the upper end of the femur (thighbone), not the pelvis. A fractured hip usually is caused by a fall. Elderly people, especially women, are susceptible to this type of injury because of brittle bones (*osteoporosis*). Often, the bone actually fractures while the victim is walking, resulting in a fall (rather than the fall causing the fracture).

Recognizing a Hip Fracture

- Severe pain in the groin area
- Inability to lift the injured leg
- Leg may appear shortened and be rotated with the toes pointing abnormally outward or inward

Care for a Hip Fracture

1. Treat for shock.
2. Stabilize the injured leg against movement.
3. Monitor the ankle pulse (posterior tibial).
4. Seek immediate medical care. This injury is best transported by EMS personnel.

Thigh Injuries

▶ Femur Fracture

Because the femur (thighbone) is the largest bone in the body, considerable force is required to break it. Femur injuries can occur in any part of the femur, from the hip to just above the knee joint. A fracture of the femur usually is caused by a fall or a direct blow.

Femur fractures often include open wounds and external bleeding may be severe. If the blood vessels are damaged, the victim may lose 1 or 2 quarts of blood into the thigh. There may be loss of blood circulation to the lower part of the extremity or nerve damage, especially with lower third femur fractures.

Recognizing a Femur Fracture

- Severe pain at the injury site
- Deformity may occur; the leg may appear shorter
- Swelling comes from severe damage to blood vessels
- Victim may report having heard or felt a severe pop or snap at the time of injury

Care for a Femur Fracture

1. Assess and treat for shock if indicated.
2. Cover a wound with a sterile dressing.

3. Stabilize the injured leg against movement.
4. Monitor the ankle pulse (posterior tibial).
5. Seek immediate medical care. This injury is best transported by EMS personnel.

▶ Muscle Contusion

The muscle group on the front of the thigh is the *quadriceps group* and often gets bruised. Depending on the force of impact and the muscles involved, the contusion may be of varying degrees of severity.

Recognizing a Muscle Contusion

The victim received a direct hit producing:
- Swelling
- Pain and tenderness
- Tightness or firmness of the site when pressed
- Visible bruise that may appear hours later

Care for a Muscle Contusion

1. Follow the RICE procedures. Apply an ice pack for 20 minutes, three to four times daily for the next 48 hours.
2. Stretch the muscle by bending the knee toward the victim's chest.

FYI

Thigh Muscle Injuries: Strain or Contusion?

Athletes often injure the large quadriceps muscles of their thighs. According to one report, strains (pulling of the muscle, which causes tears) should be treated first with ice, compression, elevation of the limb, nonsteroidal anti-inflammatory drugs, and use of crutches. After several days, the athlete can start gentle stretching and knee extension but should avoid straight-leg raises. For thigh contusions (direct blow, causing bruising), the knee should be immediately flexed and immobilized in that position for 24 hours. Ice should be applied for the first half hour and intermittently thereafter to slow bleeding and prevent swelling.

Source: Kaeding C C, et al. 1995. Quadriceps strains and contusions. *Phys Sportsmed* 23(1):59.

FYI

Charley Horse

The term *charley horse* came about in the 1880s among baseball players. At that time, the outfield grass of some major league ballparks was mowed by horses pulling lawn mowers. At Ebbet's Field in New York, the horse that did this chore—Charley—had a continual limp. When a baseball player was hit in the leg with a ball or received a blow to his leg muscle that caused him to limp, he was said to be walking like Charley. The muscle blow and the contusion that caused the pain and limping were referred to as a *charley horse*. The term remains popular in the United States.

▶ Muscle Strain

When a muscle is overstretched, it can result in a tear, called a *strain*. Different degrees of strains occur, but first aiders will be unable to determine their degree.

Recognizing a Muscle Strain

While running or jumping, the victim:
- Feels a pop or pulling sensation

And later has:
- Tenderness
- Stiffness and pain during movement
- Swelling
- A visible bruise appearing days later

Care for a Muscle Strain

1. Follow the RICE procedures. Apply an ice pack for 20 minutes, three to four times daily for the next 48 hours.
2. Stretch the muscle but do not force stretching.

Knee Injuries

Knee injuries, of which there are many types, are among the most serious joint injuries. Their severity is difficult to determine, thus medical care is necessary if the injury is from being hit or twisted and not from overuse. You probably have seen a physician or an athletic trainer performing stress tests on a player's knee on the sidelines at a football game. Controversy exists about the exact meaning and interpretation of many of the ligament stress tests. First aiders should not perform such tests.

▶ Knee Fracture

A fracture of the knee generally occurs as a result of a fall or a direct blow.

Recognizing a Knee Fracture

Fractures about the knee may occur at the end of the femur, at the end of the tibia, or in the *patella* (knee-cap). Determining whether a fracture exists is difficult. Some fractured knees may look like a dislocation. Other signs include:
- Deformity
- Tenderness
- Swelling

Care for a Knee Fracture

1. If a pulse can be felt in the ankle (posterior tibial) with no deformity, splint the leg with the knee straight.
2. If a pulse can be felt in the ankle with significant deformity, splint the knee in the position found.
3. Seek medical care. However, if a pulse is absent in the ankle, immediately seek medical care.

▶ Knee Dislocation

A knee dislocation is a serious injury. Deformity will be grotesque.

Recognizing a Knee Dislocation

- Excruciating pain
- Deformity
- Pulse may be absent in the ankle (posterior tibial)
- Do not confuse a knee dislocation with a patella dislocation; a knee dislocation is a much more serious injury

Care for a Knee Dislocation

1. Stabilize the knee in the position found.
2. Seek medical care immediately.

▶ Patella Dislocation

A dislocated patella (kneecap) can be a very painful injury and must be treated immediately. Some people have repeated kneecap dislocations, just as others have a tendency for shoulder dislocations. A dislocated patella most commonly occurs in teenagers and young adults who are engaged in athletic activities.

Recognizing a Patella Dislocation

A blow or twisting causes the kneecap to be moved to the outside of the knee joint and there is:
- Possible swelling
- An inability to bend or straighten the knee
- Pain
- Deformity; compare it with the other kneecap

Care for a Patella Dislocation

1. Follow the RICE procedures (except compression).
2. Do not try to relocate a dislocated kneecap (sometimes the kneecap replaces itself).
3. Splint the knee in the position found.
4. Seek medical care.

▶ Knee Sprain

Ligament injuries occur most often in sports. The knee is very prone to ligament injury, ranging from mild sprains to complete tearing. The knee will be swollen and painful and usually cannot be used normally.

Recognizing a Knee Sprain

At the time of injury, the victim has:
- Severe pain
- The feeling of a pop or snap
- A locking sensation

OR the victim:
- May not be able to walk without limping
- May not be able to bend or straighten the knee

Later, there may be:
- Swelling in the knee
- Bruising

Care for a Knee Sprain

1. Follow the RICE procedures.
2. Seek medical care.

▶ Knee Contusion

Contusions of the knee are caused by a direct blow or by falling on the knee.

Recognizing a Knee Contusion

After a direct blow to the kneecap, the victim has:
- Pain
- Swelling
- Tenderness
- Bruise marks (black-and-blue discoloration)

Care for a Knee Contusion

Follow the RICE procedures.

Lower Leg Injuries

▶ Tibia and Fibula Fractures

Tibia and fibula injuries can occur at any place between the knee joint and the ankle joint. When both bones are broken, there may be marked deformity of the leg. When only one bone is broken, the other acts as a splint, and little deformity may be present. Some victims with a fibula fracture can walk on the injured leg. When the tibia (shin bone) is broken, an open fracture and severe deformity are likely to exist. Injuries to the blood vessels, caused by the extreme deformity, are common with injuries of the tibia and the fibula, and the pain usually is severe.

Recognizing Tibia and Fibula Fractures

A direct blow or twisting forces produce:
- Severe pain
- Swelling
- Visible deformity
- Tenderness when touched

Muscle Injuries

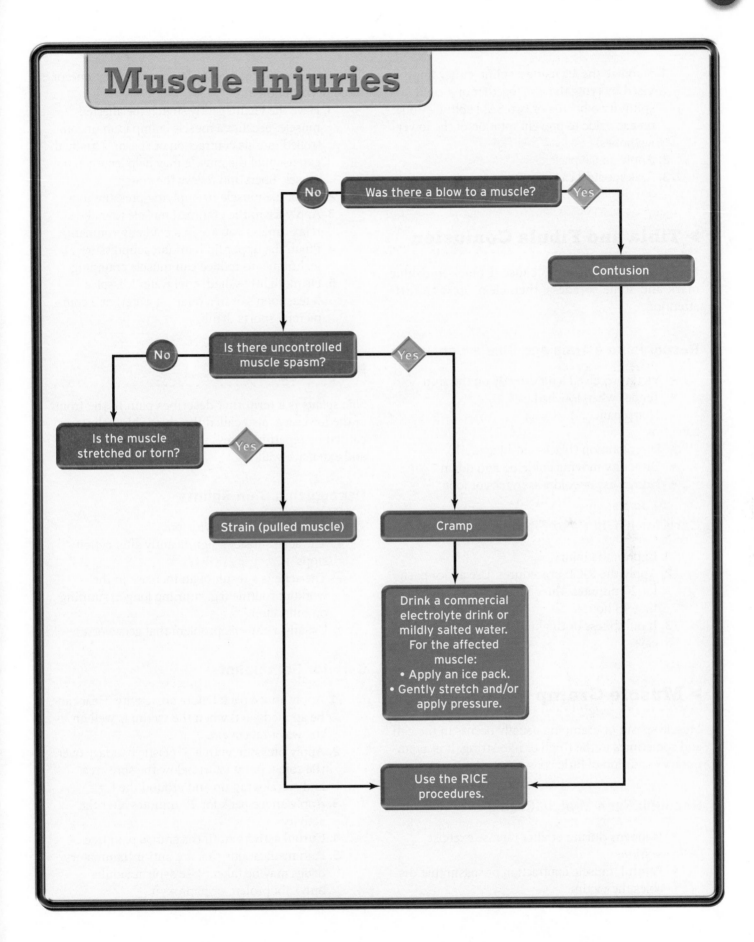

Was there a blow to a muscle?

No → Is there uncontrolled muscle spasm?

Yes → Contusion

No → Is the muscle stretched or torn?

Yes → Cramp

Yes → Strain (pulled muscle)

Cramp → Drink a commercial electrolyte drink or mildly salted water. For the affected muscle:
• Apply an ice pack.
• Gently stretch and/or apply pressure.

Contusion → Use the RICE procedures.

Strain (pulled muscle) → Use the RICE procedures.

Care for Tibia and Fibula Fractures

1. Stabilize the leg using a splint, either improvised by tying the legs together or a rigid splint (two boards or two SAM splints—one on each side to prevent rotation of the lower leg bones).
2. Apply an ice pack.
3. Seek medical care.

▶ Tibia and Fibula Contusion

Many contusions simply cause a black-and-blue mark and some soreness, then clear up with little attention.

Recognizing a Tibia and Fibula Contusion

- Victim received a hit directly on the shin
- Tender when touched
- Sharp pain

Later has:

- Discoloration (black-and-blue mark)
- Difficulty moving ankle up and down
- Numbness or coldness in toes or foot

Care for a Tibia and Fibula Contusion

1. Expose the injury.
2. Apply the RICE procedures. Use an ice pack for 20 minutes, three to four times daily, for first 48 hours.
3. If numbness or tingling exists, seek medical care.

▶ Muscle Cramp

Muscle spasm or cramping usually occurs in the calf and sometimes in the thigh or hamstring. It is a temporary condition of little consequence.

Recognizing a Muscle Cramp

- Happens during or after intense exercise sessions
- Painful, muscle contraction or spasm that disables the victim

Care for a Muscle Cramp

There are many treatments for cramps. Try one or more of the following:

1. Have the victim gently stretch the affected muscle. Because a muscle cramp is an uncontrolled muscle contraction or spasm, a gradual extension of the muscle may help lengthen the muscle fibers and relieve the cramp.
2. Relax the muscle by applying pressure to it.
3. Apply ice to the cramped muscle to make it relax (unless you are in a cold environment).
4. Pinch the upper lip hard (an acupressure technique) to reduce calf muscle cramping.
5. Drink lightly salted, cool water (dissolve ¼ teaspoon salt in a quart of water) or a commercial sports drink.

▶ Shin Splints

Shin splints is a term that describes pain in the front of the lower leg, also called the shin. Shin splints are caused by repetitive stress in the leg such as running and extensive walking.

Recognizing Shin Splints

The shin aches during activity, but:

- The ache subsides significantly after activity stops
- The ache is a result of an increase in the workout routine (eg, running longer, running on hills, etc.)
- Usually a chronic problem that gets worse

Care for Shin Splints

1. Apply an ice pack before an activity. Heat can be applied later, when the victim is well on the way to recovery.
2. Apply pressure with a 3″ elastic bandage over the sorest point (start below the sore area and spiral wrap up and around the leg).
3. Apply an ice pack for 20 minutes after the activity.
4. Curtail activity until the shin is pain free.
5. Pain medications that are anti-inflammatory drugs may be taken: Use aspirin (adults only), ibuprofen, or naproxyn.

▶ Ankle and Foot Injuries

The ankle and the foot frequently are injured, mainly by twisting, which stretches or tears the supporting ligaments. Incorrect treatment can have consequences that include lifelong disability. In some cases, the damage requires surgical correction. Most ankle injuries are sprains; about 85% of sprains involve the outside (lateral) ligaments and are caused by the ankle having turned or twisted inward **Figure 15-4**.

Recognizing Foot and Ankle Injuries

It is difficult to tell the difference between a severely sprained ankle and a fractured ankle. A useful two-part test can help determine whether an X-ray of the ankle or midfoot is needed:

1. Press along the bones. Pain and tenderness over the back edge or the tip of either of the ankle knob bones (malleolus bones) or the midfoot's outside bone (fifth metatarsal) or inside bone (navicular) may indicate a broken bone.
2. Ask the victim, "Have you tried standing on it?" Putting some weight on the foot may hurt a little, but if the victim is able to do that and take four or more steps, most likely the ankle or foot is sprained. If it is broken, the victim will not want to put any weight on it and will not be able to take more than four steps.
3. A few additional signs and symptoms may help determine whether an injured ankle or foot is sprained or fractured. These indicators are not hard-and-fast rules but useful guidelines to help you treat foot and ankle injuries.
   - If the victim hops on the good foot and the injured ankle cannot tolerate the jarring, suspect a fracture.
   - Foot injuries usually lead to substantial swelling. It has been observed that ankle sprains tend to swell on only one side of the foot (usually the lateral or outer side), whereas swelling on both sides of the foot usually accompanies fractures.

Care for Foot and Ankle Injuries

Controversy exists about whether to remove a shoe from an injured foot. Those who favor leaving the shoe on believe it acts as a splint and helps retard swelling. However, taking off the shoe allows for a better examination, better checking of the CSM, and better care. A shoe that is left on often does not cover and, thus, cannot compress the injured area that is swelling. If a shoe acts as a compression device, it could also reduce blood circulation in the foot as the swelling increases. In addition, footwear left in place will thwart efforts to apply an ice pack and an elastic bandage. Use the RICE procedures to limit swelling.

Aftercare of an Ankle Injury

1. First 24 to 48 hours: Use the RICE treatment.
2. Within 3 to 7 days: Use a contrast bath if swelling persists. Submerge the ankle for 1 minute in cold water (45° F to 60° F) and then for 4 minutes in warm water (100° F to 105° F). Continue to alternate cold and warm submersions for 15 minutes. Gently move the foot up and down for mobility. This should be done once or twice a day for 1 to 2 weeks.
3. Once the initial swelling has decreased, discontinue immobilization and start range-of-motion exercises, even if the injured ankle cannot bear weight. Joint motion decreases swelling and stiffness and prevents fluid accumulation.

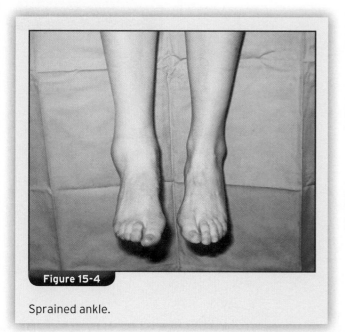

Figure 15-4

Sprained ankle.

Sprains, Strains, Contusions, Dislocations

Ankle Injuries

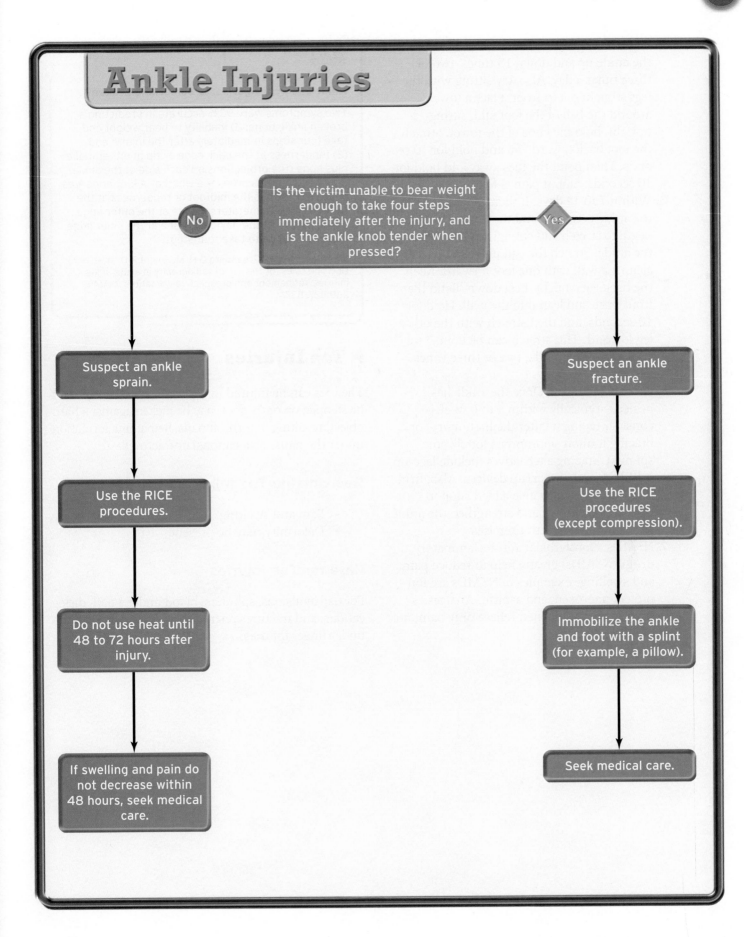

Is the victim unable to bear weight enough to take four steps immediately after the injury, and is the ankle knob tender when pressed?

No

Suspect an ankle sprain.

Use the RICE procedures.

Do not use heat until 48 to 72 hours after injury.

If swelling and pain do not decrease within 48 hours, seek medical care.

Yes

Suspect an ankle fracture.

Use the RICE procedures (except compression).

Immobilize the ankle and foot with a splint (for example, a pillow).

Seek medical care.

4. Begin with gentle exercises such as bending the ankle up and down 15 times, two or three times a day. Also, try sitting with the legs straight out in front. Place a towel around the ball of the foot and, sitting upright, hold the ends of the towel. Stretch the foot back toward you and hold for 10 seconds. Then point the toes away and hold for 10 seconds. Stop if pain is felt.

5. Within 7 to 14 days: If there is no pain when the ankle is rotated and there is no swelling, begin to stretch and strengthen the calf and the ankle. Stretch the calf muscles by leaning against a wall with one foot forward. Keep the back leg straight, heel down. Bend the front knee and lean into the wall. Hold for 10 seconds, and then stretch with the other leg forward. This stretch can be done 5 to 10 times on each side, two or three times a day.

6. Avoiding reinjury: Once the ankle has healed—typically within 4 to 6 weeks—consider taping it (after the first injury) or bracing it (more appropriate for chronic sprains). Bracing alternatives include lace-up, gel-filled, and air-stirrup devices. Also, firm high-top shoes may give added support. Continue to stretch and strengthen the ankle and calf muscles with exercises.

7. NSAIDs: Nonsteroidal anti-inflammatory drugs (NSAIDs) greatly help to reduce pain and swelling. Examples of NSAIDs are ibuprofen, naproxen, and aspirin. Analgesics such as acetaminophen relieve only pain, not swelling.

FYI

Ankle and Foot Injuries: Is Something Broken?

Two symptoms were 93% accurate in predicting a broken ankle bone: (1) inability to bear weight and take four steps immediately after the injury; and (2) tenderness at the back edge or tip of either malleolus bone (the projections on each side of the ankle). Similar symptoms predicted whether a foot bone was broken: (1) pain in the midfoot or tenderness at the base of the fifth metatarsal bone at the outer edge of the foot or at the navicular bone at the inner edge, plus (2) inability to take four steps.

Sources: Stiell I G, Greenberg G H, McKnight R D, et al. 1993. Decision rules for the use of radiography in acute ankle injuries: refinement and prospective validation; *JAMA* 269:1127-1132.

▶ Toe Injuries

The toes can be injured in various ways. The toes can be stepped on or the foot may be kicked against a hard object, resulting in torn-off nails, hematoma formation under the nails, dislocations, or fractures.

Recognizing Toe Injuries

- Pain and swelling
- Deformity may be present

Care for Toe Injuries

For nail avulsions, splinters, blood under a nail, dislocations, and fractures refer to the appropriate sections under finger injuries.

prep kit

▶ Ready for Review

- Injuries to the extremities are common.
- There are many types of injuries to the extremities, ranging from simple contusions to complex open fractures.
- RICE is the acronym for Rest, Ice, Compression, and Elevation.
- Shoulder injuries include:
  - Shoulder dislocation
  - Clavicle fracture
  - Contusion
  - Tendinitis
- Elbow injuries include:
  - Elbow fracture and dislocation
  - Tennis elbow
  - Golfer's elbow
- Hand injuries include:
  - Crushed hand
- Finger injuries include:
  - Finger fracture
  - Finger dislocation
  - Sprained finger
  - Nail avulsion
  - Splinters
  - Blood under a nail
  - Ring strangulation
- Hip joint injuries include:
  - Hip dislocation
  - Hip fracture
- Thigh injuries include:
  - Femur fracture
  - Muscle contusion
  - Muscle strain
- Knee injuries include:
  - Knee fracture
  - Knee dislocation
  - Patella dislocation
  - Knee sprain
  - Knee contusion
- Lower leg injuries include:
  - Tibia and fibula fracture
  - Tibia and fibula contusion
  - Muscle cramp
  - Shin splints
  - Ankle and foot injuries
  - Toe injuries

▶ Vital Vocabulary

contusion A bruise; an injury that causes a hemorrhage in or beneath the skin but does not break the skin.

dislocations Bones are displaced from their normal joint alignment, out of their sockets, or out of their normal positions.

fracture A break or crack in the bone.

sprain A trauma to the joint that injures the ligaments.

strain An injury to a muscle caused by a violent contraction or an excessive, forcible stretching.

tendinitis Inflammation of a tendon caused by overuse.

▶ Assessment in Action

During a flag football game at a neighborhood park, your teammate is going back for a sure interception. He jumps for the ball, catches it, and comes down, twisting his ankle in a small hole on the field. Your teammate is in pain and is feeling nauseous.

Directions: Circle Yes if you agree with the statement; circle No if you disagree.

Yes   No   **1.** It is difficult to distinguish between a severely sprained ankle and a fractured ankle.

Yes   No   **2.** If the victim cannot walk at least four steps and reports tenderness when you press on the ankle knob bone (malleous), suspect a fractured ankle.

Yes   No   **3.** Heat should be applied immediately to a sprained ankle to increase blood flow and decrease pain.

Yes   No   **4.** Swelling on both sides of the ankle usually indicates a sprained ankle.

prep kit

▶ Check Your Knowledge

Directions: Circle Yes if you agree with the statement; circle No if you disagree.

Yes No **1.** Injuries heal faster if rested.

Yes No **2.** Compression increases internal bleeding, helping the injury to heal faster.

Yes No **3.** Tennis elbow results from sharp, quick twists of the wrist.

Yes No **4.** The three bones in the fingers are very strong and do not break easily.

Yes No **5.** The hip joint is easily dislocated.

Yes No **6.** Considerable force is required to break the femur.

Yes No **7.** A strain is actually a tear in the muscle.

Yes No **8.** Knee injuries are not serious.

Yes No **9.** Shin splints are a pain that runs down the back of the leg.

Yes No **10.** Most ankle injuries are not fractures.

16

Splinting Extremities

Splinting Extremities

Injured extremities should be stabilized by splinting the extremity in the position in which it was found. To stabilize means to minimize further injury by holding a body part to prevent movement. All fractures should be stabilized before a victim is moved. The reasons for splinting to stabilize an injured area are to:

- Reduce pain.
- Prevent damage to muscles, nerves, and blood vessels.
- Prevent a closed fracture from becoming an open fracture.
- Reduce bleeding and swelling.

All fractures are complicated to some degree by damage to the soft tissue and structures surrounding the bone. The major cause of tissue damage at a fracture site is movement by the end of the broken bone. The end of a broken bone is sharp, and it is important to prevent a fractured bone from moving into soft tissues.

▶ Types of Splints

A **splint** is any device used to stabilize a fracture or a dislocation. Such a device can be improvised (for example, a folded newspaper), or it can be one of several commercially available splints (for example, SAM splint). Lack of a commercial splint should never prevent you from properly stabilizing an injured extremity. Splinting sometimes requires improvisation.

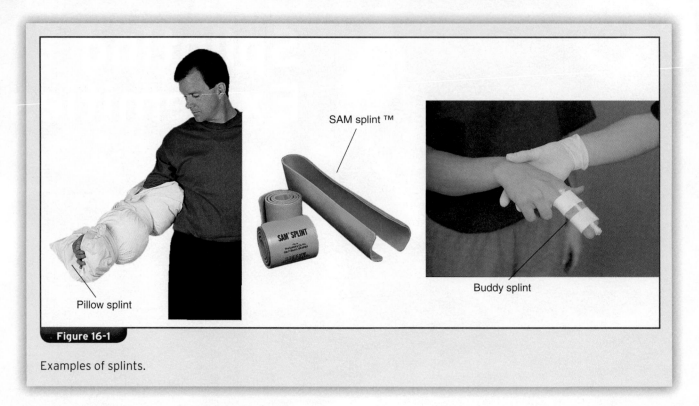

SAM splint ™

Pillow splint

Buddy splint

Figure 16-1

Examples of splints.

A rigid splint is an inflexible device attached to an extremity to maintain stability. It can be a padded board, a piece of heavy cardboard, or a SAM splint molded to fit the extremity. Whatever its construction, a rigid splint must be long enough to be secured well above and below the fracture site. A soft splint, such as a pillow, is useful mainly for stabilizing fractures of the lower leg or the forearm **Figure 16-1**.

A self-splint, or anatomic splint, is almost always available because it uses the body itself as the splint. A self-splint is one in which the injured extremity is tied to an uninjured part (for example, an injured finger to the adjacent finger, the legs together, or an injured arm to the chest).

▶ Splinting Guidelines

All fractures and dislocations should be stabilized before the victim is moved. When in doubt, apply a splint. To apply a splint:

1. Cover any open wounds with a sterile dressing before applying a splint.
2. Check the CSM in the extremity. If pulses are absent and medical help is hours away, gently line up a fracture or a dislocation to restore blood flow. Support the limb and move gently to line up the parts. Joints may be left in a position of comfort. Line up the limb above and below the joint, do not force anything into position. Any movement of a fracture is expected to cause pain; you should be aware of this and warn the victim. You do not have to align the limb perfectly, just align it enough to allow the return of circulation.
3. Determine what to splint by using the rule of thirds. Imagine each long bone as being divided into thirds. If the injury is located in the upper or lower third of a bone, assume that the nearest joint is injured. Therefore, the splint should extend to stabilize the bones above and below the unstable joint. For example, for a fracture of the upper third of the tibia (shinbone), the splint must extend above the knee to include the upper leg, as well as the lower leg, because the knee is unstable. For a fracture of the middle third of a bone, stabilize the joints above and below the fracture (for example, the wrist and elbow for a fractured radius or ulna; the shoulder and elbow for a fractured humerus; the knee and ankle for a fractured tibia or fibula). In addition to splinting an upper extremity fracture, place the injured arm in an arm sling and a swathe (binder).

4. If two first aiders are present, one should support the injury site and minimize movement of the extremity until splinting is completed.

5. When possible, place splint materials on both sides of the injured part, especially when two bones are involved, such as the radius and ulna in the lower arm or the tibia and fibula in the lower leg. This sandwich splint prevents the injured extremity from rotating and keeps the two bones from touching. With rigid splints, use extra padding in natural body hollows and around any deformities.

6. Apply splints firmly but not so tightly that blood flow into an extremity is affected. Check the CSM before and periodically after the splint is applied. If the pulse disappears, loosen the splint enough so you can feel the pulse. Leave the fingers or toes exposed so the CSM can be checked easily.

7. Use RICE (rest, ice, compression, and elevation) on the injured part. When practical, elevate the injured extremity after it is stabilized to promote drainage and reduce swelling. Do not, however, apply ice packs if a pulse is absent.

If the victim has a possible spinal injury and an extremity injury, the spinal injury takes precedence. Splinting the spine is always a problem. Tell the victim not to move. Then stabilize the spine with rolled blankets or similar objects placed on each side of the neck and torso. In most cases, it is best to wait until EMS personnel arrive with proper equipment to handle spinal injuries.

Most fractures do not require rapid transportation. An exception is an arm or a leg without a pulse, which means there is insufficient blood flow to the injured extremity. In that case, immediate medical care is necessary.

Seek medical care for the following injuries or situations:

- Any open fracture
- Any dislocation (injury that causes joint deformity)
- Any joint injury with moderate to severe swelling
- Any injury in which there is deformity, tenderness, or swelling over the bone
- If the victim is unable to walk or bear weight after a lower extremity injury

CAUTION

DO NOT straighten dislocations or fractures of the spine, elbow, wrist, hip, or knee because of the proximity of major nerves and arteries. Instead, if the CSM assessment findings are normal, splint joint injuries in the position in which you find them.

DO NOT apply traction on open fractures. Instead, cover the wound with a sterile dressing and apply a splint.

- If a snap, crackle, or pop was heard at the time of injury
- If the injured area, especially a joint, becomes hot, tender, swollen, or painful
- If you are unsure whether a bone was broken
- If the injury does not improve rapidly, especially over the first few days

▶ Slings

An open triangular bandage can be used as a **sling**. A folded triangular bandage known as a cravat can be used as a **swathe** (binder) in conjunction with a sling. A cravat may also be applied using the same procedures as an open triangular sling but placed around the wrist when long splints on an upper arm or forearm may be in the way. To apply an arm sling to the upper arm, forearm, or hand/wrist injuries, follow the steps in **Skill Drill 16-1**:

Hold the victim's arm slightly away from the chest, with the wrist and hand slightly higher (about 4″) than the tip of the elbow. Place a triangular bandage between the forearm and chest with the point of the triangular bandage toward the elbow and stretch the bandage well beyond the elbow. Pull the upper end of the bandage over the uninjured shoulder (**Step ❶**).

8. Bring the lower end of the bandage over the forearm (**Step ❷**).

9. Bring the end of the bandage around the neck to the uninjured side and tie to the other end at the hollow above the clavicle on the uninjured side. If possible, secure the point of the bandage at the elbow with a safety pin or twist it into a pigtail, which can be tied into a knot or tucked inside the sling (**Step ❸**).

skill drill

16-1   Arm Sling for Arm Injury

1 Place the bandage between the forearm and chest with the point of the bandage toward the elbow and stretch beyond the elbow. Pull the upper end of the bandage over the uninjured shoulder.

2 Bring the lower end of the bandage over the forearm.

3 Bring the end of the bandage around the neck to the uninjured side and tie to the other end at the hollow above the clavicle on the uninjured side.

4 Place a swathe around the upper arm and body. The center of the swathe should be placed over the arm. The hand should be in thumb-up position within the sling and slightly above the level of the elbow.

Place a swathe (binder) around the upper arm and body. The center of the swathe (binder) should be placed over the arm. The hand should be in thumb-up position within the sling and slightly above the level of the elbow (about 4″). Place padding underneath both knots for comfort. Adjust the sling to support the hand and wrist; only the fingers should be exposed (**Step ④**).

To apply a sling for clavicle or shoulder injuries, follow the steps in **Skill Drill 16-2**:

1. Hold arm slightly away from the chest, with the wrist and hand slightly higher (about 4″) than the tip of the elbow. Place a triangular bandage between the forearm and chest with its point toward the elbow and stretching well beyond it. Pull the upper end over the shoulder on the uninjured side. Bring the other end of the bandage over the forearm and tuck it under the armpit (between the arm and body) on the injured side (**Step ①**).

2. Continue bringing the lower end of the bandage around the victim's back where it is tied to the upper end of the bandage (**Step ②**).

3. Place a swathe (binder) around the chest and forearm rather than the upper arm (**Step ③**). The center of the swathe (binder) should be placed over the forearm. The hand should be in a thumb-up position within the sling and slightly above the level of the elbow (about 4″) (**Step ④**).

If bandages or other resources are unavailable, you may need to improvise a sling **Figure 16-2**.

- Place the hand inside a buttoned jacket.
- Use a belt, necktie, or other clothing item looped around the neck and the injured arm.
- Pin the sleeve of the shirt or jacket to the clothing in the desired position.
- Turn up the lower edge of the victim's jacket or shirt over the injured arm and pin it to the upper part of the jacket or shirt.

▶ Splinting Specific Areas

Shoulder

Shoulder injuries involve the clavicle (collarbone), the scapula (shoulder blade), or the head of the humerus (upper arm). To stabilize the shoulder and upper arm against movement with a shoulder sling, follow these steps:

1. Support the injured arm slightly away from the chest, with the wrist and hand higher than the elbow.

2. Place an open triangular bandage between the forearm and the chest, with the point stretching well beyond the elbow.

3. Pull the upper end of the bandage over the shoulder on the uninjured side.

4. Bring the lower end of the bandage over the forearm, under the armpit on the injured side, and around the victim's back.

5. Tie the upper and lower ends of the triangular bandage.

6. Check the pulse and fingernail color for signs of circulation loss.

7. The hand should be in a thumb-up position in the sling and slightly above the level of the elbow **Figure 16-3**.

To further stabilize the arm, fold another triangular bandage to make a swathe that measures 3″ to 4″ wide. Tie one or two swathes (binders) around the upper arm and chest of the victim. This stabilizes the clavicle (collarbone) and most shoulder injuries, as well as upper humerus (upper arm) fractures.

Most shoulder dislocations (about 95%) are anterior, meaning that the top of the humerus pops out in front of the shoulder joint. The victim will hold the arm in a fixed position away from the chest wall. In these cases, the most comfortable splinting method is to place a pillow or rolled blanket between the involved arm and the chest. This fills the space created; you can then use cravats or a roller bandage to secure the arm against the chest. If the injury

skill drill

16-2   Sling for Clavicle or Shoulder Injury

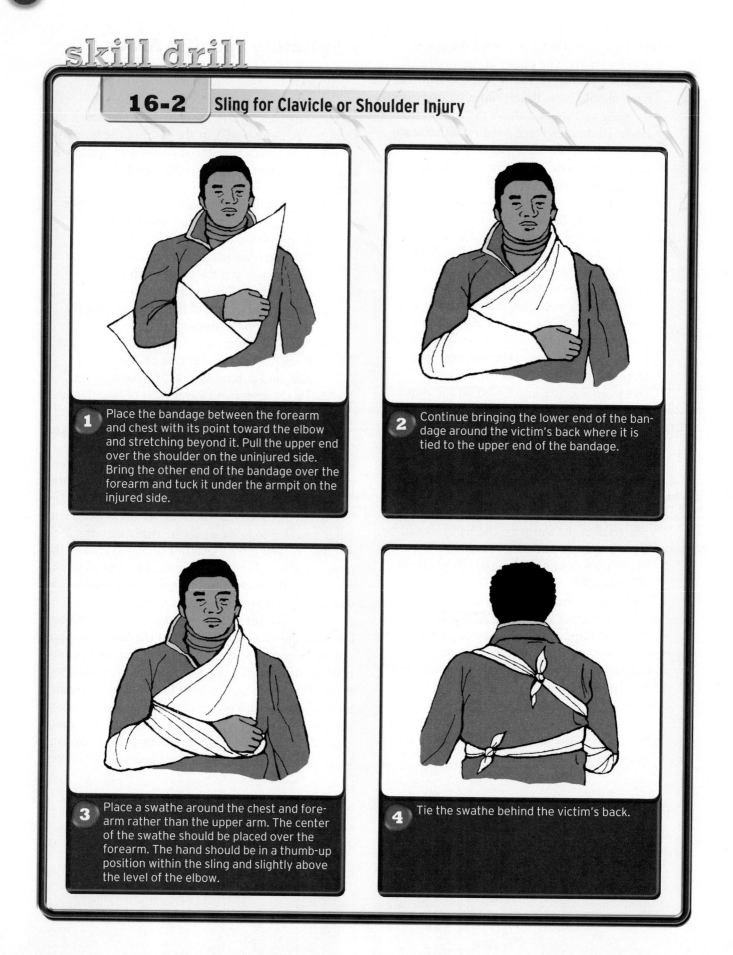

1 Place the bandage between the forearm and chest with its point toward the elbow and stretching beyond it. Pull the upper end over the shoulder on the uninjured side. Bring the other end of the bandage over the forearm and tuck it under the armpit on the injured side.

2 Continue bringing the lower end of the bandage around the victim's back where it is tied to the upper end of the bandage.

3 Place a swathe around the chest and forearm rather than the upper arm. The center of the swathe should be placed over the forearm. The hand should be in a thumb-up position within the sling and slightly above the level of the elbow.

4 Tie the swathe behind the victim's back.

Figure 16-2A

Figure 16-2B

Figure 16-2C

Figure 16-2D

Improvised slings. **A.** A buttoned jacket. **B.** A belt, necktie, or other clothing item looped around the neck and the injured arm. **C.** Sleeve of the jacket or shirt pinned to the clothing. **D.** Lower edge of the victim's jacket or shirt pinned up over the injured arm.

occurs in a remote setting (hours from medical care), use one of the methods described in Chapter 24, *Wilderness First Aid*, to reduce an anterior shoulder dislocation.

Humerus (Upper Arm)

Fractures of the humerus (upper arm) should be stabilized with a rigid splint. Extend the splint along the outside of the humerus. Then apply a sling and a swathe over the rigid splint, using the chest wall as an additional splint Skill Drill 16-3 .

1. Gently place the injured arm across the chest. If available, tie a rigid splint to the outside of the arm. (**Step ❶**). If a rigid splint is not available, go to Step 2.
2. Loop a cravat bandage or strap around the wrist and neck to allow the arm to hang in the sling position. Gravity will then provide gentle traction (**Step ❷**).

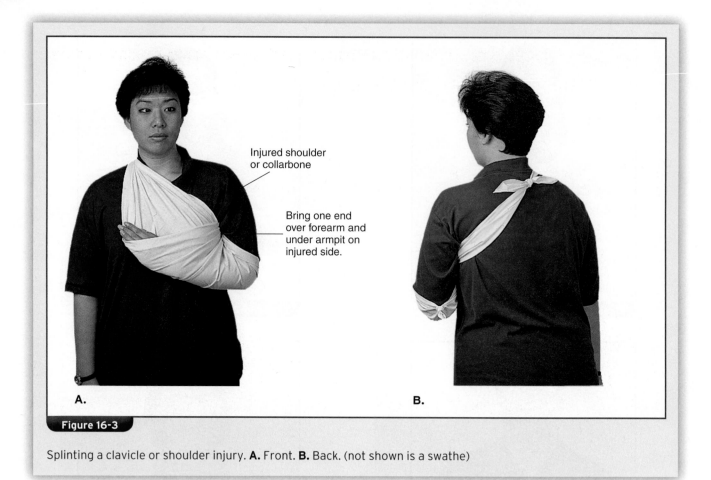

Injured shoulder
or collarbone

Bring one end
over forearm and
under armpit on
injured side.

A.   B.

Figure 16-3

Splinting a clavicle or shoulder injury. **A.** Front. **B.** Back. (not shown is a swathe)

3. Secure the arm to the chest with a swathe (folded triangular bandage) (**Step** ❸).

Elbow

An elbow must be stabilized in the position in which it is found—if bent, splint it bent; if straight, splint it straight (Skill Drill 16-4 and Skill Drill 16-5). If the injured elbow is straight, place a rigid splint along the inside of the arm from the hand to the armpit. Secure the splint with a roller bandage or several cravat bandages. For a bent elbow, apply a rigid splint diagonally, so that it extends from the humerus (near the armpit) to the wrist, to prevent motion of the elbow. Depending on how bent the elbow is, you can also use a sling and a swathe (binder) for a bent elbow.

To splint an elbow in the bent position, follow the steps in **Skill Drill 16-4** :

1. If the injured elbow is bent, place a rigid splint from the upper arm to the wrist (**Step** ❶).
2. Tie a rigid splint onto the arm with cravat bandages (**Step** ❷).

3. Place the arm in a sling and check CSM (**Step** ❸).

To splint an elbow in the straight position, follow the steps in **Skill Drill 16-5** :

1. If the injured elbow is straight, place a rigid splint along the inside of the arm from the hand to the armpit (**Step** ❶).
2. Secure with a roller bandage or several cravat bandages (**Step** ❷).
3. Check CSM (**Step** ❸).

Forearm

To stabilize a forearm fracture, use one rigid splint extending from the palm of the hand out past the elbow and a second one on the opposite side of the arm. Placing splints on both sides of the injured part (sandwich splint) keeps the forearm from twisting or rotating **Figure 16-4** .

Keep the victim's thumb in an upright position so that the two bones in the forearm (the radius and the ulna) do not touch each other (Skill Drill 16-6). Secure the splint with a roller bandage or several cravats. A

skill drill

16-3 Splinting Upper Arm (Humerus)

1 Gently place injured arm across the chest. If available, tie a rigid splint to the outside of the arm. If a rigid splint is not available, go to step 2.

2 Loop a cravat or strap around the neck and wrist to allow the arm to hang in the sling position.

3 Secure the arm to the chest with a swathe (folded triangular bandage).

skill drill

16-4   Splinting Elbow in Bent Position

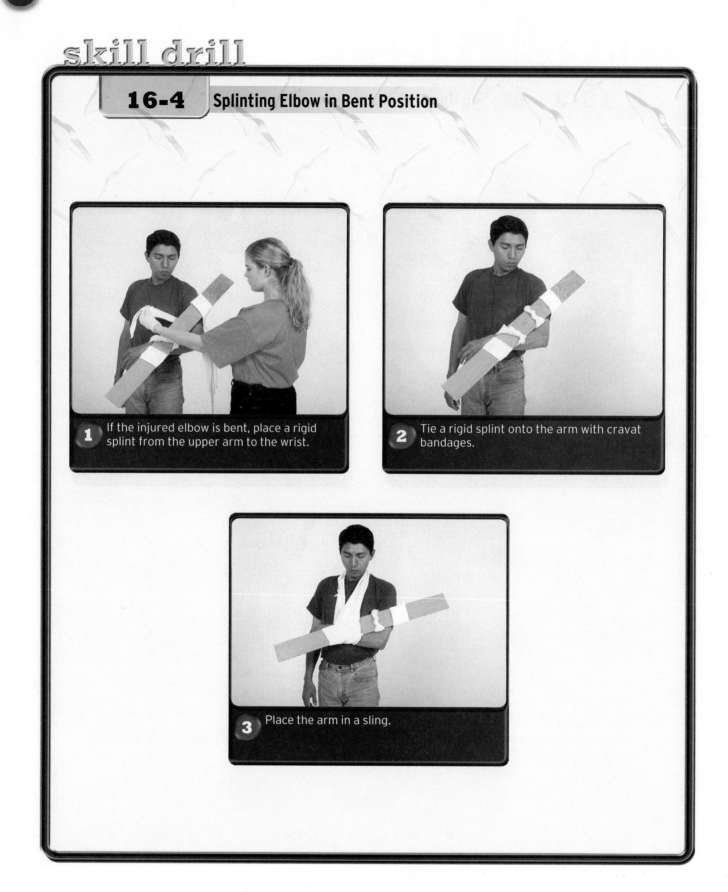

1 If the injured elbow is bent, place a rigid splint from the upper arm to the wrist.

2 Tie a rigid splint onto the arm with cravat bandages.

3 Place the arm in a sling.

skill drill

16-5   Splinting Elbow in Straight Position

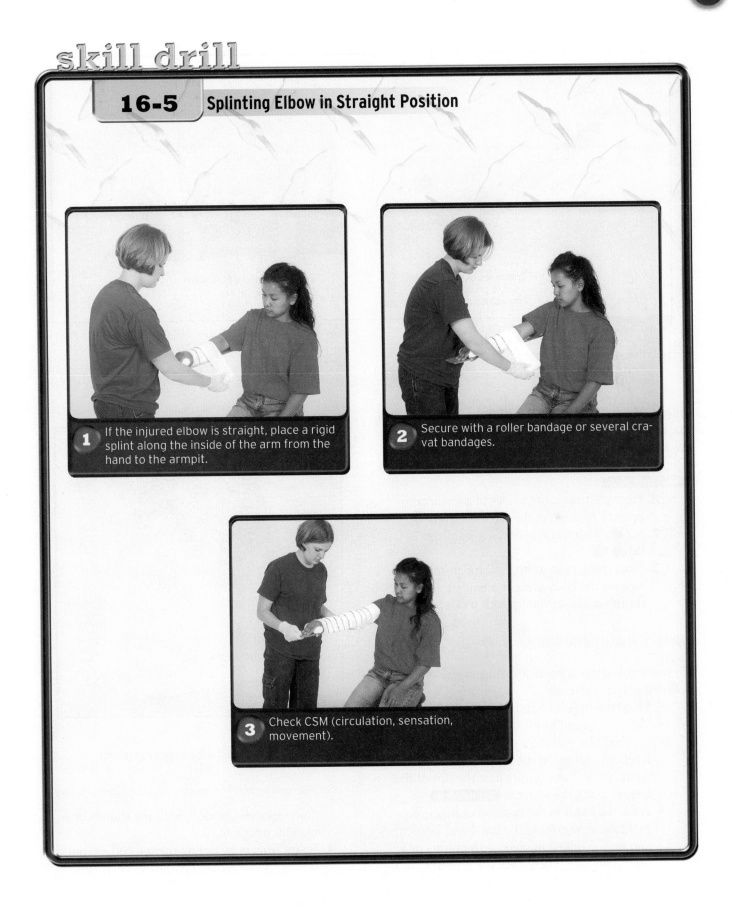

1 If the injured elbow is straight, place a rigid splint along the inside of the arm from the hand to the armpit.

2 Secure with a roller bandage or several cravat bandages.

3 Check CSM (circulation, sensation, movement).

Splints should be on both
sides to prevent rotation
(shows use of cardboard).

Keep
thumb
upright.

Rigid splint from palm
out past elbow.

Figure 16-4

Splinting a forearm fracture.

pillow or a rolled, folded blanket also can be secured to the arm. Put the arm in a sling and secure it with a swathe (binder) around the body **Figure 16-5**.

To splint the forearm, follow the steps in **Skill Drill 16-6**:

1. Place splints on both sides of a forearm to prevent rotation of the forearm (**Step ❶**).
2. Secure with a cravat or roller bandage (**Step ❷**).
3. Place the arm in a sling. A binder or swathe around the body is recommended. Keep the thumb in the upright position (**Step ❸**).

Wrist, Hand, and Fingers

To stabilize the wrist, hand, and fingers, use one of the following three methods:

- Place the injured hand in the position of function (hand looks like it is holding a baseball) by placing a rolled pair of socks or a roller bandage in the palm. Then attach a rigid splint that extends past the tips of the fingers along the forearm **Figure 16-6**.
- Place the hand in the position of function, mold a pillow around the hand and forearm, and tie the pillow in place with cravats or a roller bandage. Then place the arm in a sling

Figure 16-5

An arm sling can help stabilize upper extremity injuries.

and a swathe (binder), with the thumb in an upright position.
- Splint fingers by taping them together (buddy taping), with gauze separating the fingers.

skill drill

16-6   Splinting Forearm (Radius/Ulna)

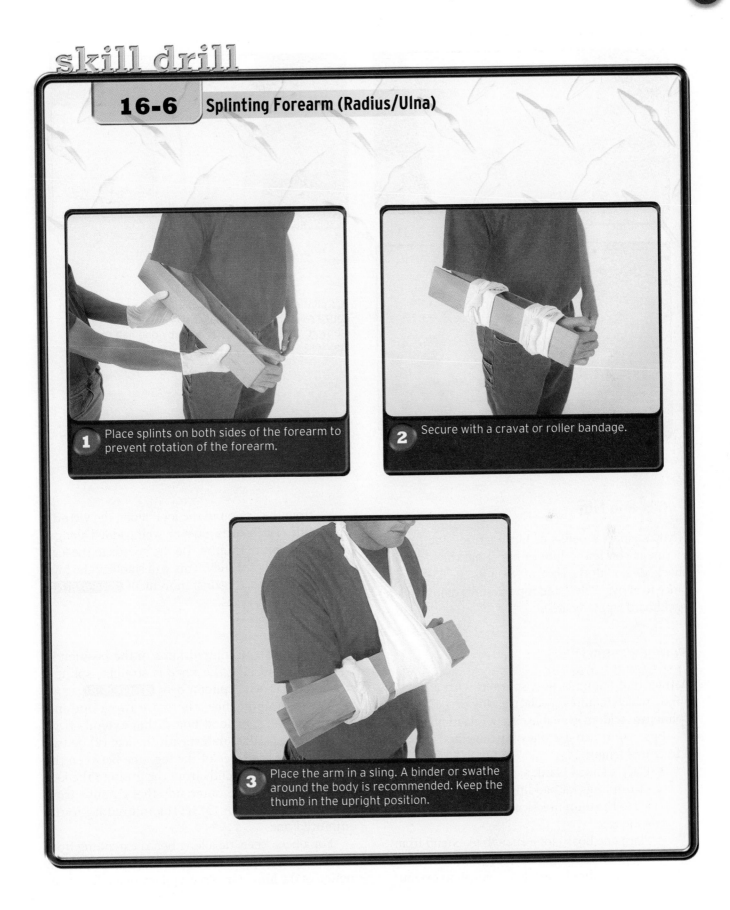

1 Place splints on both sides of the forearm to prevent rotation of the forearm.

2 Secure with a cravat or roller bandage.

3 Place the arm in a sling. A binder or swathe around the body is recommended. Keep the thumb in the upright position.

Figure 16-6A

Figure 16-6B

Figure 16-6C

A. Splinting a wrist, hand, or finger fracture. **B.** Use gauze roller bandage. Apply roller working up to the elbow. **C.** Overlap previous layer by one half to three quarters.

Pelvis and Hip

If you suspect a pelvis or hip fracture, stabilize the victim as you found him or her. Treat the victim for shock, do not lift the legs, and wait for the EMS ambulance to arrive. Pelvis and hip fractures require a long backboard (spine board).

Femur (Thigh)

A fractured femur is best splinted with a traction splint, which requires special training to use. Traction splints are seldom available except on ambulances.

First aiders can use one of two methods to splint a fractured femur:

- Place a folded blanket or pillows between the victim's legs for padding, then tie the injured leg to the uninjured leg with several cravats or bandages.
- Place one board long enough to extend from the groin to the foot between the victim's legs. Place another board, long enough to extend

from the armpit to the foot, along the victim's side. The boards must be well padded along their entire lengths. Tie the boards to the leg and body securely. This will stabilize the hip and the knee against movement **Figure 16-7**.

Knee

Always stabilize an injured knee in the position in which you find it. If the knee is straight, splint it straight; if it is bent, splint it bent **Figure 16-8**.

For a straight knee, there are three options: (1) tie one long, padded board that extends from the hip to the ankle underneath the leg; (2) tie two boards along the sides of the leg, one between the victim's legs that extends from the groin to the foot and the other on the outer side that extends from the hip to the foot; or (3) tie the injured leg to the uninjured one.

For a bent knee, tie a long board extending from just below the hip to just above the ankle to prevent motion of the knee. Or, place a pillow or a rolled blan-

One splint should reach from the armpit to past the heel.

The other splint should be long enough to reach from the groin to past the heel.

Tie the splints on snugly. The knots should not press the body.

Figure 16-7

Splinting a femur fracture.

A.

B.

Figure 16-8

Splint knee in position found. **A.** If the knee is bent, splint it bent. **B.** If the knee is straight, splint it straight.

ket beneath the knee and tie the injured leg to the uninjured leg.

To splint a knee in the straight position, follow the steps in **Skill Drill 16-7**:

1. Carefully lift the injured leg and place a rigid splint (long board) under the leg that extends from the buttocks to beyond the foot (**Step ❶**).
2. Place cravat bandages under the rigid splint and place soft padding under the knee and ankle (**Step ❷**).
3. Tie the cravat bandages. Do not tie the knots over the injured area (**Step ❸**).

To splint a knee in the bent position, follow the steps in **Skill Drill 16-8**:

1. Place a rigid splint (long board) against the injured leg. Do not place the splint against the knee (**Step ❶**).
2. Tie a cravat bandage around the splint and lower leg (**Step ❷**).
3. Tie a cravat bandage around the splint and thigh (**Step ❸**).
4. Tie knots over the splint, not over the leg (**Step ❹**).

Lower Leg

Stabilize the lower leg with two boards that extend from the upper thigh to the bottom of the foot. Or, place a folded blanket or pillow between the victim's legs for padding, and then tie the injured leg to the uninjured leg with several swathes, cravats, or bandages **Figure 16-9**.

To splint the lower leg using the self-splint method, follow the steps in **Skill Drill 16-9**:

1. Place padding (such as a folded blanket) between the legs. Push the cravat bandages under the leg with a thin board (**Step ❶**).
2. Tie the legs together (**Step ❷**).
3. Tie knots between the legs, over the padding (folded blanket) (**Step ❸**).

To splint the leg using rigid splints, follow the steps in **Skill Drill 16-10**:

skill drill

16-7   Splinting a Knee in the Straight Position

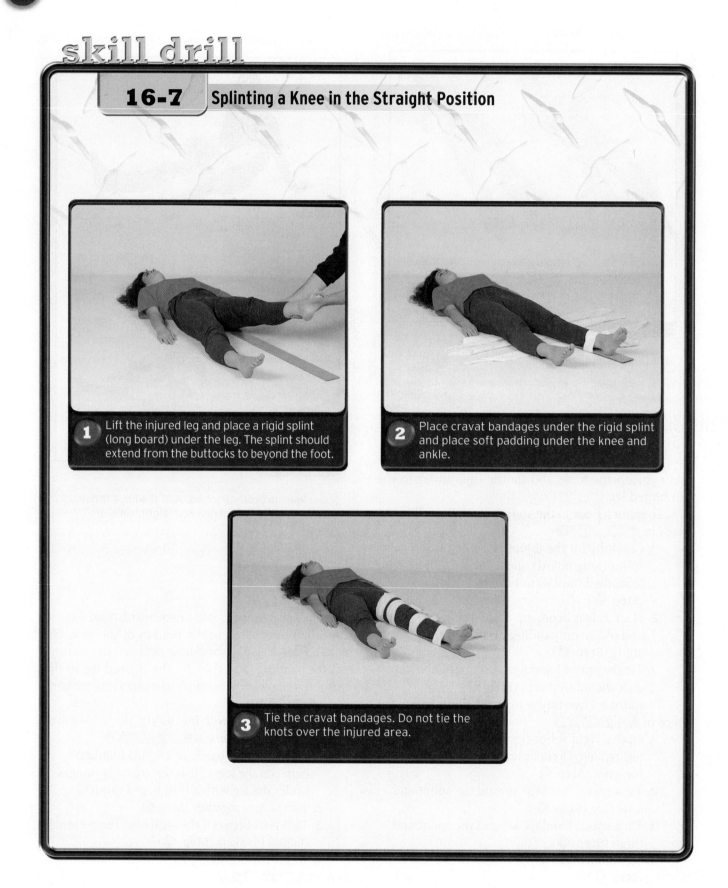

1 Lift the injured leg and place a rigid splint (long board) under the leg. The splint should extend from the buttocks to beyond the foot.

2 Place cravat bandages under the rigid splint and place soft padding under the knee and ankle.

3 Tie the cravat bandages. Do not tie the knots over the injured area.

skill drill

16-8   Splinting a Knee in the Bent Position

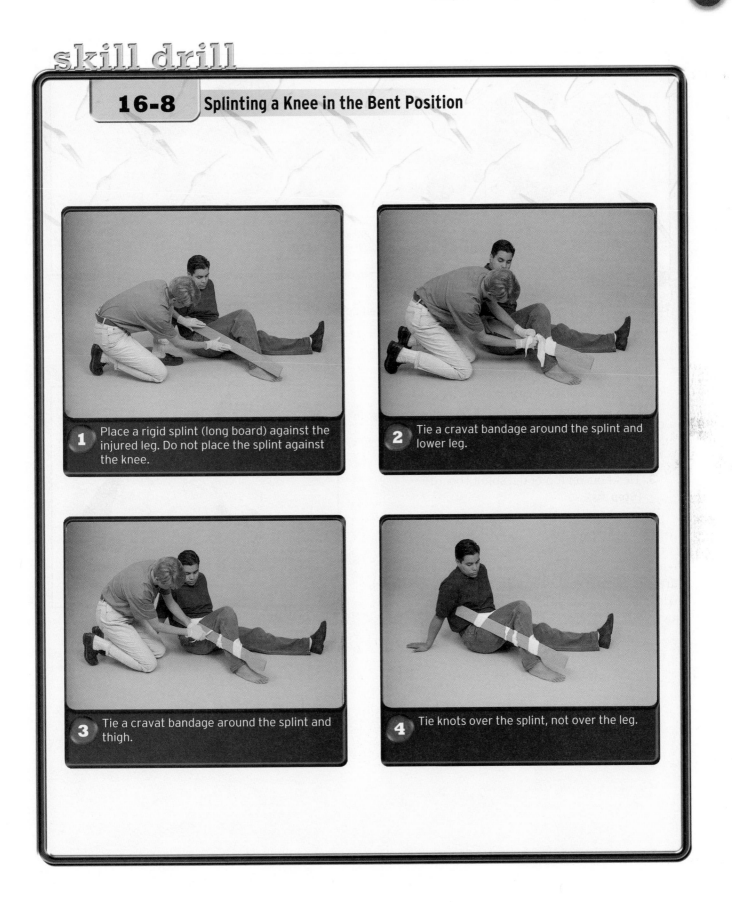

1 Place a rigid splint (long board) against the injured leg. Do not place the splint against the knee.

2 Tie a cravat bandage around the splint and lower leg.

3 Tie a cravat bandage around the splint and thigh.

4 Tie knots over the splint, not over the leg.

Figure 16-9

Place padding between legs.
A.

Tie legs together.

Place padded boards on each side of leg.
B.

Tie boards on snugly.

Two methods of splinting tibia and fibula fractures: **A.** Self-splint, **B.** Two boards.

1. Place one rigid splint (board) on the outside (lateral) and another inside (medial). Push the cravat bandages under the leg and splints with a thin board (**Step ❶**).
2. Tie both splints and leg together with cravat bandages (**Step ❷**).
3. Tie knots on top of the splint (board) (**Step ❸**).

Ankle and Foot

Treat ankle and foot injuries with the RICE procedures. To further stabilize an ankle, wrap a pillow or folded blanket around the ankle and foot and tie with cravats **Figure 16-10**.

Elastic bandages holding U-shaped cloth under pillow

Fold a pillow around ankle and tie it in place.

Figure 16-10

Splinting an ankle and foot.

skill drill

16-9   Splinting Lower Leg (Self Splint)

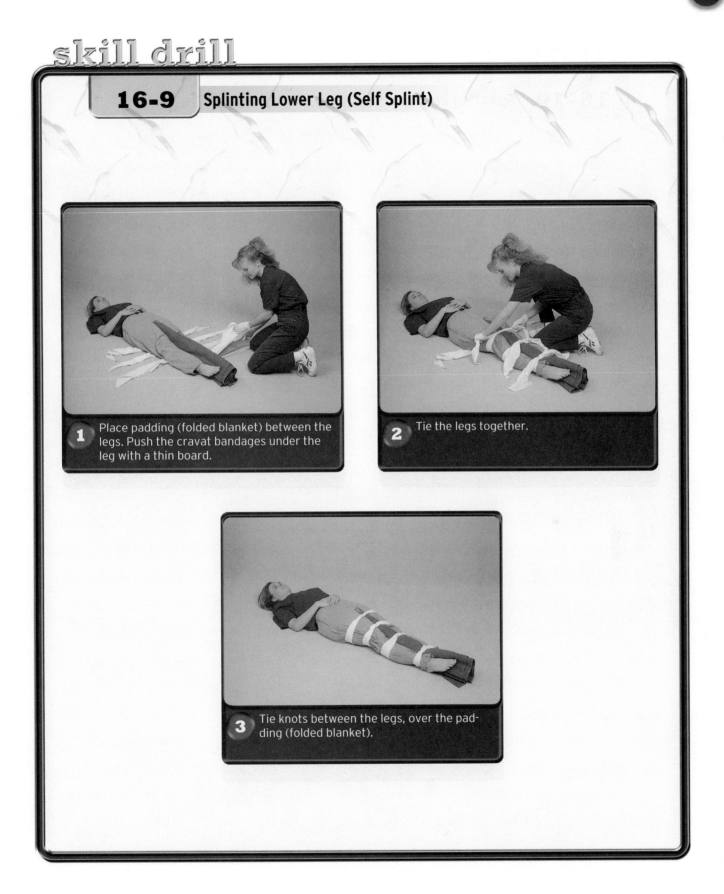

1 Place padding (folded blanket) between the legs. Push the cravat bandages under the leg with a thin board.

2 Tie the legs together.

3 Tie knots between the legs, over the padding (folded blanket).

skill drill

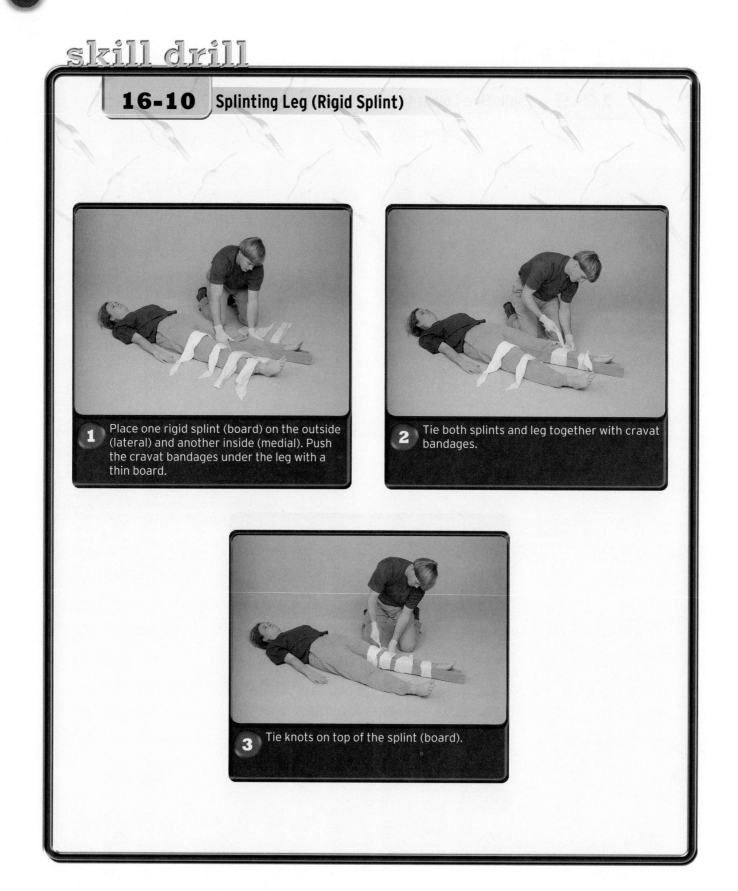

16-10 Splinting Leg (Rigid Splint)

1 Place one rigid splint (board) on the outside (lateral) and another inside (medial). Push the cravat bandages under the leg with a thin board.

2 Tie both splints and leg together with cravat bandages.

3 Tie knots on top of the splint (board).

prep kit

▶ Ready for Review

- Until medical care is available, stabilize the injury by splinting the extremity in the position found.
- A splint is any device used to stabilize a fracture or dislocation.
- When in doubt, apply a splint.
- A sling is any bandage or material that helps support the weight of an injured area.

▶ Vital Vocabulary

<u>sling</u> A triangular bandage applied around the neck to support an injured upper extremity; any material long enough to suspend an upper extremity by passing the material around the neck; used to support and protect an injury of the arm, shoulder, or clavicle.

<u>splint</u> Any support used to immobilize a fracture or to restrict movement of a part.

<u>swathe</u> A cravat tied around the body to decrease movement of a part.

▶ Assessment in Action

You are out with your best friend at a dog park, walking her Irish wolfhound. Your friend is animated and engrossed in your conversation. Suddenly, a rabbit leaps out of the hedges and the dog lurches forward, pulling your friend and causing her to trip and let go of the leash. You call to the dog, which becomes obedient again, and then your friend complains about pain in one of her fingers that appears to be deformed.

Directions: Circle Yes if you agree with the statement; circle No if you disagree.

Yes   No   **1.** You should stabilize the finger until medical care becomes available.

Yes   No   **2.** You should splint the finger to prevent a possible closed fracture from becoming an open fracture.

Yes   No   **3.** Splinting increases blood flow to the fracture, thus speeding up the healing process.

Yes   No   **4.** If you do not have a commercial splint, you could improvise one.

▶ Check Your Knowledge

Directions: Circle Yes if you agree with the statement; circle No if you disagree.

Yes   No   **1.** All fractures are complicated to some degree by damage to the soft tissue and structures surrounding the bone.

Yes   No   **2.** A rigid splint should never be used on an extremity.

Yes   No   **3.** All fractures and dislocations should be stabilized before the victim is moved.

Yes   No   **4.** Always check the CSM in the extremity.

Yes   No   **5.** Shoulder injuries can involve the clavicle, the scapula, and the tibia.

Yes   No   **6.** An elbow must be stabilized in the position in which it is found.

Yes   No   **7.** Always straighten an injured knee before splinting it.

Yes   No   **8.** First aiders should always use traction splints on leg fractures.

Yes   No   **9.** Buddy taping is when you tape two fingers together with gauze separating the fingers.

Yes   No   **10.** You can make a temporary sling by pinning a shirt or coat sleeve to the front of the coat or shirt.

17 Sudden Illnesses

Unexplained Change in Responsiveness

Victims can be fully alert (responsive), completely unresponsive, or can range anywhere between these two. Not all responsive victims are fully alert and they may respond to different levels of stimulation (eg, respond to your voice or squeezing of shoulder muscle). The level of responsiveness and mental status indicate how well the brain is functioning.

The main causes for a decrease in a person's alertness and responsiveness are brain injury and lack of either oxygen or glucose reaching the brain. The mnemonic STOP offers clues to the cause(s) of changes in responsiveness Table 17-1.

Heart Attack

Heart muscle needs oxygen to survive. A coronary attack (heart attack) occurs when the blood flow that brings oxygen to the heart muscle is severely reduced or cut off completely. This happens when coronary arteries that supply the heart with blood slowly become thicker and harder from a buildup of plaque (ie, fat, cholesterol, and other substances). This slow process is known as atherosclerosis Figure 17-1A. When plaque in a heart artery breaks free, a blood clot forms around the plaque. This blood clot can block the artery and shut off blood flow

Table 17-1 STOP Mnemonic

S	Sugar	Blood glucose too low (insulin reaction) or too high (diabetic coma)
	Seizures	
	Stroke	
	Shock	
T	Temperature	Too high (heatstroke) or too low (hypothermia)
O	Oxygen	Inadequate oxygen
P	Poisoning	Drug/alcohol overdose
		Carbon monoxide poisoning
	Pressure on brain	Head injury

FYI

Risk Factors for Heart Disease

Several factors contribute to an increased risk of heart attack and stroke. The more risk factors present, the greater the possibility that a person will develop heart disease.

Risk Factors You Cannot Change

- *Heredity:* Tendencies appear in family lines.
- *Sex:* Men have a greater risk, although heart attack is still the leading cause of death among women.
- *Age:* Most heart attack victims are 65 years or older.

Risk Factors You Can Change or Control

- *Cigarette smoking:* Smokers have more than twice the risk of heart attack as nonsmokers.
- *High blood pressure:* This condition adds to the heart's workload.
- *High blood cholesterol level:* Too much cholesterol in the blood can cause a buildup on the walls of the arteries.
- *Diabetes:* This condition affects the blood's cholesterol and triglyceride levels.
- *Obesity:* Being overweight influences blood pressure and blood cholesterol, can result in diabetes, and can place added strain on the heart.
- *Physical inactivity:* Inactive people have twice the risk of heart attack as active people.
- *Stress:* All people feel stress but react in different ways. Excessive, long-term stress can lead to physical problems in some people.

to the heart muscle. When the heart muscle is starved for oxygen and nutrients, it is called ischemia. When damage or death of part of the heart muscle occurs as a result of ischemia, it is called a **heart attack** or myocardial infarction (MI) **Figure 17-1B** .

Heart and blood vessel disease is America's number one killer. About half of the deaths from heart and blood vessel disease are from coronary heart disease, which includes heart attack. About 325,000 people a year die of coronary attack before they get to a hospital emergency department.

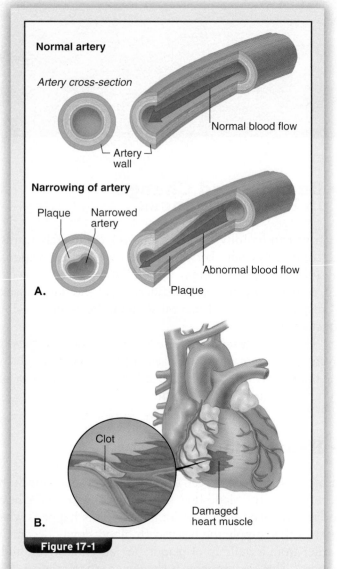

Normal artery

Artery cross-section

Normal blood flow

Artery wall

Narrowing of artery

Plaque   Narrowed artery

Abnormal blood flow

A.   Plaque

Clot

B.   Damaged heart muscle

Figure 17-1

A. A normal artery with normal blood flow and an artery with plaque buildup. **B.** A heart attack occurs when a clot prevents blood flow to a part of the heart.

Difference Between Heart Attack and Cardiac Arrest

The conditions *heart attack* and *cardiac arrest* confuse many people. The two are very different, and so is the first aid and emergency care for them.

- **Heart attack.** When one or more of the arteries delivering blood to the heart becomes blocked, a heart attack results. Oxygen-rich blood cannot reach the heart muscle, and the heart muscle becomes damaged. This damage to the heart muscle can lead to disturbances of the heart's electrical system and can lead to a cardiac arrest.
- **Cardiac arrest.** Cardiac arrest occurs when either the heart stops beating (asystole) or when the heart's lower chambers (ventricles) suddenly develop a rapid irregular rhythm (ventricular fibrillation), causing the ventricles to quiver rather than contract. The quivering motion of the ventricles renders the heart an ineffective pump that can no longer supply the body and brain with oxygen-rich blood. Within seconds, the victim becomes unresponsive and has no pulse. Only immediate action such as cardiopulmonary resuscitation (CPR) and external defibrillation can offer hope of survival.

Recognizing a Heart Attack

Some heart attacks are sudden and intense, leaving no doubt about what is happening. Most heart attacks, however, start slowly, with mild pain or discomfort. Heart attack victims are often not sure what is wrong and wait too long before getting help.

The National Heart, Lung and Blood Institute offers these signs of a possible heart attack:

- **Chest discomfort.** Most heart attacks involve discomfort in the center of the chest that lasts more than a few minutes or that goes away and comes back. It can feel like uncomfortable pressure, squeezing, fullness, or pain.
- **Discomfort in other areas of the upper body.** Symptoms can include pain or discomfort in one or both arms, the back, neck, jaw, or stomach.
- **Shortness of breath** with or without chest discomfort.
- **Other signs** may include breaking out in a cold sweat, nausea, or lightheadedness.

The most common heart attack symptom for both men and women is chest pain or discomfort. However,

---

FYI

No Chest Pain in One Third of Heart Attacks

A study of hundreds of thousands of heart attack victims found that as many as one third had no chest pain and that they were less likely to seek help and twice as likely to die.

The study found that women, people of color, people older than 75 years, and people with previous heart failure, stroke, or diabetes were most likely to have painless heart attacks. Although doctors have long known about painless heart attacks, many said they did not realize the number was so high.

Patients with chest pain were more than twice as likely to be diagnosed at admission and to receive clot-busting drugs or undergo angioplasty to open clogged arteries.

Source: Canto JG, Shlipak MG, Rogers WJ, et al. Prevalence, clinical characteristics, and mortality among patients with myocardial infarction presenting without chest pain. *JAMA.* 2000. 283:3223-3229.

---

women are somewhat more likely than men to experience some of the other symptoms, especially shortness of breath, nausea/vomiting, and back or jaw pain.

Care for Heart Attack

Treat a suspected heart attack in the following manner:

1. Immediately call 9-1-1 if a heart attack is suspected or if the chest pain does not go away in a victim taking nitroglycerin. Medications to dissolve a clot must be given early. Do not drive yourself or anyone else to the hospital.
2. Monitor breathing. If the victim becomes unresponsive and stops breathing, begin CPR.
3. Help the victim to the most comfortable resting position, usually sitting Figure 17-2. Loosen clothing around the neck and waist. Be calm and reassuring.
4. If the victim is alert, able to swallow, and not allergic to aspirin, help the victim take one adult aspirin (325 mg) or two chewable children's aspirin (81 mg each). Pulverize them or have the victim crunch them with his or her teeth before swallowing.

Find out if the victim is using nitroglycerin. Nitroglycerin tablets, spray, or ointment can relieve chest pain from angina but not always from a heart attack. Nitroglycerin dilates the

Half-sitting position.

Support back.

Knees bent.

Place padding under knees.

Figure 17-2

Help the victim into a relaxed position to ease strain on the heart.

coronary arteries, which increases blood flow to the heart muscle. It also lowers blood pressure and dilates the veins, thus decreasing the work of the heart and the heart muscle's need for oxygen.

Caution: Because nitroglycerin lowers blood pressure, the victim should sit or lie down once it is taken. Let the victim take one pill or one spray under the tongue. If necessary, help him or her take it. If the chest pain or discomfort does not improve within 5 minutes after the one dose, call 9-1-1. Previously, victims were told to take up to three doses, 5 minutes apart.

FYI

Dangerous Morning Hours

Studies in the 1990s demonstrated diurnal variation in the onset of acute cardiovascular disorders (such as heart attack and cardiac death). The results consistently show an increased incidence of acute cardiac events in the morning hours (6:00 AM to noon) and a low incidence at night. Some data suggest another late afternoon or evening peak of incidence.

Source: Peckova M, et al. 1998. Circadian variation in the occurrence of cardiac arrests. *Circulation* 98(1):31–39.

▶ Angina

Chest pain called <u>angina pectoris</u> can result from coronary heart disease just as a heart attack does Table 17-2 . Angina occurs when coronary arteries supplying the heart muscle with oxygen-rich blood become narrow and cannot carry sufficient blood to meet the demands during:

- Physical exertion
- Excitement
- Emotional upset
- Eating of a heavy meal
- Extreme hot or cold temperature exposure
- Cigarette smoking

Table 17-2 Chest Pain

Cause of Pain	Characteristics	Care
Muscle or rib pain from exercise or injury	Reproduced by movement Tender spot when pressed	Rest Aspirin or ibuprofen
Respiratory infection (eg, pneumonia, bronchitis, pleuritis)	Cough Fever Sore throat Production of sputum	Antibiotics
Indigestion	Belching Heartburn Nausea Sour taste	Antacids
Angina pectoris	Lasts less than 10 minutes (but pain is similar to that of a heart attack)	Rest Victim's nitroglycerin
Heart attack (myocardial infarction)	Lasts more than 10 minutes Pressure, squeezing, or pain near center of the chest Pain spreads to shoulders, neck, or arms Lightheadedness, fainting, sweating, nausea, shortness of breath	Call 9-1-1 Check breathing Resting position Victim's nitroglycerin

Recognizing Angina

It can be difficult to differentiate a heart attack from angina, even for physicians. Chest pain from a heart attack is as likely to happen at rest as during activity, the pain lasts longer than 10 minutes, and it is not relieved by nitroglycerin. Differentiate angina from a heart attack by these signs and symptoms:

- Chest pain is described as crushing, squeezing, or like somebody standing on the victim's chest.
- Pain can spread to the jaw, the arms (frequently the left arm), and the mid-back.
- Pain usually lasts from 3 to 10 minutes, but rarely longer than 10 minutes.
- The pain is almost always relieved by the victim's prescribed nitroglycerin.
- Pain can be associated with shortness of breath, nausea, or sweating.
- Victim feels anxious.

Care for Angina

Angina can be treated with drugs that affect the blood supply to the heart muscle, the heart's demand for oxygen, or both. Drugs that affect the blood supply are coronary vasodilators; they cause blood vessels to relax. When this happens, the opening inside the vessels (the lumen) gets bigger. Then blood flow improves, letting more oxygen and nutrients reach the heart muscle.

Nitroglycerin mainly relaxes the veins and relaxes the coronary arteries a little. By relaxing the veins, it reduces the amount of blood that returns to the heart and eases the heart's workload. By relaxing the coronary arteries, it increases the heart's blood supply. Physicians often prescribe nitroglycerin for those with angina.

1. Have the victim stop what he or she is doing and sit down. Keep bystanders away. Provide calm reassurance to help reduce the victim's anxiety.
2. If the victim has medically prescribed nitroglycerin, either tablets or a spray, let the victim use it. This is one pill or one spray under the tongue. Follow the prescription label's directions. If necessary, help him or her use it.
3. If the chest pain or discomfort does not improve within 5 minutes after taking one dose of nitroglycerin, call 9-1-1. Previously, victims were told to take up to three

---

FYI

Other Causes of Chest Pain

Not all causes of chest pain relate to the heart, including:

- Muscle or rib pain due to exercise, excessive coughing, or injury. The victim can reproduce the pain by movement, and often the area of complaint is tender when pressed. Rest and aspirin or ibuprofen relieves the pain.
- Respiratory infections such as pneumonia, bronchitis, pleuritis, or lung injury. Chest pain due to these conditions usually worsens when the victim coughs or breaths deeply. Fever and colored sputum might be present. The victim needs medical care and may require prescribed medications.
- Indigestion, usually accompanied by belching, heartburn, nausea, and a sour taste in the mouth. This type of pain is relieved by antacids.

FYI

Why Don't They Call?

A study asked heart attack victims who waited for more than 20 minutes before getting help why they delayed. Their answers included the following:

- They thought the symptoms would go away.
- The symptoms were not severe enough.
- They thought it was a different illness.
- They were worried about medical costs.
- They were afraid of hospitals.
- They feared being embarrassed.
- They wanted to wait for a better time.
- They did not want to find out what was wrong.

The average time that elapsed between symptom onset and hospital arrival was 2 hours; 28% waited at least 1 hour, 33% waited 1 to 3 hours, 15% waited 3 to 6 hours, and 23% waited more than 6 hours. Most victims reported they were not sure their symptoms were severe enough to merit action as drastic as calling 9-1-1.

The same study concluded that one way to shorten out-of-hospital delay is to encourage victims with heart-related symptoms to use EMS rather than slower transportation methods.

Source: Meischke H, Eisenberg MS, Schaeffer SM, Larsen MP. 1995. Reasons patients with chest pain delay or do not call 911. *Ann Emerg Med.* 25(2):193-197.

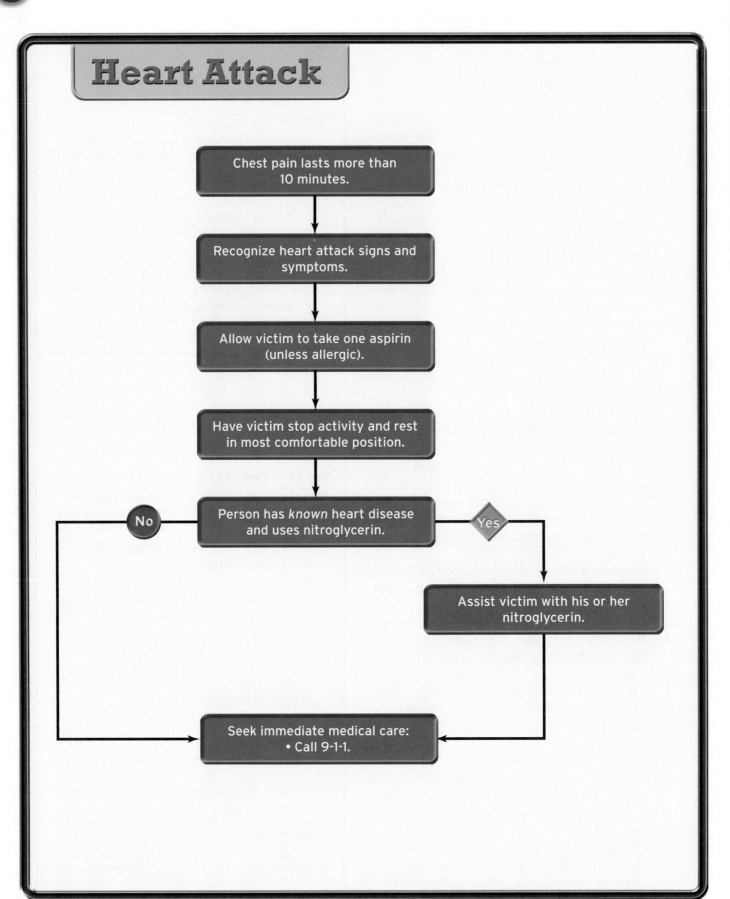

Heart Attack

Chest pain lasts more than 10 minutes.

↓

Recognize heart attack signs and symptoms.

↓

Allow victim to take one aspirin (unless allergic).

↓

Have victim stop activity and rest in most comfortable position.

↓

No ← Person has *known* heart disease and uses nitroglycerin. → **Yes**

Assist victim with his or her nitroglycerin.

Seek immediate medical care:
• Call 9-1-1.

nitroglycerin tablets, 5 minutes apart, when they had chest pain or discomfort. This procedure has been changed so that if there is no improvement within 5 minutes after taking one dose, 9-1-1 should be called.

▶ Stroke (Brain Attack)

A <u>stroke</u>, also called a brain attack, occurs when there is a sudden interruption of blood flow to the brain. This occurs when arteries in the brain rupture or become blocked so part of the brain does not receive the blood flow it needs **Figure 17-3**. Deprived of oxygen-rich blood, nerve cells in the affected area of the brain cannot function and die within minutes. Because dead brain cells are not replaced, the devastating effects of strokes often are permanent. When nerve cells do not function, the part of the body they control cannot function either. Each year, about 800,000 Americans suffer a new or recurrent stroke, and about one fourth of these victims die, making it the third leading cause of death.

Strokes are classified as ischemic or hemorrhagic:

- **Ischemic stroke.** This type of stroke occurs when blood vessels to the brain become narrowed or clogged with fatty deposits called plaque, cutting off blood flow to brain cells. High blood pressure is the most important risk factor for ischemic stroke and can be controlled. Ischemic strokes are the most common type of stroke and account for about 85% of all strokes. Ischemic strokes usually occur at night or first thing in the morning.

  Because tissue plasminogen activators (tPA) and other clot-busting drugs must be given as soon as possible after stroke onset (within 3 hours), it is important to recognize a stroke and to seek immediate medical care.

- **Hemorrhagic stroke.** About 15% of all strokes happen when a blood vessel ruptures in or near the brain. This kind of stroke is often associated with a very severe headache, nausea, and vomiting. Usually the symptoms appear suddenly.

Immediately seek medical care if there is a possibility of stroke. Any or all of the following procedures might be needed:

- Medication to control high blood pressure
- Medication to reduce brain swelling
- Surgery to repair an aneurysm or remove a blood clot

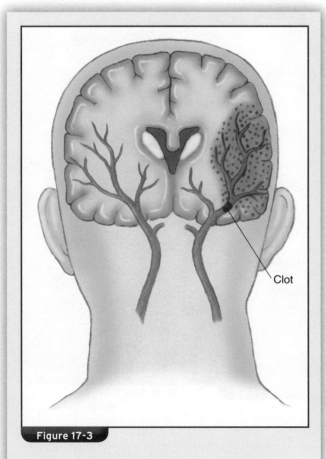

Figure 17-3

A blood clot can block the brain's blood supply.

FYI

Give Me 5 for Stroke

The American Academy of Neurology, the American College of Emergency Physicians, and the American Heart Association/American Stroke Association formed a joint campaign known as "Give Me 5" for Stroke. Women especially need to know the warning signs, because they account for over 60% of the deaths from stroke. They are also often the health information keepers for their families. Give Me 5 for Stroke uses easy-to-remember words to help identify the five signs of stroke. The key words are:

- Walk: Is their balance off?
- Talk: Is their speech slurred or face droopy?
- Reach: Is one side weak or numb?
- See: Is their vision all or partly lost?
- Feel: Is their headache severe?

Recognizing Stroke

Symptoms of stroke include the following:

- Weakness, numbness, or paralysis of the face, an arm, or a leg on only one side of the body
- Blurred or decreased vision, especially in one eye
- Problems speaking or understanding
- Dizziness or loss of balance
- Sudden, severe, and unexplained headache
- Deviation of the eyes from PEARL (pupils equal and reactive to light), which might mean the brain is being affected by lack of oxygen

The Cincinnati Stroke Scale is a proven method for quickly identifying stroke victims. When you suspect a stroke, apply these three simple tests Table 17-3 :

- Facial droop
- Arm drift
- Speech

CAUTION

DO NOT give a stroke victim anything to drink or eat. The throat can be paralyzed, which restricts swallowing.

A. A normal smile. B. Facial droop.

A. Normal arm position. B. Arm droop.

Table 17-3 Cincinnati Prehospital Stroke Scale

Test	Normal	Abnormal
Facial droop **Figure 17-4** (Ask victim to show teeth or smile.)	Both sides of face move equally well.	One side of the face does not move as well as the other.
Arm drift **Figure 17-5** (Ask victim to close eyes and hold out both arms with palms up.)	Both arms move the same, or both arms do not move.	One arm does not move, or one arm drifts down compared with the other side.
Speech (Ask victim to say, "The sky is blue in Cincinnati.")	Victim uses correct words with no slurring.	Victim slurs words, uses inappropriate words, or is unable to speak.

Care for a Stroke Victim

First aid for a stroke victim is limited to supportive care:

1. Call 9-1-1 immediately. Minimize brain damage by getting the victim to medical care.
2. Check the time at which the first signs appeared. A physician can use the information to determine whether a clot-busting drug can be given.
3. Monitor breathing. If the victim becomes unresponsive and stops breathing, begin CPR.
4. If the victim is unresponsive and breathing, place the victim in the recovery position to keep the airway open and to permit possible secretions and vomit to drain from the mouth.
5. If the victim is responsive, get the victim into a comfortable position with the head elevated. Be sure that the victim does not exert himself or herself.
6. Do not give the victim anything to drink or eat.
7. Reassure and keep the victim warm until EMS arrives.

▶ Asthma

Asthma is a chronic (long-term) lung disease that inflames and narrows the airways. Asthma causes recurring periods of wheezing (a whistling sound when a person breathes), chest tightness, shortness of breath, and coughing. The coughing often occurs at night or early in the morning.

Asthma affects people of all ages, but it most often starts in childhood and has the highest prevalence rate in those ages 5 to 17 years. In the United States, about 23 million people are known to have asthma.

The airways are tubes that carry air into and out of the lungs. People who have asthma have inflamed airways. This makes the airways swollen and very sensitive. They tend to react strongly to certain substances that are breathed in.

When the airways react, the muscles around them tighten. This causes the airways to narrow, allowing less air to flow to the lungs. Swelling makes the airways even narrower. Cells in the airways may make more mucus than normal **Figure 17-6**. Mucus is a sticky, thick liquid that can further narrow a person's airways.

A. Normal   **B.** Narrowed

Figure 17-6

A. A cross-section of a normal airway. **B.** A cross-section of an airway during asthma symptoms, with the airway narrowed and inflamed, a thickened airway wall, and mucus.

This chain reaction can result in asthma symptoms. Symptoms can happen each time the airways are irritated. Sometimes symptoms are mild and go away on their own or after minimal treatment with an asthma medicine. At other times, symptoms continue to get worse. An asthma attack is when symptoms get more intense and/or additional symptoms appear.

It is important to treat symptoms when they are first noticed. This helps prevent the symptoms from worsening and causing a severe asthma attack. Severe asthma attacks may require medical care, and they can cause death.

Some of the known triggers of asthma are listed in **Table 17-4**.

Recognizing an Asthma Attack

Asthma varies a great deal from one person to another. Symptoms can range from mild to moderate to severe and can be life threatening. The episodes can come occasionally or often. Between episodes, the person has no breathing difficulties.

The common asthma signs and symptoms include:

- **Excessive coughing.** Coughing from asthma is often worse at night or early in the morning.
- **Wheezing.** Wheezing is a whistling or squeaky sound that occurs when the victim breathes.
- **Chest tightness.** This may feel like something is squeezing or sitting on the chest.
- **Shortness of breath.** Some people who have asthma say they cannot catch their breath or they feel out of breath.

Table 17-4 Common Asthma Triggers

Environmental	Drugs or Chemicals	Conditions or Events
• Cold air	• Aspirin	• Gastroesophageal reflux
• House dust mites	• Beta blocker medicine	• Allergic rhinitis
• Cockroaches	• Food or drug preservatives	• Panic attacks
• Animals (eg, cats, dogs, rodents)	• Seafood, shellfish	• Menstruation, pregnancy
• Indoor irritants (eg, wood-burning stoves)	• Occupational exposure to chemicals	• Viral respiratory infections
• Outdoor air pollution (eg, vehicle emissions)	• Household cleaning agents	• Emotional stress, excitement
• Indoor or outdoor molds and fungi	• Perfumes	• Exercise
• Tobacco smoke		
• Pollen (eg, grass, trees)		

- **Sitting in the tripod position.** This position involves leaning forward with hands on knees or other support, trying to breathe.
- **Inability to speak in complete sentences** without pausing for breath.
- **Nostrils flaring** with each breath.

Not all people who have asthma have these symptoms. Likewise, having these symptoms does not always mean that the person has asthma.

Care for an Asthma Attack

1. Place the victim in a comfortable, upright position, leaning slightly forward (tripod position).
2. Ask the victim about any asthma medication he or she uses. Most asthmatics have some form of medication, usually administered through physician-prescribed, handheld inhalers or a device (nebulizer) that turns liquid medicine into a mist for inhalation **Figure 17-7**.

   Asthma is treated with two types of medicines: long-term control and quick-relief medicines. Quick-relief, or "rescue," medicines relieve asthma symptoms that may flare up; a first aider should know about these medications.

   All people who have asthma need a quick-relief medicine to help relieve asthma symptoms that may flare up. Inhaled

Asthma medication for an attack.

Keep victim sitting up.

Figure 17-7

Most asthmatics have some form of medication that may assist them during an asthma attack.

short-acting beta-agonists are the first choice for quick relief. These inhaled medicines act quickly to relax tight muscles around the airways during a flare-up, allowing the airways to open up so air can flow through them. Asthma symptoms should respond to inhaled medicine quickly (within 1 hour).

The quick-relief medicine should be taken when the first asthma symptoms are noticed. The quick-relief inhaler should be with the person at all times. Most people who have asthma can safely manage their symptoms using their medications.

Using a Physician-Prescribed Quick-Relief Inhaler (Metered-Dose Inhaler)

1. Check the inhaler's expiration date.
2. The inhaler should be at room temperature.
3. If there is a spacer/holding chamber, attach the inhaler to it.
4. Shake the inhaler several times.
5. The victim should blow out the air in the lungs.
6. The victim's lips should be placed around the inhaler and the victim should begin to inhale deeply.
7. The victim depresses the handheld inhaler to release the medicine as he or she breathes in slowly until the lungs are full.
8. If using a spacer/holding chamber, the victim should press down on the inhaler and then wait 5 seconds before breathing in.
9. The victim should hold his or her breath for at least 10 seconds, allowing the medication to be absorbed into the lungs.
10. Wait for several breaths before taking a second dose.

Who gets asthma?

Asthma is very common, affecting more than 23 million people in the United States, including almost 7 million children. No one knows for sure why some people have asthma and others do not. People who have family members with allergies or asthma are more likely to have asthma.

In young children, boys are nearly twice as likely as girls to develop asthma, but this sex difference tends to disappear in older age groups. Obesity is a newly identified risk factor for asthma.

What causes asthma?

People generally think of asthma in terms of episodes or attacks. Actually, the asthmatic condition is always present, but symptoms may be dormant until triggered by an allergen, respiratory infection, or cold weather. Other triggers may include aspirin, environmental irritants, physical exertion, and, less commonly, food additives and preservatives.

Source: American College of Allergy, Asthma and Immunology, http://www.acaai.org/allergist/asthma/Pages/what_causes_asthma.aspx

3. If asthma signs and symptoms (eg, coughing, wheezing, tight chest) begin, the victim can take two puffs of the quick-relief medicine. If the victim's condition does not improve but symptoms are mild, call the victim's physician for advice and administer up to four more puffs over 30 minutes.
4. If the medicine is not helping, breathing is hard and fast, the nose opens wide during breathing, or the victim cannot walk or talk well, call 9-1-1 or take the victim to the nearest emergency department if that would be faster. The victim can take four more puffs of the quick-relief medicine (two puffs at a time, waiting 15 minutes between each set of two puffs) while awaiting EMS or traveling to the hospital.

▶ Hyperventilation

Fast, deep breathing, called hyperventilation, is common during emotional stress. The victim might be hysterical or quite calm. Other factors that can cause rapid breathing include untreated diabetes, severe shock, certain poisons, and brain swelling due to injury or high altitude.

Recognizing Hyperventilation

Signs of hyperventilation include:
- Shortness of breath
- Fast breathing (more than 40 breaths per minute)
- Tingling or numbness of the hands, feet, and around the mouth
- Dizziness or lightheadedness

Breathing Into a Paper Bag

A popular remedy for anxiety-related hyperventilation is to breathe into a paper bag. Do not do this. Tests on healthy people show that bag rebreathing rarely restores blood-gas balance but often causes dangerous stress to the heart and respiratory system, especially in people with a chronic respiratory disease.

Source: Callaham M. 1989. Hypoxic hazards of traditional paper bag rebreathing in hyperventilating patients. *Ann Emerg Med.* 18(6):622-628.

Care for Hyperventilation

If you encounter someone who is hyperventilating, these steps can help:

1. Calm and reassure the victim.
2. Take the victim to a quiet place or ask bystanders to leave. Have the victim sit down.
3. Encourage the person to breathe slowly, using the abdominal muscles: inhale through the nose, hold the full inhalation for 1 to 2 seconds, then exhale slowly through pursed lips.

▶ Chronic Obstructive Pulmonary Disease

Chronic obstructive pulmonary disease (COPD) is a broad term applied to emphysema, chronic bronchitis, and related lung diseases. The incidence of COPD is very high in North America, and the most common causative factor is cigarette smoking.

Chronic obstructive pulmonary disease describes a disease that makes it hard for a person to breathe because the normal flow of air into and out of the person's lungs is partially obstructed.

Because COPD takes many years to develop before a person notices difficulty breathing, COPD is usually considered a disease of older adults and is most commonly diagnosed in people older than 60 years.

Chronic bronchitis is caused by chronic infection, which can be brought on by irritations such as tobacco smoke. The bronchi become thick, unable to stretch, and partially blocked. Early symptoms include a cigarette cough or a cough due to a cold. Later, more severe symptoms include difficulty breathing, increased sputum, and severe coughing.

Emphysema often occurs with chronic bronchitis. The alveoli of the lungs are partially destroyed, and the lungs have lost their elasticity, making it difficult for the victim to exhale. Common symptoms include coughing, wheezing, and shortness of breath. Breathing is extremely difficult for people with emphysema.

Recognizing Chronic Obstructive Pulmonary Disease

The signs and symptoms of COPD are similar to those of asthma. Most victims will wheeze; coughing and shortness of breath might be more prominent in people with COPD than in asthma. Many people with COPD depend on a constant low level of artificially supplied oxygen to maintain breathing.

Care for Chronic Obstructive Pulmonary Disease

Use the following guidelines when caring for someone with COPD:

1. Persons with COPD usually will have their own physician-prescribed medications. Assist the victim to take any prescribed medications.
2. Place the victim in the sitting position that provides the greatest comfort.
3. Encourage the victim to cough up any secretions.
4. For acute breathing distress, obtain immediate medical assistance. The victim might need oxygen, which is available from EMS and at hospital emergency departments.

▶ Fainting

A sudden, brief loss of responsiveness not associated with a head injury is known as <u>syncope</u> (fainting) or <u>psychogenic shock</u>.

Simple fainting is common and benign and can have physical or emotional causes. Fainting can happen suddenly when blood flow to the brain is interrupted. The nervous system dilates blood vessels to three to four times their normal size and allows blood to pool in the legs and lower body.

Syncope, or simple fainting, can be precipitated by unpleasant emotional stimuli such as the sight of blood or strong fear. It usually occurs when the victim is in the upright position.

Most fainting episodes are associated with decreased blood flow causing deficient oxygen or glucose in the brain. The decreased blood flow can be caused by a slow heart rate (vagal reaction, in which the vagus nerve, which slows the heart rate, is overstimulated by fright, anxiety, drugs, or fatigue), heart-rhythm disturbances, dehydration, heat exhaustion, anemia (low hemoglobin), or bleeding. Decreased glucose (<u>hypoglycemia</u>) can be caused by diabetes, medications used to treat diabetes, or infections.

Sitting or standing for a long time without moving, especially in a hot environment, can cause blood to pool in dilated vessels, which results in a

Fainting

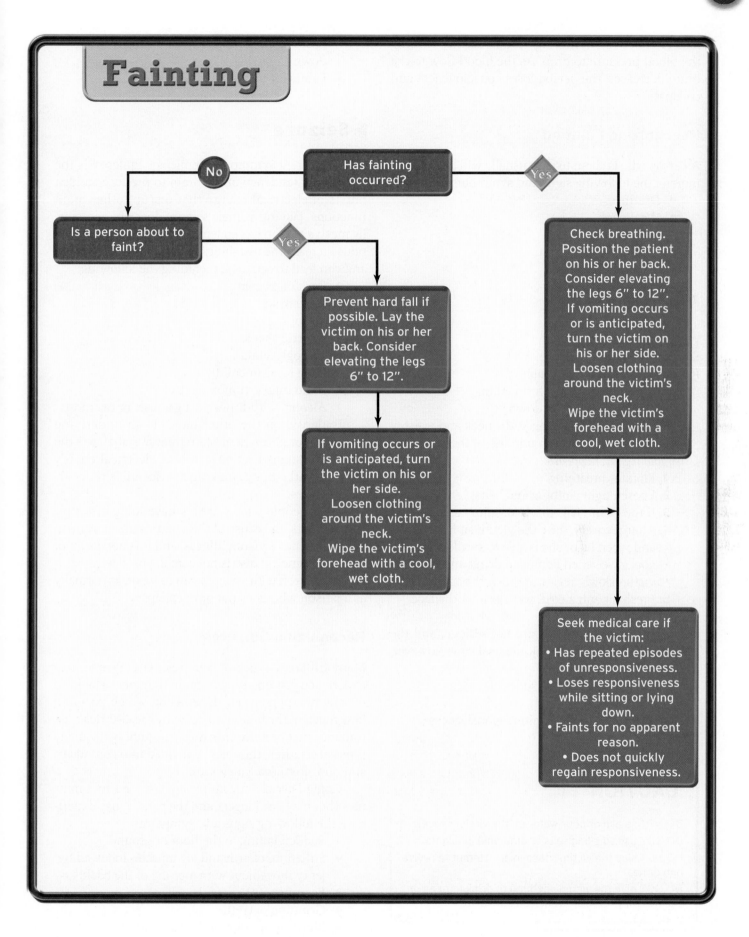

No ← **Has fainting occurred?** → **Yes**

Is a person about to faint? — **Yes** →

Prevent hard fall if possible. Lay the victim on his or her back. Consider elevating the legs 6" to 12".

↓

If vomiting occurs or is anticipated, turn the victim on his or her side.
Loosen clothing around the victim's neck.
Wipe the victim's forehead with a cool, wet cloth.

Check breathing. Position the patient on his or her back. Consider elevating the legs 6" to 12". If vomiting occurs or is anticipated, turn the victim on his or her side. Loosen clothing around the victim's neck. Wipe the victim's forehead with a cool, wet cloth.

Seek medical care if the victim:
• Has repeated episodes of unresponsiveness.
• Loses responsiveness while sitting or lying down.
• Faints for no apparent reason.
• Does not quickly regain responsiveness.

loss of effective circulating blood volume, causing the blood pressure to drop. As the blood flow to the brain decreases, the person loses consciousness and collapses.

Recognizing Fainting

A person who is about to faint usually will have one or more of the following signs and symptoms:

- Dizziness
- Weakness
- Seeing spots
- Visual blurring
- Nausea
- Pale skin
- Sweating

Care for Fainting

If a person appears about to faint:

1. Prevent the person from falling.
2. Help the person lie down.
3. Loosen tight clothing at the neck and waist.
4. Stay with the victim until he or she recovers.

If fainting has happened:

1. Monitor breathing.
2. Loosen tight clothing and belts.
3. If the victim fell, check for injuries.
4. After recovery, have the victim sit for a while, and when he or she is able to swallow, give cool, sweetened liquids to drink and help the victim slowly regain an upright posture.
5. Fresh air and a cold, wet cloth for the face usually aid recovery.

Most fainting episodes are not serious, and the victim recovers quickly. Seek medical care, however, if the victim:

- Has had repeated episodes of unresponsiveness
- Does not quickly regain responsiveness

CAUTION

DO NOT splash or pour water on the victim's face.
DO NOT use smelling salts or ammonia inhalants.
DO NOT slap the victim's face in an attempt to revive him or her.
DO NOT give the victim anything to drink until he or she has fully recovered and can swallow.

- Loses responsiveness while sitting or lying down
- Faints for no apparent reason

▶ Seizure

Seizures are a symptom of epilepsy. Epilepsy is the underlying tendency of the brain to produce sudden bursts of electrical energy that disrupt other brain functions. Having a single seizure does not necessarily mean a person has epilepsy. Several medical conditions increase the instability or irritability of the brain and can lead to seizures, including the following:

- Lack of oxygen
- Heatstroke
- Poisoning
- Electric shock
- Hypoglycemia
- High fever in children
- Brain injury, tumor, or stroke
- Alcohol withdrawal, drug abuse, or overdose

Epilepsy, on the other hand, is an underlying condition (or permanent brain injury) that affects the delicate systems that govern how electrical energy behaves in the brain, making it susceptible to recurring seizures.

Most people with seizures have idiopathic epilepsy; that is, the cause of the seizures is not known. Epilepsy is not a mental illness, and it is not a sign of low intelligence. It also is not contagious. Between seizures, a person with epilepsy can function as normally as a person who does not have epilepsy.

Recognizing Seizures

Many different types of seizures exist. People may experience just one type or more than one. The kind of seizure a person has depends on which part and how much of the brain is affected by the electrical disturbance that produces seizures. To simplify the many types of seizures, they can be divided into convulsive and nonconvulsive categories.

Convulsive seizures typically last for 1 to 2 minutes (but may last longer), and the person may experience the following signs and symptoms:

- Sudden falling to the floor or ground
- Stiffening of arm and leg muscles followed by jerky movement with arching of the back
- Foaming at the mouth
- Grinding of teeth
- Bluish-gray color of the face and lips

- Eyes roll upward
- Loss of bladder and bowel control

Nonconvulsive seizures last only a few seconds, and the person may experience the following signs and symptoms:

- Staring, confused, or inattentive
- Frequent eye blinking
- Involuntary movements (eg, lip smacking, picking at clothes, fumbling)

Nonconvulsive seizures are so brief that they often escape detection.

FYI

Knowledge of Epilepsy

A survey found that about half of all persons have witnessed an epileptic seizure either in person or on television; about one third of all persons know someone with epilepsy, but relatively few are familiar with epilepsy, how to respond to a seizure, or the Epilepsy Foundation.

Source: Kobau R, Price P. 2003. Knowledge of epilepsy and familiarity with this disorder in the U.S. population. *Epilepsia.* 44(11):1449-1454.

Status Epilepticus

Most seizures end after a few seconds or a few minutes. If they are prolonged, or occur in a series, it is called **status epilepticus**. This is an emergency situation and requires immediate medical care. Repeated, uncontrolled seizures can lead to brain damage, fractures, severe dehydration, and aspiration. In adults, the most common cause of status epilepticus is failure to take prescribed medicines for epilepsy.

CAUTION

DO NOT restrain the victim.

DO NOT put anything between the victim's teeth during the seizure.

DO NOT splash or pour water or any other liquid on the victim's face.

DO NOT move the victim to another place (unless it is the only way to protect the victim from injury).

DO NOT leave a victim until he or she is fully alert and recovered.

Caring for a Seizure

The following information is adapted from the Epilepsy Foundation and can be used for seizure victims with a known seizure disorder.

First Aid for a Convulsive Seizure

- Do not restrain or hold the person down or try to stop his or her movements.
- Clear the area around the person of anything hard or sharp. Remove glasses.
- Loosen ties, scarves, or anything around the neck that could interfere with breathing.
- Place something flat and soft, like a folded jacket, under the head.
- Turn him or her gently onto one side to help keep the airway open.
- Do not try to force the mouth open with any hard implement or with fingers. Efforts to hold the tongue down can injure the teeth or jaw. A person having a seizure cannot swallow his or her tongue.
- Stay with the person until the seizure ends naturally. Do not leave him or her alone until the person is fully conscious, alert, and able to speak normally.
- Ask if there is anyone who should be called to help him or her get home.
- Look for a medical ID (although its absence does not rule out a seizure).

This may not be a medical emergency, even though it looks like one. It stops naturally after a few minutes. The average person with a known seizure disorder who has a typical seizure should rest and then continue about his or her activities. The person will need limited assistance, if any, unless he or she needs to be driven home. People who have just seized should not be permitted to drive. If this is a person's first seizure or if it represents a change in a person's seizure disorder (eg, more frequent, different kind), call 9-1-1.

First Aid for a Nonconvulsive Seizure

- Watch the person carefully and explain to others what is happening. They may think that the dazed person is drunk or on drugs.
- Guide the person gently away from any danger (eg, steps, highway, hot stove). Do not grab and hold them because they may struggle or lash out.
- Stay with the victim until he or she has fully recovered.

When to Call 9-1-1

- A seizure lasts more than 5 minutes.
- A second seizure starts soon after the first has ended.
- Alertness does not start to return after shaking has stopped.

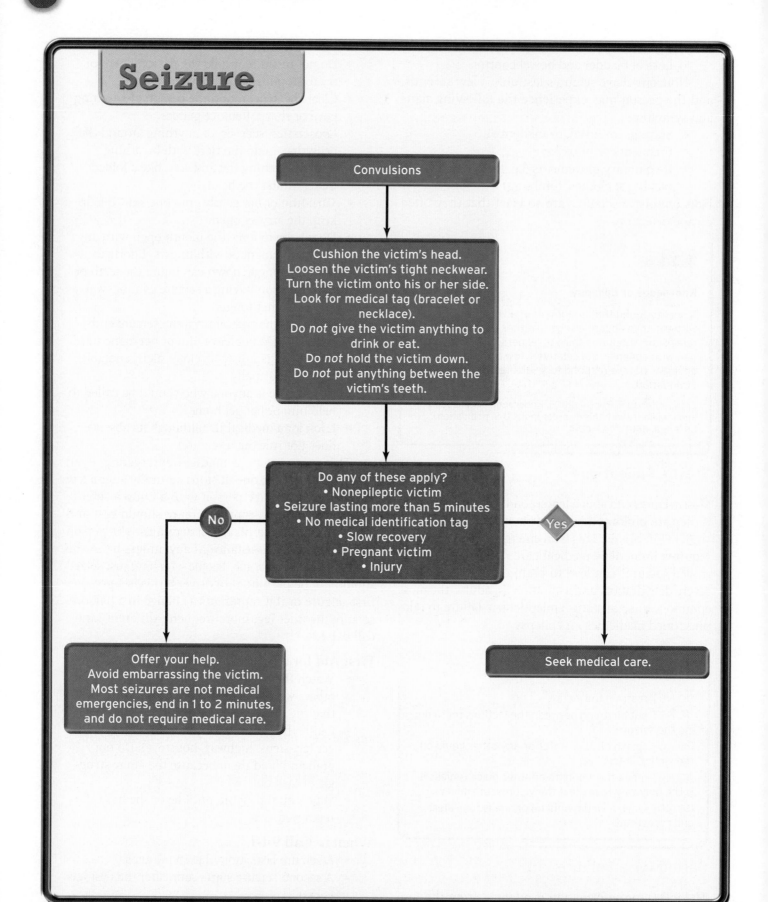

Seizure

Convulsions

Cushion the victim's head.
Loosen the victim's tight neckwear.
Turn the victim onto his or her side.
Look for medical tag (bracelet or necklace).
Do *not* give the victim anything to drink or eat.
Do *not* hold the victim down.
Do *not* put anything between the victim's teeth.

Do any of these apply?
• Nonepileptic victim
• Seizure lasting more than 5 minutes
• No medical identification tag
• Slow recovery
• Pregnant victim
• Injury

No

Yes

Offer your help.
Avoid embarrassing the victim.
Most seizures are not medical emergencies, end in 1 to 2 minutes, and do not require medical care.

Seek medical care.

- The seizure happened in water.
- The victim is injured (eg, bleeding from the head, unequal pupils, vomiting), diabetic, or pregnant.
- No medical identification tag is found, and there is no way of knowing whether the seizure is caused by epilepsy.
- The victim has never had a seizure before.

FYI

Seizures in Medical TV Dramas

About half the time, the doctors and nurses on popular fictional TV medical shows give improper seizure first aid that, in reality, could lead to broken teeth, bruises, or dislocations, according to a study presented at the American Academy of Neurology's annual meeting.

In the study, around 280 hours of recent medical dramas were watched, and when a clip showing a seizure was found, it was reviewed and compared with the Epilepsy Foundation's first aid guidelines for seizures. Fifty-nine seizures were found, and 46% of the actions by the doctor and nurse actors were considered inappropriate. They noted such poor medical actions as holding a patient down, attempting to stop involuntary movement, and putting something in a patient's mouth while a seizure was in progress. In about 29% of the cases, the action was medically correct. The remaining seizure incidents were on the screen too briefly to judge.

Source: Moeller A, et al. Depiction of seizure first aid management in medical television drama. American Academy of Neurology. Abstract 1105. http://www.medpagetoday.com/tbprint.cfm?tbid=18468

▶ Diabetic Emergencies

Insulin is a hormone produced by the pancreas that assists the body in using energy from food **Figure 17-8**. Insulin takes glucose from the blood and then carries it into the cells where it is used. When excess glucose remains in the blood and is not transferred to the cells, they must rely on fat for fuel. Because blood glucose is a major source of fuel used by the body, when it cannot be used it will build up in the blood. The blood glucose then overflows into the urine, passing through the body unused and discarded. When this occurs, a condition called <u>diabetes</u> develops **Table 17-5**. Insulin is either ineffective or lacking in the body. Diabetes is not contagious and in most cases special diet and/or medication can control it.

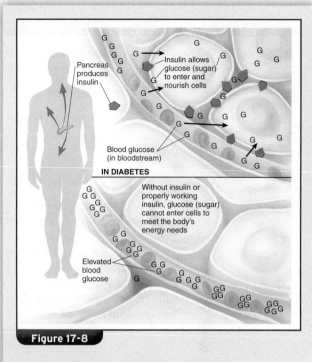

Figure 17-8

Normal metabolism (top) and diabetes (bottom).

The body is continuously balancing glucose and insulin. Too much insulin and not enough glucose leads to low blood glucose and possibly insulin reaction. Insulin reaction results from severe low blood glucose, causing unconsciousness and possibly death. Too much glucose and not enough insulin leads to high blood glucose, the production of ketones, and possibly diabetic coma. Ketones cause a sweet or fruity odor on the breath.

Types of Diabetes

Type 1 Diabetes

Type 1 diabetes (formerly called juvenile-onset or insulin-dependent diabetes) is most commonly diagnosed in childhood, but it may present at any age in life. About 2 million of the individuals with diabetes have type 1 diabetes. This type of diabetes requires external insulin (not made by the body), which enables the glucose to enter the cells. External insulin is necessary because the body is unable to produce the insulin the cells require. When a person with type 1 diabetes is deprived of external insulin, he or she will become very ill. Type 1 diabetics will usually be thin or not overweight.

Table 17-5 Diabetic Emergencies

	Diabetic Coma (high blood glucose)	Insulin Shock (low blood glucose)
Cause	Not enough insulin; too much glucose	Too much insulin; not enough glucose
Insulin level	Insufficient	Excessive
Onset of symptoms	Gradual	Sudden
Skin	Flushed, dry, warm	Pale, clammy
Breath	Fruity odor	Normal
Thirst	Severe	Normal
Urination	Frequent	Normal
Behavior	Normal to disorientation, drowsiness, and change in mood	Appearance of intoxication: combativeness, bad temper, anger, confusion, disorientation
Other symptoms	Drowsiness, vomiting, heavy breathing, eventual stupor or unconsciousness	Sudden hunger, eventual stupor, or unresponsiveness
First aid	• If in doubt, give sugar. • Give fluids to fight dehydration. • Take victim to hospital.	Give sugar. Seek medical care.

Type 2 Diabetes

Type 2 diabetes used to be known as non-insulin-dependent or adult-onset diabetes. The incidence of type 2 diabetes is reaching epidemic proportions in the United States. More than 21 million people currently have type 2 diabetes. Excess body weight and a sedentary lifestyle are widely recognized risk factors, especially because type 2 diabetes is being diagnosed in a growing number of children and adolescents. Other risk factors include a family history of type 2 diabetes and age older than 45 years. The age of onset is usually over the age of 40 years, but it can occur at any age. This type of diabetes may require insulin replacement and other medication.

Gestational Diabetes

Gestational diabetes occurs in some pregnancies. It usually ends after a baby is born, but when women who had gestational diabetes get older, type 2 diabetes can develop. Gestational diabetes results from the body's resistance to the action of insulin. This resistance is caused by hormones produced during pregnancy. Gestational diabetes is usually treated with diet, but some women need insulin.

Recognizing Low Blood Glucose (Hypoglycemia)

The condition of low blood glucose, called hypoglycemia, is sometimes referred to as an insulin reaction.

This condition occurs in a diabetic for several reasons: too much insulin, too little or delayed food intake, exercise, alcohol, or any combination of these factors.

The American Diabetes Association lists the following signs and symptoms in insulin reaction and hypoglycemia as diabetic emergencies requiring first aid:

- Sudden onset
- Staggering, poor coordination, clumsiness
- Anger, bad temper
- Pale face color
- Confusion, disorientation
- Sudden hunger
- Excessive sweating
- Trembling, shakiness
- Seizure
- Eventual unconsciousness

Care for Low Blood Glucose (Hypoglycemia)

The best course of action is giving sugar to the victim using the rule of 15s.

1. The diabetic should check his or her blood glucose. If it is not within a proper range, he or she should eat 15 g of sugar. If the diabetic is not able to test his or her blood glucose, and you strongly suspect that the victim has

Table 17-6 Fast-Acting Sugar (10 to 15 grams)

- Two to five glucose tablets
- One tube of glucose gel
- 4 oz of regular soda (not diet)
- 4 oz of orange or apple juice
- 2 Tbsp of raisins
- Five to seven Lifesavers candy
- 6 to 8 oz of skim or 1% milk
- Two tsp of honey or corn syrup

low blood glucose, give the victim 10 to 15 g of fast-acting sugar if all the following conditions are present (Table 17-6):

- The victim is a known diabetic.
- The victim's mental status is not altered.
- The victim is alert enough to swallow.

2. Wait 15 minutes for the sugar to get into the blood.
3. If the diabetic is able, check the blood glucose level again. If it is still low, he or she should consume 15 more grams of sugar. If testing is not available, and there is no improvement in 15 minutes, give the victim 15 more grams of sugar.
4. If there is no improvement, seek immediate medical care.

If the victim is or becomes unresponsive, call 9-1-1 immediately. In all cases, seek medical care following a diabetic episode and advise the victim's physician of the incident. Hypoglycemia can be a life-threatening emergency.

Another emergency procedure uses an injected medication called glucagon, available by a physician's prescription, to raise blood glucose quickly. Glucagon works the opposite of insulin. It mobilizes glucose stored in the muscles and liver as glycogen. Be aware that many people vomit after receiving glucagon. A family member or friend should learn when and how to inject glucagon in an emergency.

Recognizing High Blood Glucose (Diabetic Coma, Hyperglycemia)

The opposite reaction of hypoglycemia is called diabetic coma or **hyperglycemia**. This condition occurs when a diabetic has too much glucose in their blood. There are several scenarios that can cause this medical condition, such as insufficient insulin, overeating, illness, inactivity, stress, or a combination of these factors.

The American Diabetes Association lists the following signs and symptoms as warranting first aid in the case of a diabetic emergency involving hyperglycemia and diabetic coma:

- Gradual onset
- Drowsiness
- Extreme thirst
- Very frequent urination
- Flushed skin
- Vomiting
- Fruity breath odor
- Heavy breathing
- Eventual unconsciousness

Care for High Blood Glucose (Diabetic Coma, Hyperglycemia)

If you are uncertain whether the victim has a high or low blood glucose level and the victim is responsive and able to drink, give him or her a beverage or food containing sugar. If there is no improvement in the victim's condition within 15 minutes, seek medical care immediately.

FYI

Summary of the Rule of 15s for Low Blood Glucose

The diabetic should check his or her blood glucose level. If it is not within the appropriate range, he or she should eat 15 g of sugar, wait 15 minutes, check the blood glucose again and, if low, eat 15 more grams of sugar, wait 15 minutes and check the blood glucose again. If still low, seek immediate medical care.

Q&A

How can you tell the difference between hypoglycemia (insulin reaction) and hyperglycemia (diabetic coma)?

It is difficult to determine whether a person has hypoglycemia or hyperglycemia. Sugar helps the person with hypoglycemia, but not the person with hyperglycemia. However, do not debate whether to give sugar; sugar will cause no harm in either condition.

Ask the diabetic two questions: "Have you eaten today?" and "Have you taken your insulin today?" If the diabetic has taken his or her insulin but has not eaten, suspect hypoglycemia. If the diabetic has eaten but has not taken insulin, suspect hyperglycemia. If you are unsure which condition exists, give sugar.

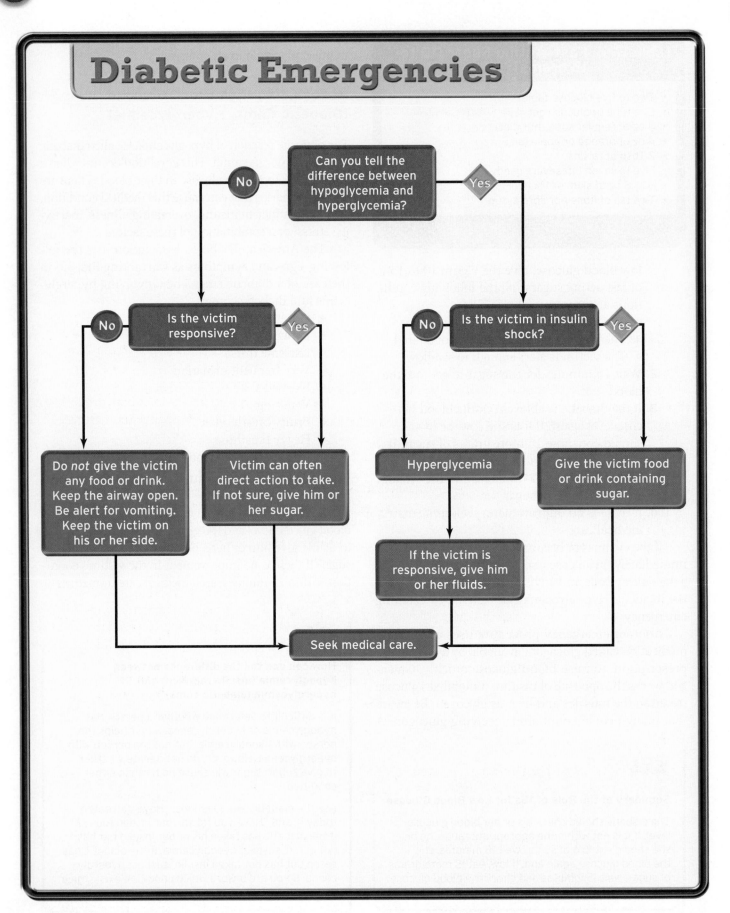

Diabetic Emergencies

No ← Can you tell the difference between hypoglycemia and hyperglycemia? → **Yes**

No ← Is the victim responsive? → **Yes**

No ← Is the victim in insulin shock? → **Yes**

Do *not* give the victim any food or drink. Keep the airway open. Be alert for vomiting. Keep the victim on his or her side.

Victim can often direct action to take. If not sure, give him or her sugar.

Hyperglycemia

Give the victim food or drink containing sugar.

If the victim is responsive, give him or her fluids.

Seek medical care.

▶ Abdominal Complaints

People with gastrointestinal problems usually complain about one or more of the following symptoms:

- **Abdominal pain that is aching, cramping, sharp, or dull.** It might be constant, or it can come and go. The pain could indicate a mild problem or an acute problem requiring immediate surgery.
- **Nausea and vomiting.** Vomiting is the ejection of the stomach's contents through the mouth. Nausea is a feeling of the need to vomit.
- **Diarrhea or constipation.** Diarrhea is the frequent passage of loose, watery stools. Constipation is the opposite of diarrhea; stools are infrequent, hard, and difficult to pass.

▶ Abdominal Pain

The abdomen is the area between the diaphragm and the groin. Abdominal organs are either hollow or solid. Hollow organs are tubes, such as the stomach and the intestines, through which material passes, conducting food through the body. Solid organs are solid masses of tissue in which much of the chemical work of the body takes place. The liver, spleen, and gallbladder are solid organs. The peritoneum is a thin membrane lining the entire abdominal cavity. Inflammation of the peritoneum is called peritonitis.

There are many possible causes of abdominal pain—some not so serious and some life threatening. They often can be serious enough to require emergency surgery.

Abdominal problems are so difficult to diagnose that even skilled physicians can have trouble pinpointing an exact cause. It is neither feasible nor useful for a first aider to distinguish among the many causes of abdominal pain because first aid usually will be similar regardless of the cause.

Recognizing Abdominal Pain

A first aider should ask the following questions:

- When did the pain start? Where is it located?
- Is the pain constant, or does it come and go? Constant pain can be more serious than a cramping pain. Constant abdominal pain suggests inflammation of an organ; cramping suggests obstruction of a hollow organ.
- Does belching or passing gas relieve the pain? If so, the intestine might be affected.
- Does the victim feel nauseated, or does he or she have a good appetite?
- Is there diarrhea or vomiting?
- Does the victim feel warm (feverish)?
- Does anyone near the victim have similar symptoms?
- For a female, is there any chance of pregnancy? Any pain with pregnancy should be treated as an emergency.
- Is the abdomen rigid to the touch? A rigid abdomen can be a sign of an emergency condition.

Care for Abdominal Pain

Care for people with abdominal complaints includes the following:

1. Give the victim only clear fluids (anything you can see through, except alcohol and caffeinated beverages). Have the victim slowly sip the fluids.
2. Give the victim an antacid.
3. If practical, place a hot-water bottle against the victim's abdomen or have the victim soak in a warm bath.
4. Recognize the possibility of vomiting and be prepared for it. Keep the victim on the left side to help prevent vomiting.
5. Keep the victim in a comfortable position, usually lying down with knees bent (unless the victim is nauseated).
6. Seek medical care if any of the following applies:
   - Pain is constant and severe.
   - The victim is unable to drink fluids.
   - The victim is or might be pregnant.
   - The abdomen is rigid and painful.
   - The abdomen is swollen.
   - More pain occurs after you press your fingers on the victim's abdomen and suddenly release them.

CAUTION

DO NOT give enemas and laxatives, which can worsen the condition or cause complications such as ruptured bowel.

DO NOT give fluids other than clear fluids as long as the pain continues.

DO NOT give solid foods.

DO NOT give milk products.

- There is bloody, blood-stained, or black stool or vomit.
- The victim has a fever.
- There is lightheadedness or fainting.
- Pain began around the belly button and later moved to the lower right part of the abdomen. This is a sign of appendicitis.

▶ Nausea and Vomiting

Nausea (upset stomach) and vomiting (throwing up) often occur with conditions such as mild altitude sickness, motion sickness, brain injury, intestinal viruses, eating or drinking too much, and being emotionally upset. In minor illnesses, nausea and vomiting should clear up in a day. Persistent nausea and vomiting can signal more serious illnesses such as appendicitis, food poisoning, or bowel obstruction. In general, if the condition lasts longer than 1 or 2 days, or if the victim vomits multiple times in a short period, the victim could become dehydrated (lose too much fluid). Young children and elderly people can be more seriously affected.

Recognizing Nausea and Vomiting

First aiders should determine the answers to the following questions:
- Is there abdominal pain?
- Is there blood or brown, grainy material in the vomit?
- Is there diarrhea? Vomiting and diarrhea together usually indicate a self-limited viral infection.
- Are there signs of dehydration (for example, the victim is dizzy when standing; has dry, cracked lips; is very thirsty)?
- Does anyone else near the victim have similar symptoms?
- Has the victim had a recent head injury?

Care for Nausea and Vomiting

Caring for someone with nausea and vomiting includes the following steps:
1. Give the victim small amounts of clear fluids (eg, sports drinks, clear soups, flat decaffeinated soda, apple or cranberry juice), except alcohol and caffeinated beverages.
2. If the victim is able to keep fluids down, offer carbohydrates (eg, bread, cereal, pasta)

first—they are easier to digest. Avoid milk products and meats for 48 hours.
3. Have the victim rest and avoid exertion until he or she is able to eat solid foods easily.
4. Prevent inhalation of vomit by positioning the victim on his or her side to allow drainage. Inhaled vomit can result in severe pneumonia.
5. Seek medical care if:
   - Blood or brown, grainy material appears in the vomit.
   - There is constant abdominal pain.
   - The victim faints when standing.
   - The victim is unable to keep fluids down for more than 24 hours.
   - The victim has severe, projectile vomiting (vomit shoots out in large quantities).
   - The vomiting follows a recent head injury.

Recognizing Motion Sickness

Signs of motion sickness include:
- Nausea
- Pale skin
- Cold sweats
- Vomiting
- Dizziness
- Headache
- Fatigue

Care for Motion Sickness

1. If the victim is prone to motion sickness, he or she should sit near the midsection of a plane, boat, bus, train, or car. People susceptible to motion sickness should not read; should look far ahead to the horizon, not to the sides; and should avoid overeating.
2. A person prone to motion sickness should try taking an antihistamine 1 hour before traveling (follow label directions).

▶ Diarrhea

Diarrhea is the passage of loose, watery, or unformed stools (usually more than four times a day). Diarrhea can be a symptom of intestinal infection (bacterial, viral, or parasitic), food poisoning, or food sensitivity or allergy, among other ailments. Dehydration can occur if the body loses too much fluid through the stool and the victim cannot drink enough fluid to keep up with the fluid losses from the diarrhea. Elderly and very young people are especially prone to dehydration, which can result in dangerous chemical imbalances. Replacing fluids and electrolytes such as sodium and potassium is of primary importance for any person with diarrhea. Diarrhea flushes bacteria and parasites out of the body. Letting diarrhea run its course is best because then bacteria or parasites are not trapped in the intestines.

Recognizing Diarrhea

First aiders treating persons with diarrhea should determine the answers to the following questions:

- Was the victim recently exposed to untreated, possibly contaminated water or food?
- Is there blood or mucus in the stool? Their presence can signal more serious problems.
- Are there signs of dehydration (for example, the victim is dizzy when standing; has dry, cracked lips; is very thirsty)?
- Does the victim have cramping abdominal pain?
- Does the victim lose bowel control (sometimes)?
- Is the victim feverish (sometimes)?
- Does anyone else near the victim have similar symptoms?

Care for Diarrhea

Care for people with diarrhea includes the following steps:

1. Have the victim drink lots of clear fluids (8 to 10 eight-oz glasses daily). This is the single most important treatment.
2. When the victim can tolerate clear fluids, give mild foods such as soup and gelatin. Later, the BRAT diet—bananas, rice, applesauce, toast—is recommended.
3. Bismuth can help in most cases (follow label directions). Be aware that bismuth can turn the stool and the tongue black. People sensitive to aspirin should not use it. If the person cannot let the diarrhea run its course, over-the-counter medications will calm the bowel, reducing movement of food through the intestines.
4. Seek medical care if:
   - The victim has bloody stools, which might appear black. (Keep in mind that bismuth preparations can cause black stools.)
   - There is no improvement after 24 hours.
   - The victim has a fever.
   - The victim has severe, constant abdominal pain.
   - The victim is severely dehydrated.

CAUTION

DO NOT give milk products and meats for 48 hours after diarrhea stops.

DO NOT give caffeine, which stimulates the intestine and causes urination, furthering dehydration.

DO NOT give excessive amounts of sugary beverages.

▶ Constipation

Constipation is the passage of hard, dry stools. Most physicians define constipation as two or fewer bowel movements a week, of which 25% require straining. Constipation is rarely more than a passing discomfort in otherwise healthy people. Normal bowel movements can occur three times a day or once every 3 days. Minor changes in diet, fluid intake, activity, or emotional state can cause bowel movement changes. Rectifying any of those changes will also relieve constipation in most cases. Bowel stimulants or laxatives are rarely needed.

Recognizing Constipation

The following are signs of constipation:

- **Bloating sensation of abdomen.** A very painful or visibly swollen abdomen is a more serious problem than simple constipation.
- **Hard, dry stools.** Small strings of blood are not unusual if the stool was painful to evacuate.

Care for Constipation

Care for those with constipation includes the following:

1. Have the victim eat more fiber (fresh or dried fruits, vegetables, bran). Fiber causes the colon to contract. Over-the-counter fiber products such as Metamucil and Citrucel can be used, but the label directions should be followed.
2. Make sure the victim drinks plenty of fluids (8 to 10 eight-oz glasses daily). Excessively

hard stools often are the result of dehydration.

3. Encourage the victim to remain active. Activity such as walking stimulates colon contractions.

4. If there is no improvement, try one of the following:
   - A stool softener (docusate sodium)
   - Caffeine, which stimulates colon contractions

5. Seek medical care if the victim experiences any of the following:
   - Severe abdominal pain
   - Visibly swollen or very painful abdomen
   - Fever
   - Vomiting

CAUTION

DO NOT give laxatives such as Epsom salts to people with severe abdominal pain or vomiting.

DO NOT give alcohol.

DO NOT give binding foods, such as bananas, cheese, and applesauce.

▶ Emergency Care Wrap-up

Condition	What to Look For	What to Do
Heart Attack	• Chest pressure, squeezing, or pain • Pain spreading to shoulders, neck, jaw, or arms • Dizziness, sweating, nausea • Shortness of breath	1. Help victim take his or her prescribed medication. 2. Call 9-1-1. 3. Help victim into a comfortable position. 4. Give one adult or two children's aspirin. 5. Monitor breathing.
Angina	• Chest pain similar to a heart attack • Pain seldom lasts longer than 10 minutes	1. Have victim rest. 2. If victim has his or her own nitroglycerin, help the victim use it. 3. If pain continues beyond 10 minutes, suspect a heart attack and call 9-1-1.
Stroke	• Sudden weakness or numbness of the face, an arm, or a leg on one side of the body • Blurred or decreased vision • Problems speaking • Dizziness or loss of balance • Sudden, severe headache	1. Call 9-1-1. 2. If responsive, help victim into a comfortable position with head and shoulders slightly raised. 3. If unresponsive, move onto his or her side.
Breathing Difficulty	• Abnormally fast or slow breathing • Abnormally deep or shallow breathing • Noisy breathing • Bluish lips • Need to pause while speaking to catch breath	**Unknown Reason** 1. Help victim into a comfortable position. 2. Call 9-1-1. **Asthma Attack** 1. Help victim into a comfortable position. 2. Help victim use inhaler. 3. Call 9-1-1 if victim does not improve. **Hyperventilation** 1. Encourage victim to inhale, hold breath a few seconds, then exhale. 2. Call 9-1-1 if condition does not improve.
Hyperventilation	• Fast breathing (> 40 breaths per minute)	1. Calm and reassure victim. 2. Inhale slowly through nose, hold for 1–2 seconds, exhale slowly through pursed lips.
COPD	• Similar to asthma—wheeze, cough, short of breath	1. Help in taking prescribed medicine. 2. Place in comfortable sitting position. 3. Drink clear fluids. 4. Might need medical care for oxygen.
Fainting	• Sudden, brief unresponsiveness • Pale skin • Sweating	1. Check breathing. 2. Check for injuries if victim fell. 3. Consider raising feet 6 to 12 inches. 4. Call 9-1-1 if needed.

▶ Emergency Care Wrap-up

Condition	What to Look For	What to Do
Seizures	• Sudden falling • Unresponsiveness • Rigid body and arching of back • Jerky muscle movement	1. Prevent injury. 2. Loosen any tight clothing. 3. Roll victim onto his or her side. 4. Call 9-1-1 if needed.
Diabetic Emergencies	**Low blood glucose** • Develops very quickly • Anger, bad temper • Hunger • Pale, sweaty skin **High blood glucose** • Develops gradually • Thirst • Frequent urination • Fruity, sweet breath odor • Warm and dry skin	1. If uncertain about high or low blood glucose level, give sugar. 2. Repeat in 15 minutes if no improvement. 3. Call 9-1-1 if victim does not improve.
Abdominal Pain	• Pain between the nipple line and groin	1. Give clear fluids. 2. Give antacid. 3. Soak in warm bath or apply hot-water bottle against abdomen. 4. Keep in comfortable position.
Nausea and Vomiting	• Upset stomach, throwing up food	1. Give small amount of clear fluids. 2. When able to keep down fluids, offer carbohydrates (ie, bread, cereal, pasta).
Diarrhea	• Loose, watery stools	1. Drink lots of clear fluids. 2. Give mild foods. 3. Give bismuth (follow label's directions).
Constipation	• Hard, dry stools	1. Eat more fiber. 2. Drink more fluids.

▶ Ready for Review

- A heart attack occurs when the heart muscle tissue dies because its blood supply is reduced or stopped.
- Angina pectoris can result from coronary heart disease just as a heart attack does.
- A stroke occurs when part of the blood flow to the brain is suddenly cut off.
- Asthma is chronic, inflammatory lung disease characterized by repeated breathing problems. Hyperventilation is fast, deep breathing and is common during emotional stress.
- Chronic obstructive pulmonary disease (COPD) is a broad term applied to emphysema, chronic bronchitis, and related lung diseases.
- Fainting is a sudden brief loss of responsiveness not associated with head injury.
- A seizure results from an abnormal stimulation of the brain's cells causing uncontrollable muscle movements.
- Diabetes is a condition in which insulin is lacking or ineffective.
- Hypoglycemia is very low blood glucose and can be caused by too much insulin, too little or delayed food intake, exercise, alcohol, or a combination of these factors.
- Hyperglycemia occurs when the body has too much glucose in the blood and can be caused by insufficient insulin, overeating, inactivity, illness, stress, or a combination of these factors.
- People with gastrointestinal problems usually report pain, nausea, vomiting, diarrhea, or constipation.
- Nausea (upset stomach) and vomiting (throwing up) often occur with conditions such as mild altitude sickness, motion sickness, brain injury, intestinal viruses, eating or drinking too much, and being emotionally upset.
- Diarrhea is the frequent passage of loose, watery, or unformed stools and can be a symptom of intestinal infection, food poisoning, food allergy, or other ailments.
- Constipation is the passage of hard, dry stools and is rarely more than a passing discomfort in otherwise healthy people.

▶ Vital Vocabulary

angina pectoris A spasmodic pain in the chest, characterized by a sensation of severe constriction or pressure on the anterior chest; associated with insufficient blood supply to the heart, aggravated by exercise or tension, and relieved by rest or medication.

asthma A condition marked by recurrent attacks of breathing difficulty, often with wheezing, due to spasmodic constriction of the air passages, often as a response to allergens or to mucus plugs in the bronchioles.

diabetes A condition that develops when glucose builds up in the blood, overflows into the urine, and passes through the body unused.

heart attack Lay term for a condition resulting from blockage of a coronary artery and subsequent death of part of the heart muscle; an acute myocardial infarction; sometimes called simply a coronary.

hyperglycemia An abnormally increased concentration of glucose in the blood.

hypoglycemia An abnormally diminished concentration of glucose in the blood.

psychogenic shock A shock-like state due to severe emotional distress; may result in a fainting spell resulting from a transient decrease in blood flow to the brain.

seizure Generalized, uncoordinated muscular activity associated with a loss of responsiveness; a convulsion; an attack of epilepsy.

status epilepticus The occurrence of two or more seizures without a period of complete consciousness between them.

stroke A brain injury due to bleeding in the brain tissue or to a blockage of blood flow, causing permanent damage.

syncope Fainting; a brief period of unresponsiveness.

prep kit

▶ Assessment in Action

You are on a 5-day backpack trip in the mountains with your friends. On day three, and after several tough miles into the hike, your friend seems to be disoriented and is stumbling over rocks and tree roots on the trail. He falls to the ground and is responsive. You know that this friend has type 1 diabetes and did take his insulin in the morning.

Directions: Circle Yes if you agree with the statement; circle No if you disagree.

Yes   No   **1.** This person is very likely suffering from hyperglycemia.

Yes   No   **2.** Low blood glucose levels can be caused by too much insulin, too little or delayed food intake, exercise, and alcohol.

Yes   No   **3.** To give sugar in this scenario, the victim must be a known diabetic, have an altered mental status, and must be awake enough to swallow.

Yes   No   **4.** You should follow the rule of 15s when giving sugar to the victim in this scenario.

▶ Check Your Knowledge

Directions: Circle Yes if you agree with the statement; circle No if you disagree.

Yes   No   **1.** Heart attack victims can experience chest pain.

Yes   No   **2.** You can help the victim of chest pain take his or her nitroglycerin.

Yes   No   **3.** A responsive stroke victim should lie down with his or her head slightly raised.

Yes   No   **4.** Asthma victims may have a prescribed inhaler.

Yes   No   **5.** A victim who is breathing fast (hyperventilation) should be encouraged to breathe slowly by holding inhaled air for several seconds and then exhaling slowly.

Yes   No   **6.** Immobilize the spine of a victim having a seizure.

Yes   No   **7.** Some seizure victims display a rigid arching of the back.

Yes   No   **8.** A person having seizures always requires medical attention.

Yes   No   **9.** If in doubt about the type of diabetic emergency a victim is experiencing, give sugar to a responsive victim who can swallow.

Yes   No   **10.** Nitroglycerin can relieve chest pain associated with angina.

Poisoning

Poison

▶ What Is a Poison?

The American Association of Poison Control Centers defines a **poison** (also known as a toxin) as anything that can harm someone if it is: (1) used in the wrong way, (2) used by the wrong person, or (3) used in the wrong amount.

Poisons can be classified by how they enter the body:

- Ingested (swallowed)—through the mouth
- Inhaled (breathed)—through the lungs
- Injected—through needlelike device (eg, snake's fangs, bee's stinger)
- Absorbed (direct contact)—through the skin or eyes

Poisons come in four forms: solids (such as pain medicine pills or tablets), liquids (such as household cleaners, including bleach), sprays (such as spray cleaners), and gases (such as carbon monoxide [CO]).

Most consumer products are safe if label directions are followed, but some can be poisonous if used incorrectly. The most common poisons are not necessarily the most dangerous ones. Some of the more dangerous poisons that could be found in a home include the following:

- Antifreeze and windshield washer products
- Some medicines
- Corrosive cleaners such as drain openers, oven cleaners, toilet bowl cleaners, and rust removers
- Fuels such as kerosene, lamp oil, gasoline
- Pesticides

chapter
at a glance

- ▶ **Poison**

- ▶ **Alcohol Emergencies**

- ▶ **Drug Emergencies**

- ▶ **Carbon Monoxide Poisoning**

- ▶ **Plant-Induced Dermatitis: Poison Ivy, Poison Oak, and Poison Sumac**

Q&A

Are some poisons absorbed through the skin?

Chemical substances, including some medicines and poisons, are absorbed through the skin. Heavy metals such as mercury and lead pass through the skin and can result in chronic poisoning. Chlordane, malathion, and other pesticides cross the skin barrier and can cause acute and chronic problems. Cyanide readily absorbs through the skin and can be very deadly.

▶ Ingested (Swallowed) Poisons

Ingested poisoning occurs when the victim swallows a toxic substance. Fortunately, most poisons have little toxic effect or are ingested in such small amounts that severe poisoning rarely occurs. However, the potential for severe or fatal poisoning is always present. About 80% of all poisonings happen by ingesting a toxic substance.

Swallowing nonfood substances is so common among children that it is unusual for a child to reach the age of 5 years without ingesting a nonfood substance at least once. Although many nonfood substances such as dirt and paper are not harmful, others present definite health threats. Some have the potential to block the airway. Others are poisonous. Hundreds of thousands of poisonings occur in the United States each year, but only a small percentage progress to severe or life-threatening conditions. Over 50% of all poison cases occur in children younger than six years.

Analgesics (pain medications) account for the largest category of poisoning exposures. Basically, any substance that is accessible to a child is a potential poison. Analgesic products that contain acetaminophen, for example, are involved in poisoning incidents more often than other analgesics, not because acetaminophen is more toxic but because products that contain acetaminophen outsell products that contain other analgesics .

It is important not to confuse poisoning frequency with poisoning severity. Plants and mushrooms, for example, account for about 2.5% (about 65,000 cases) of the total poisoning exposures reported each year. However, plant and mushroom ingestion result in only 0.02% of serious poisonings and 1 death each year. Therefore, most exposures to plants are minor, with harmless effects. On the other hand, gun-blueing

Figure 18-1

Sources of poisons.

products (agents containing selenious acid that are used to maintain the blue color of gun barrels) were involved in 100 poisoning episodes and resulted in 4 deaths (death rate of 4%). So despite fewer episodes of exposure, the potential for harm is much greater. Fortunately, most poison ingestions involve products with minor toxic effects or amounts so small that severe poisoning rarely occurs **Table 18-1**.

Recognizing Ingested Poisoning

The following are signs of ingested poisoning:
- Abdominal pain and cramping
- Nausea or vomiting
- Diarrhea
- Burns, odor, or stains around and in the mouth

Table 18-1 Substances Most Frequently Involved in Human Exposures

Substance	Annual Number	Percentage of Total Exposures*
Analgesics	331, 123	13.3
Cosmetics/personal care products	224,884	9.0
Cleaning substances (household)	213,595	8.6
Sedatives/hypnotics/antipsychotics	165,539	6.6
Foreign bodies/toys/miscellaneous	130,244	5.2
Topical preparations	114,024	4.6
Antidepressants	102,510	4.1
Cold and cough preparations	98,636	4.0
Pesticides	93,998	3.8
Cardiovascular drugs	91,421	3.7
Antihistamines	89,287	3.6
Alcohols	86,588	3.5
Bites and envenomations	73,229	2.9
Antimicrobials	68,982	2.8
Vitamins	68,911	2.8
Plants	63,362	2.5
Hormones and hormone antagonists	58,274	2.3
Gastrointestinal preparations	57,667	2.3
Hydrocarbons	46,418	1.9
Stimulants and street drugs	46,411	1.9
Anticonvulsants	45,995	1.8
Chemicals	44,736	1.8
Arts/crafts/office supplies	38,940	1.6
Electrolytes and minerals	34,507	1.4
Fumes/gases/vapors	34,361	1.4

*Percentages are based on the total number of exposures (2,491,049)
Source: American Association of Poison Control Centers.

- Drowsiness or unconsciousness
- Seizure
- Poison container nearby

Care for Ingested Poisoning Victims

If you think someone has been poisoned:

1. Check the condition of the victim. Call 9-1-1 immediately if the person:
   - Has collapsed (is unresponsive)
   - Is having trouble breathing; monitor for breathing and, if absent, begin CPR
   - Has severe pain in the chest
   - Shows other life-threatening signs

2. Call **Poison Help** (1-800-222-1222) even if there are no signs of poisoning Figure 18-2 . Try to identify what poison is involved. If possible, bring its container to the phone.

3. A nurse, pharmacist, or other poison expert will answer your call. Be ready to tell the person:
   - The name of the product (found on the container's label)
   - The amount of product involved (eg, half the bottle, a dozen tablets)
   - How long ago the poison contacted the victim
   - The age and weight of the victim
   - What signs of poisoning you notice

Poison Help logo.

Figure 18-3

The left-side position delays the advance of the poison into the small intestine.

FYI

Poisoning: Where Can You Call for Help?

If someone swallows poison, do not call the hospital emergency department. Call the poison center. Researchers who made 156 test calls to 52 hospital emergency departments in Illinois found that the advice given was correct only 64% of the time. Calls to the same emergency department on different days for the same problem did not consistently produce the same advice. In contrast, poison centers gave correct advice in 17 (94%) of 18 test calls.

Source: Wigder H N, Erickson T, Morse T, Saporta V. 1995. Emergency department poison advice telephone calls. *Ann Emerg Med* 25:349-352.

CAUTION

DO NOT give water or milk to dilute poisons other than caustic or corrosive substances (acids and alkalis) unless told to do so by staff at a poison center. Fluids can dissolve a dry poison such as tablets or capsules more rapidly and fill up the stomach, forcing the stomach contents (the poison) into the small intestine, where it will be absorbed faster. Vomiting and aspiration could occur.

CAUTION

DO NOT gag or tickle the back of the victim's throat with a finger or a spoon handle. This method is usually ineffective in causing vomiting, and any vomiting produced is not very forceful.

DO NOT give dish soap, raw eggs, or mustard powder. They are not effective.

DO NOT use syrup of ipecac.

4. A poison expert will decide whether the person is in danger. The poison expert will give you the advice you need and may stay on the phone with you while you get help or call you later to follow up.
5. Most calls (about 70%) can be handled outside of a hospital. If you need a physician or an ambulance, the poison expert will tell you right away.
6. Place the victim on his or her left side (recovery position) . For ingested poisoning, the left side is best because it positions the end of the stomach where it enters the small intestine (pylorus) straight up. Gravity will delay (by as much as 2 hours) the advance of the poison into the small intestine, where absorption into the victim's circulatory system is faster. The side position also helps prevent aspiration (inhalation) into the lungs if vomiting begins.
7. Save poison containers, plants, and the victim's vomitus to help medical personnel identify the poison.

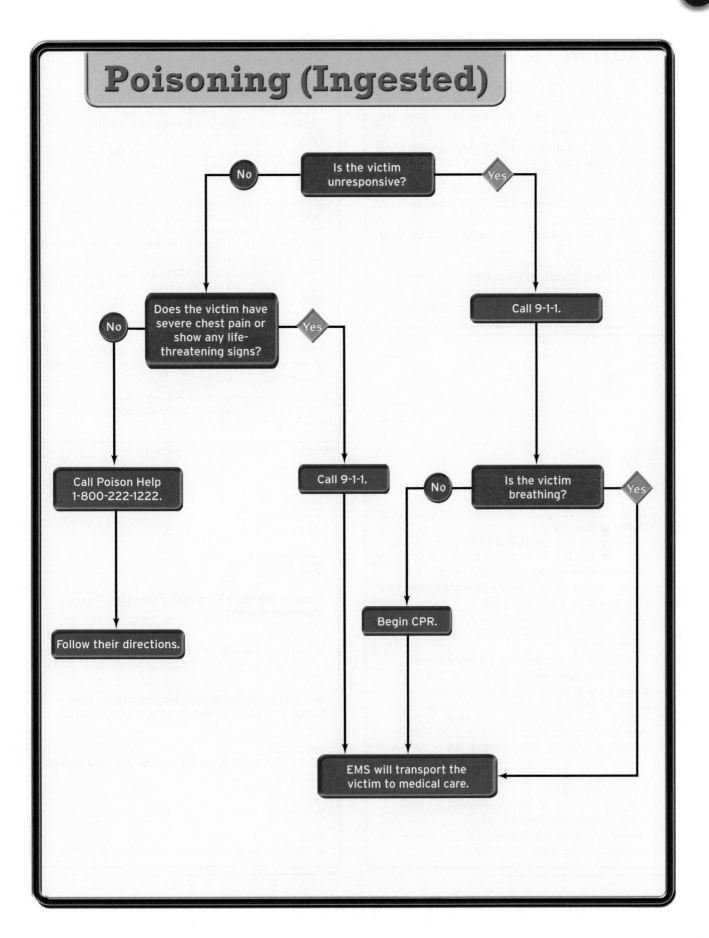

Poisoning (Ingested)

CAUTION

DO NOT follow the first aid procedures or recommendations on a container label without first getting confirmation from a medical source. Many labels are incorrect or out of date.

DO NOT try to neutralize a poison. Giving weak acids, such as lemon juice or vinegar, is not safe, contrary to the advice given on many drain cleaner and lye product labels. Chemical neutralization releases large quantities of heat that can burn sensitive tissues.

DO NOT think that a specific antidote exists for most poisons. An antidote is a substance that counteracts a poison's effects. Few poisons have specific antidotes that will effectively block their toxic effects.

DO NOT think that there is a universal antidote. No product is effective in treating most or all poisons.

FYI

Poison Center History

The idea for a poison center came from a part-time secretary at the American Academy of Pediatrics during the early 1950s. She called hospitals in Chicago to find out why children were in the emergency department with certain problems. What had they eaten? What did they drink?

At the time, companies did not have to tell people much about the ingredients in their products. The secretary asked companies what ingredients in their products might be making children sick. She then asked a group of medical professionals to set treatment guidelines. When doctors had questions, they would call her, and she would read medical advice to them off note cards.

Soon after, the US Surgeon General ordered copies of her 1,000 index cards to be sent to health departments across the country. From this, the first poison center was founded, and the idea spread throughout the nation.

Source: US Department of Health and Human Services http://www.poisonhelp.hrsa.gov/poison-centers/about-poison-centers/index.html

FYI

About Poison Control Centers

- Sixty accredited poison control centers exist in the United States.
- They provide free assistance by phone to anyone in the 50 states, Puerto Rico, The Federated States of Micronesia, American Samoa, and Guam.
- All centers can be reached by calling the same telephone number: 1-800-222-1222.
- Centers are staffed by pharmacists, physicians, nurses, and other poison experts who are toxicology specialists.
- All calls to a center are answered by a trained medical professional.
- About 70% of all the calls to a center about a potential poisoning are managed onsite and outside of a health care facility. This saves costly emergency department visits. The other 30% of the calls are from a health care facility requesting advice.
- All calls are kept confidential and can be translated into 161 languages.
- Calls are free and can be made 24 hours a day, 7 days a week, 365 days a year.
- They also provide educational outreach poison prevention programs.

FYI

Some of the More Frequently Ingested Plants (Common Names)

Philodendron
Symptoms: Burning sensation in lips, mouth, throat; contact dermatitis; remote risk of mouth and throat swelling

Dieffenbachia, Dumbcane, Mother-in-Law Plant
Symptoms: Same as philodendron, speech may be impaired

Poinsettia
Symptoms: Possible contact dermatitis, mild nausea, vomiting

Jade Plant
Symptoms: None

Holly
Symptoms: Nausea, persistent vomiting, diarrhea

Alcohol Emergencies

▶ Alcohol Intoxication

Alcohol is a depressant, not a stimulant. It affects a person's judgment, vision, reaction time, and coordination. In very large amounts, it can cause death by paralyzing the respiratory center of the brain.

Alcohol is the most commonly used and abused drug in the United States, possibly even the world. It is also one of the most lethal because it is implicated as a cofactor in up to 40% of drownings, over 40% of traffic deaths **Figure 18-4**, 67% of homicides, and 33% of suicides. It directly affects more than 12 million people annually (10% of all males and 3% of all females) and causes more than 200,000 deaths. Alcohol abuse is a major national health problem, ranking with heart disease and cancer. Lack of data makes it difficult to assess the actual number of alcohol-related injuries. It is estimated, however, that about 25% of the patients treated in hospital emergency departments were for intoxication alone. Nearly 50% of patients in trauma centers were injured while under the influence of alcohol.

Helping an intoxicated person is often difficult because the person could be belligerent and combative. However, it is important that people who abuse alcohol be helped and not labeled as drunks. Their condition can be quite serious, even life threatening.

Occasionally, a person will have consumed so much alcohol that there are signs of central nervous system depression. In such cases, complete respiratory support might be necessary. Death can result from the excessive consumption of alcohol.

The consumption of alcohol is deeply embedded in our society. Because of the widespread use of alcohol, people whose lives are affected directly or indirectly by alcohol abuse should be educated so they can recognize problems and know what to do in an emergency.

Recognizing Intoxication

Although the following signs indicate alcohol intoxication, some might also mean illness or injury other than alcohol abuse, such as diabetes or heat injury:

- The odor of alcohol on a person's breath or clothing
- Unsteady, staggering walking
- Slurred speech and the inability to carry on a conversation
- Nausea and vomiting
- Flushed face

Seizures can result from alcohol ingestion or alcohol withdrawal. Any seizures related to alcohol require medical evaluation. Diabetic coma can mimic alcohol intoxication, as can poisoning and neurologic problems.

Care for Intoxicated Individuals

First aid for an intoxicated person includes these steps:

1. Look for any injuries. Alcohol can mask pain.
2. Monitor breathing and treat accordingly.
3. If the intoxicated person is lying down, place him or her in the recovery (left-side) position to reduce the likelihood of vomiting and aspiration of vomit and to delay the absorption of alcohol into the bloodstream. Be sure to check that the victim is breathing and does not have a spinal injury before you move him or her. The recovery position can be used for responsive and unresponsive persons.
4. Call the poison center for advice or the local emergency number for help. It might be best to let EMS personnel decide whether the police should be alerted.
5. If the victim becomes violent, leave the scene and find a safe place until police arrive.
6. Provide emotional support.

Figure 18-4

Drunk driving test.

Preventing Poisoning

Follow these precautions to reduce the risk of poisoning:

1. Household products and medicines should be kept out of reach and out of sight of children, preferably in a locked cabinet or closet. When an adult who is using household products or taking medicine leaves the room, even briefly, he or she should move the containers to a safe place.
2. Medicines should be stored separately from other household products and kept in their original containers—never in cups or soft-drink bottles.
3 All products should be properly labeled, and the label should be read before use.
4. A light should be turned on when giving or taking medicine.
5. Because children tend to imitate adults, adults should avoid taking medications in their presence.
6. Medicines should be referred to by their correct names. Do not tell children that medicines are candy; they are not.
7. Use household substances in child-resistant packaging. Prescription medicines should be kept in safety packaging.

To avoid poisonings among elderly persons:

1. Always read the label and follow instructions when taking medicine.
2. Turn on a light at night when taking medicine.
3. Never mix medicines and alcohol, and never take more than the prescribed amount of medicine.
4. Do not borrow a friend's medicine or take old medicines.
5. Inform the physician what other medicines are being taken to avoid the risk of adverse drug interactions.

Source: US Consumer Product Safety Commission.

DO NOT let an intoxicated person sleep on his or her back.

DO NOT leave an intoxicated person alone unless he or she becomes violent.

DO NOT try to handle a hostile intoxicated person by yourself. Find a safe place, and then call the police for help.

---

7. Assume that an injured or unresponsive victim has a spinal injury and needs to be stabilized against movement. Because of decreased pain perception, an intoxicated victim cannot be assessed reliably. If you suspect a spinal injury, wait for EMS personnel to arrive. They have the proper equipment and training to stabilize and move a victim.

8. Because many intoxicated people have been exposed to the cold, suspect hypothermia (dangerously low body temperature) and move the person to a warm place whenever possible. Remove wet clothing and cover the person with warm blankets. Handle a hypothermic victim gently because rough handling could induce a deadly heart rhythm.

Drug Emergencies

Drugs are classified according to their effects on the user:

- Uppers are stimulants of the central nervous system. They include amphetamines, cocaine, and caffeine **Figure 18-5** .
- Downers (sedative-hypnotic) are depressants of the central nervous system. They include barbiturates, tranquilizers, marijuana, and narcotics **Figure 18-6** .
- Hallucinogens alter and often enhance the sensory and emotional information in the brain centers. They include LSD (lysergic acid diethylamide), mescaline, peyote, and PCP (phencyclidine hydrochloride, or angel dust). Marijuana also has some hallucinogenic properties.

Figure 18-5

Cocaine.

Figure 18-6

Marijuana.

- Volatile chemicals usually are inhaled and can cause serious damage to many body organs. They include plastic model glue and cement, paint solvent, gasoline, spray paint, and nail polish remover **Figure 18-7**.

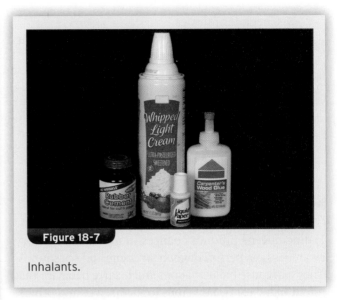

Figure 18-7

Inhalants.

▶ Sympathomimetics

Sympathomimetics are stimulants. A stimulant is any agent that produces an excited state. Amphetamine and methamphetamine (ice) are commonly taken by mouth. They are also injected in many cases. They typically are taken to make the user feel good, improve task performance, suppress appetite, or prevent sleepiness. Sympathomimetic drugs are frequently called uppers.

Cocaine can be taken in a number of different ways—through the nose, by injection, and by smoking. Crack is pure cocaine and is smoked. Smoked crack produces the most potent effect. Cocaine is one of the most addictive substances known.

Recognizing Sympathomimetic Use

Someone using sympathomimetics would exhibit the following characteristics:
- Disorganized behavior, hyperactivity, restlessness, and sometimes anxiety or great fear.
- Paranoia (which can put the user and others in danger) and delusions are common with abuse.

Care for Sympathomimetic Users

To care for someone who has used sympathomimetics, follow these steps:
1. Check breathing.
2. Call the poison center for advice or 9-1-1 for help.

3. Check for injuries.
4. Keep the person on the left side to reduce the likelihood of vomiting and aspiration of vomitus and to delay absorption of drugs.
5. Provide reassurance and emotional support.
6. If the person becomes violent, seek safety until the police arrive. Let law enforcement officers handle dangerous situations.
7. Seek medical care.

▶ Hallucinogens

Hallucinogens produce changes in mood and sensory awareness—a person might hear colors and see sounds. They can cause hallucinations and bizarre behavior that might make users dangerous to themselves and others. Acute cases need medical attention. Users should be protected from hurting themselves. The classic hallucinogen is lysergic acid diethylamide (LSD). Abuse of another hallucinogen, PCP, or angel dust, is dangerous because it causes severe behavioral changes.

Recognizing Hallucinogen Use

The user reports:
- Visual hallucinations.
- Intensity of both vision and hearing.

Care for Hallucinogen Use

To care for someone who has overdosed on hallucinogens, follow these steps:
1. Check breathing.
2. Call the poison center for advice or 9-1-1 for help.
3. Check for injuries.
4. Keep the person on the left side to reduce the likelihood of vomiting and aspiration of vomit and to delay absorption of drugs.
5. Provide reassurance and emotional support.
6. If the person becomes violent, seek safety until the police arrive. Let law enforcement officers handle dangerous situations.
7. Seek medical care.

▶ Marijuana

The flowering hemp plant called marijuana is abused throughout the world. It has been estimated that as many as 20 million people use marijuana daily in the United States.

Recognizing Marijuana Overdose

Keep the following in mind if you suspect a marijuana overdose.
- Inhaling produces euphoria, relaxation, and drowsiness.
- Short-term memory is impaired, as is capacity to do complex thinking and work.
- In some people, euphoria progresses to depression and confusion.
- Altered perception of time is common.
- Anxiety and panic can occur.
- Very high doses produce hallucinations.

Care for Marijuana Overdose Victims

To care for someone who has overdosed on marijuana, do the following:
1. Check breathing.
2. Call the poison center for advice or 9-1-1 for help.
3. Check for injuries.
4. Keep the person on the left side to reduce the likelihood of vomiting and aspiration of vomit and to delay absorption of drugs.
5. Provide reassurance and emotional support.
6. If the person becomes violent, seek safety until the police arrive. Let law enforcement officers handle dangerous situations.
7. Seek medical care.

▶ Depressants

Depressants are often prescribed as a part of legitimate medical treatment. They are easy to obtain. People sometimes solicit prescriptions from several physicians. This class of drug includes opiates (narcotics) and sedative-hypnotics (barbiturates and tranquilizers). Sedative-hypnotics are prescribed as anaesthetics, sedatives, and anti-anxiety treatments.

Recognizing Sedative-Hypnotic Drug Use

Effects of sedative-hypnotic drug overdose are similar to those of alcohol.

- Drowsiness and sleepiness
- Slurred speech
- Slow breathing rate

Opiates

The pain relievers called opiates are named for the opium in poppy seeds, the origin of heroin, codeine, and morphine. On the list of frequently abused drugs, they have been joined by a number of synthetic opiates that originated in a laboratory, with most of them having legitimate medical uses. With the exception of heroin, which is illegal in the United States, many addicts started using any of the opiates with an appropriate medical prescription.

Recognizing Opiates Overdose

Someone who has overdosed on opiates might exhibit the following signs:
- Reduced breathing rate
- Pinpoint pupils
- Sedated condition and unresponsiveness

Care for Depressant Overdose

To care for someone who has overdosed on a sedative-hypnotic drug, do the following:
1. Check breathing.
2. Call the poison center for advice or 9-1-1 for help.
3. Check for injuries.
4. Keep the person on the left side to reduce the likelihood of vomiting and aspiration of vomit and to delay absorption of drugs.
5. Provide reassurance and emotional support.
6. If the person becomes violent, seek safety until the police arrive. Let law enforcement officers handle dangerous situations.
7. Seek medical care.

▶ Abused Inhalants

Inhaling glue or other solvents (gasoline, lighter fluid, nail polish) produces effects similar to those from ingesting alcohol. Persons who sniff these substances can die of suffocation. In addition, some inhalants can cause death by changing the rhythm of the heartbeat and can cause permanent brain damage.

Recognizing Inhalant Abuse

Someone who has abused an inhalant might exhibit the following signs:
- Mild drowsiness to unresponsiveness
- Slurred speech and clumsiness
- Seizures
- Slow breathing rate
- Smell of solvents

Care for Inhalant Abuser

Someone who has abused an inhalant should be treated as follows:
1. Check breathing.
2. Call the poison center for advice or 9-1-1 for help.
3. Check for injuries.
4. Keep the person on the left side to reduce the likelihood of vomiting and aspiration of vomit and to delay absorption of drugs.
5. Provide reassurance and emotional support.
6. If the person becomes violent, seek safety until the police arrive. Let law enforcement officers handle dangerous situations.
7. Seek medical care.

Carbon Monoxide Poisoning

Carbon monoxide (CO), because of its common presence in our environment, along with its insidious nature, is the leading cause of poisoning death in the United States each year. Carbon monoxide is an odorless, colorless, nonirritating gas produced by the incomplete combustion of carbon-based fuels. According to a report from the Centers for Disease Control and Prevention, each year more than 500 Americans die of unintentional CO poisoning, and more than 2,000 commit suicide by intentionally poisoning themselves. CO poisoning sends 10,000 to the hospital annually.

People who ride long distances in older, poorly maintained cars are at increased risk. Rust is a major factor in damaging an automobile's exhaust system and creating holes in the car's body, through which CO can enter. Many deaths involve people sleeping inside a running car, often after alcohol consumption. Many deaths also involve parking in remote areas.

Persons in a closed room where there is cigarette smoking experience mild increases in the level of CO in their blood. Less familiar and, therefore, more dangerous sources of CO are faulty furnaces, water heaters, and kerosene heaters. Recreational fires, whether open-flame, charcoal, or hibachi grills, also give off CO.

Victims of CO poisoning are often unaware of its presence. The gas is invisible, tasteless, odorless, and nonirritating. It is produced by the incomplete burning of organic material such as gasoline, wood, paper, charcoal, coal, and natural gas.

FYI

Carbon Monoxide After Hurricane Katrina

Hurricane Katrina made landfall on August 29, 2005, on the Gulf Coast of the United States, causing loss of life, widespread property damage, and power outages. After hurricanes, some residents use portable generators and other gasoline-powered appliances for electrical power and cleanup. These devices produce carbon monoxide (CO), and improper use can cause CO poisoning. From August 29 through September 24, a total of 51 cases of CO poisoning were reported by hyperbaric oxygen facilities in Alabama, Louisiana, and Mississippi. CO poisoning can be prevented by reducing exposure to CO through appropriate placement and ventilation of gasoline-powered engines.

Source: CDC. *MMWR Morb Mortal Wkly Rep.* 2005. 54(39):996-998.

FYI

Carbon Monoxide Detectors Can Save Lives

The US Consumer Product Safety Commission recommends that consumers purchase and install CO detectors with labels showing they meet the requirements of the Underwriters Laboratories (UL) voluntary standard (UL 2034). The standard requires detectors to sound an alarm when the CO concentration reaches a potentially hazardous level.

Properly working CO detectors can provide an early warning before the deadly gas builds up to a dangerous level. Exposure to a low concentration during several hours can be as dangerous as exposure to a high carbon monoxide level for a few minutes. The detectors react to both conditions. Each home should have at least one CO detector in the area outside individual bedrooms. CO detectors are as important as smoke detectors to home safety.

Source: US Consumer Product Safety Commission. Carbon monoxide detectors can save lives. October 5, 2004. Available at: *http://www.cpsc.gov/CPSCPUB/PUBS/5010. html.* Accessed February 3, 2011.

Carbon monoxide causes hypoxia, or lack of oxygen, in two ways. First, the hemoglobin in red blood cells is about 200 times more likely to bind to CO than to oxygen if both are present in the blood; thus, even a small amount of CO can greatly reduce the amount of oxygen carried in the bloodstream. Second, CO does not allow the cells to use what little oxygen is delivered. In short, CO deprives the body parts that need oxygen the most—the heart and the brain.

Recognizing Carbon Monoxide Poisoning

It is difficult to determine whether a person is a victim of CO poisoning. Sometimes, a complaint of having the flu is really a symptom of CO poisoning. Although many symptoms of CO poisoning resemble those of the flu, there are differences. For example, CO poisoning does not cause low-grade fever or generalized aching or involve the lymph nodes.

The signs and symptoms of CO poisoning are as follows:

- Headache
- Ringing in the ears (tinnitus)
- Chest pain (angina)
- Muscle weakness
- Nausea and vomiting
- Dizziness and visual changes (blurred or double vision)
- Unresponsiveness
- Respiratory and cardiac arrest

The traditionally cited sign of CO poisoning is cherry-red skin and lips. This sign is uncommon, however, and occurs only at death; therefore, it is a poor initial indicator of CO poisoning. The following are earmarks of possible CO poisoning:

- The symptoms come and go.
- The symptoms worsen or improve in certain places or at certain times of the day.
- People around the victim have similar symptoms.
- Pets seem ill.

Care for Carbon Monoxide Poisoning Victims

1. Get the victim out of the toxic environment and into fresh air *immediately*.
2. Call 9-1-1, who will send EMS personnel who will be able to give the victim 100%

FYI

Carbon Monoxide Poisoning Deaths Associated With Camping

Exposure to CO is responsible for more fatal, unintentional poisonings in the United States than any other agent, with the highest incidence occurring during the cold-weather months. Although most of these deaths occur in residences or motor vehicles, two incidents among campers in Georgia illustrate the danger of CO in outdoor settings.

Case 1

A 51-year-old man, his 10-year-old son, a 9-year-old boy, and a 7-year-old girl were found dead inside a zipped-up, 10-foot by 14-foot, 2-room tent at their campsite in southeast Georgia (a pet dog also died). A propane gas stove, still burning, was found inside the tent; the stove apparently had been brought inside to provide warmth.

Case 2

A 34-year-old man and his 7-year-old son were found dead inside their zipped-up tent at a group camping site in central Georgia. They were discovered by other campers. A charcoal grill was found inside the tent; the grill apparently had been brought inside to provide warmth after it had been used outside for cooking.

During 1990 to 1994, in the United States, portable fuel-burning camp stoves and lanterns were involved in 10 to 17 CO poisoning deaths each year, and charcoal grills were involved in 15 to 27 deaths each year. During this same time, an annual average of 30 fatal CO poisonings occurred inside tents or campers.

Source: Centers for Disease Control and Prevention. *MMWR Morb Mortal Wkly Rep.* 2003. 48 (32):705-706.

oxygen, improving oxygenation and disassociating the linkage between the CO and the hemoglobin. For a responsive victim, it takes 4 to 5 hours with ordinary air (21% oxygen) or 30 to 40 minutes with 100% oxygen to reverse the effects of CO poisoning.

3. Monitor breathing.
4. Place an unresponsive breathing victim in the recovery position.
5. Seek medical care. All suspected victims of CO poisoning should obtain a blood test to determine the level of CO.

Plant-Induced Dermatitis: Poison Ivy, Poison Oak, and Poison Sumac

About 85% of the population is sensitive to poison ivy, poison oak, and poison sumac. If a person reaches adulthood without experiencing a reaction, the risk falls from 85% to 50%. With more people venturing into the outdoors, episodes of dermatitis caused by exposure to poison ivy, poison oak, and poison sumac are increasing **Figure 18-8**, **Figure 18-9**, **Figure 18-10**. (Actually, more than 60 plants can cause allergic reactions, but these three are by far the most common offenders.) Of those who do react, 15–25% will have incapacitating swelling and blistering eruptions that

Figure 18-8

Poison ivy, found in all 48 contiguous states in the United States.

require medical care **Figure 18-11**. There is no routine test to determine an individual's degree of sensitivity—a history of dermatitis is the most reliable indicator.

The resin (urushiol) of these plants is a colorless or slightly yellow, light oil. It runs in resin canals just under the surface, from the roots through the stems, into the leaves and flowers, and just under the surface of the fruit. It is not present in the nectar. The leaves of the plants are fragile and easily ruptured by high winds or by humans or animals brushing against them. The oil immediately oozes onto the surface.

Figure 18-9

Poison oak.

Figure 18-10

Poison sumac.

Figure 18-11

Poison ivy dermatitis.

The light oil generally is not visible on human skin. If present on the sole of a shoe, on the palm of a hand or glove, or on the surface of an animal's fur, it can be spread by direct contact. On some objects, the oil can stay in an active form for months or years. Urushiol can be on the handle of a rake for years and still bond to human skin within five or 10 minutes. Poison ivy leaves have been kept for up to five years with no loss of virulence. Contaminated clothing has caused rashes even after more than 1 year. Smoke from burning plants can produce severe dermatitis. People downwind from these burning leaves can be affected by airborne oil, which can be inhaled and cause airway irritation.

Most people cannot identify these irritating plants. Poison ivy and poison oak are low bushes or climbing vines with waxy, broad, green leaves in the summer that change to brown to red in the fall. The leaflets of poison ivy and poison oak grow in groups of three (three leaves radiating from a single attachment point), giving rise to the warning, "leaves of three, let them be." Poison ivy flourishes throughout most of the United States, except in Alaska and Hawaii; poison oak is found on the West and East coasts and some South Central areas of the United States. Poison sumac is found chiefly in damp, swampy areas in the eastern United States. These plants tend not to grow at elevations higher than 5,000 feet or in hot, dry deserts. A helpful method of identifying these plants is the black spot test. When the sap is exposed to the air, it turns brown in a matter of minutes and black by the next day.

People can come in contact with the urushiol of these plants from their clothes or shoes, pet fur, or the smoke from burning plants. Contrary to popular belief, no one can develop a rash by touching the fluid from the blisters (their own or others') because the fluid in the blister does not contain the oily resin. Any apparent spreading is actually a delayed reaction to contact with the resin.

Recognizing Plant-Induced Dermatitis

Most people do not realize they have come in contact with a poisonous plant until the rash erupts. Reactions can range from mild to severe.

- Mild: itching
- Mild to moderate: itching and redness
- Moderate: itching, redness, and swelling
- Severe: itching, redness, swelling, and blisters

Severity is important, but so is the amount of skin affected. The greater the amount of skin affected, the

Poison Ivy, Oak, and Sumac

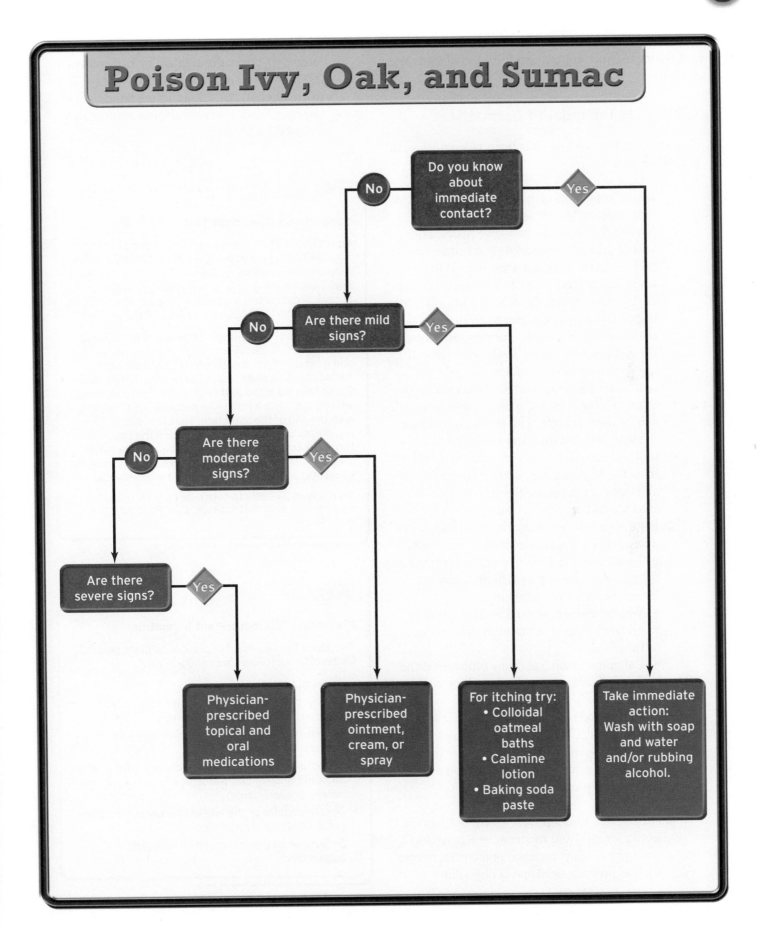

greater the need for medical care. A day or two is the usual time between contact and the onset of signs and symptoms.

Care for Plant-Induced Dermatitis

To care for someone who has been in contact with poisonous plants:

1. People who know they have been in contact with a poisonous plant should wash the skin with soap and water as soon as possible (within 5 minutes for sensitive people and within 1 hour for moderately sensitive people). Unfortunately, most victims do not know about their contact until several hours or days later, when the itching and rash begin. Use soap and water to cleanse the skin of the oily resin or apply rubbing (isopropyl) alcohol liberally (not in swab-type dabs). If too little isopropyl alcohol is used, the oil will be spread to another site and enlarge the injury. Other solvents, such as paint thinner, can be used, but they can irritate or damage the skin. Rinse with water to remove the solubilized material. Water removes urushiol from the skin, oxidizes and inactivates it, and does not penetrate the skin (as solvents do).

2. For a mild reaction, have the victim soak in a lukewarm bath sprinkled with 1 to 2 cups of colloidal oatmeal. Colloidal oatmeal makes a tub slick, so take appropriate precautions. Or, apply one of the following:
   - Wet compresses soaked with aluminum acetate for 20 to 30 minutes three or four times a day
   - Calamine lotion (calamine ointment if the skin becomes dry and cracked) or zinc oxide
   - Baking soda paste: 1 teaspoon of water mixed with 3 teaspoons of baking soda

3. For a mild to moderate reaction, care for the skin as you would for a mild reaction and use a physician-prescribed corticosteroid ointment.

4. For a severe reaction, care for the skin as you would for mild and moderate reactions and use a physician-prescribed oral corticosteroid such as prednisone. Apply a physician-

prescribed topical corticosteroid ointment or cream, cover the area with a transparent plastic wrap, and lightly bind the area with an elastic or self-adhering bandage. A physician-prescribed antihistamine can be used for itching.

FYI

Conducting a Black Spot Test

Most victims of poison ivy dermatitis do not recognize the plant. Poison ivy and poison oak leaves have three leaflets; poison sumac has 7 to 13 leaflets per leaf. The mature fruit is an off-white berry. These botanical characteristics explain the axioms, "leaflets three, let it be" and "berries white, poisonous sight!"

The black spot test is another means of identifying these plants. To check a suspicious plant, grasp a leaf and its stem where it attaches to the branch with a folded sheet of white paper (do not touch the leaf). Crush the end of the leaf stalk in the folded sheet of white paper with a rock. The paper needs to be wet with the sap of the leaf stem. The clear sap of poison ivy, poison oak, and poison sumac on the paper will turn dark brown within 10 minutes and black within 24 hours. This test is not conclusive but can strongly suggest that the plant is one of the three plants.

Source: Guin JD. 1980. The black spot test for recognizing poison ivy and related species. *J Am Acad Dermatol* 2(4):332-333.

FYI

Preventing Poisonous-Plant Dermatitis

To reduce the likelihood of poisonous-plant dermatitis developing, follow these suggestions:

- Avoid the plants.
- Wear protective clothing and use appropriate commercial barrier preparations.
- Replenish the barrier protection every 4 to 6 hours, if practical.
- Decontaminate after known exposure with liberal amounts of soap and water, and then reapply the barrier preparation.
- Decontaminate at the end of the day with isopropyl alcohol and a water rinse.
- Dispose of all contaminated clothing and equipment.

CAUTION

DO NOT use nonprescription hydrocortisone creams, ointments, and sprays in strengths of less than 1%. They offer little benefit.

DO NOT use over-the-counter anti-itch lotions that also have antihistamines because they can cause further skin irritation. Oral antihistamines often are used in conjunction with prescription creams to help decrease itching.

DO NOT let the victim rub or scratch the rash or itching skin.

▶ Stinging Nettle

The stinging nettle plant has stinging hairs on its stem and leaves. The stinging hair is a fine, hollow tube with a bladder at its base that contains a chemical irritant. When the stinging hair is touched, a fine needle-point that penetrates the skin and injects an irritating chemical is formed.

Recognizing Stinging Nettle Poisoning

Stinging nettle affects almost all people. Its effects are not an allergic response, as with poison ivy, but rather result from the direct irritant effect of the plant's sap. The effects are limited to the exposed area, and the response is usually immediate.

Stinging nettle produces some degree of redness, burning, and itching for an hour or more, depending on the area of the body exposed to the plant. For example, the thicker skin on the soles and the palms retards the stinging hairs better than areas of thinner skin, such as the backs of the hands and the arms. Humans vary in sensitivity when the plant actually contacts exposed skin.

The typical response to contact with stinging nettle is a rapid, intense burning sensation at the site of the injection. The area then might itch for an hour or more. Usually, no systemic (whole-body) effects are noted.

Care for Someone With Stinging Nettle Poisoning

Follow these guidelines to care for someone with stinging nettle poisoning:

1. Wash the exposed area with soap and water to remove irritant chemicals.
2. Apply a cold, wet pack to help soothe the painful itching. Other treatments might include a paste of colloidal oatmeal, an over-the-counter hydrocortisone cream (1%), or calamine lotion.
3. Take an over-the-counter antihistamine, if desired. Be sure to follow package directions, and be aware that antihistamines cause drowsiness.
4. The duration of the stinging nettle reaction is measured in hours, rather than days, so little therapy is needed.

▶ Emergency Care Wrap-up

Condition	What to Look For	What to Do
Ingested (swallowed) poisoning	• Abdominal pain and cramping • Nausea or vomiting • Diarrhea • Burns, odor, or stains around and in mouth • Drowsiness or unresponsiveness • Poison container nearby	1. Determine the age and size of the victim, what and how much was swallowed, and when it was swallowed. 2. If victim is responsive, call the poison control center at 1-800-222-1222. The center will advise what you should do and whether medical care is needed. 3. If the victim is unresponsive, open airway, check breathing, and treat accordingly. If breathing, place on left side in recovery position. Call 9-1-1.

Alcohol intoxication	• Alcohol odor on breath or clothing
	• Unsteadiness, staggering
	• Confusion
	• Slurred speech
	• Nausea and vomiting
	• Flushed face
		1. If the victim is responsive:
		  • Monitor breathing.
		  • Look for injuries.
		  • Place in recovery position.
		  • Call poison control center for advice (1-800-222-1222).
		  • If victim becomes violent, leave area and call 9-1-1.
		2. If victim is unresponsive, open airway, check breathing, and treat accordingly.

Drug overdose	• Drowsiness, agitation, anxiety, hyperactivity
	• Change in pupil size
	• Confusion
	• Hallucinations
		1. If the victim is responsive:
		  • Monitor breathing.
		  • Look for injuries.
		  • Place in recovery position.
		  • Call poison control center for advice (1-800-222-1222).
		  • If victim becomes violent, leave area and call 9-1-1.
		2. If victim is unresponsive, open airway, check breathing, and treat accordingly.

Carbon monoxide poisoning	• Headache • Ringing in ears • Chest pain • Muscle weakness • Nausea and vomiting • Dizziness and vision difficulties • Unresponsiveness • Breathing and heart stopped	1. Move victim to fresh air. 2. Call 9-1-1. 3. Monitor breathing. 4. Place unresponsive breathing victim in recovery position.

Plant (contact) poisoning	• Rash
	• Itching
	• Redness
	• Blisters
	• Swelling
		1. For known contact, immediately wash with soap and water.
		2. For mild reaction, use one or more:
		  • 1–2 cups of colloidal oatmeal in bathwater
		  • Calamine lotion
		  • Baking soda paste
		3. For severe reactions, perform step 2 and seek medical care.

prep kit

▶ Ready for Review

- A poison is any substance that impairs health or causes death by its chemical action when it enters the body or comes in contact with the skin.
- Poisons are classified by how they enter the body. They can be ingested, inhaled, absorbed, and injected.
- Ingested poisoning occurs when the victim swallows a toxic substance.
- Alcohol is a depressant that affects a person's judgment, vision, reaction time, and coordination.
- Drugs are classified according to their effects on the user:
  - Uppers (stimulants)
  - Downers (depressants)
  - Hallucinogens
  - Volatile chemicals
- Carbon monoxide is the leading cause of poisoning death in the United States each year.
- About 85% of the population is sensitive to poison ivy, poison oak, and poison sumac.

▶ Vital Vocabulary

carbon monoxide A colorless, odorless, poisonous gas formed by incomplete combustion, such as in fire.

ingested poisoning Poisoning caused by swallowing a toxic substance.

poison Any substance that impairs health or causes death by its chemical action when it enters the body or comes in contact with the skin; also known as a toxin.

Poison Help Medical facility providing immediate, free, expert advice any time; can be reached by calling 1-800-222-1222.

▶ Assessment in Action

You have been helping your sister paint three rooms in her home. While taking a break, your 2-year-old niece enters the room with a small cup of paint used for touch up. There is paint around and inside her mouth.

Directions: Circle Yes if you agree with the statement; circle No if you disagree.

Yes   No   1. Immediately give your niece water or milk to dilute the ingested paint.

Yes   No   2. Use syrup of ipecac to induce vomiting.

Yes   No   3. Determine how much of the paint was swallowed, when it was swallowed, and the age and size of the victim.

Yes   No   4. Call the poison control center for advice (1-800-222-1222).

▶ Check Your Knowledge

Directions: Circle Yes if you agree with the statement; circle No if you disagree.

Yes   No   1. Swallowing a poison can produce nausea.

Yes   No   2. Milk should be given to all victims of ingested poison.

Yes   No   3. A victim of alcohol intoxication does not require medical care.

Yes   No   4. Carbon monoxide has a unique smell.

Yes   No   5. Everyone who touches a poison ivy, poison oak, or poison sumac plant will have some type of skin reaction.

Yes   No   6. Causing a poisoned victim to vomit is a recommended first aid practice.

Yes   No   7. Some cases of poison ivy, poison oak, or poison sumac require medical care.

Yes   No   8. Calamine lotion can help relieve itching caused by poison ivy, poison oak, or poison sumac.

Yes   No   9. If an intoxicated or drugged person becomes violent, leave the area.

Yes   No   10. Move a victim of carbon monoxide poisoning to fresh air.

Bites and Stings

▶ Animal Bites

It is estimated that one of every two Americans will be bitten at some time by an animal or by another person. Dogs are responsible for about 80% of all animal bite injuries **Figure 19-1**. Of the nearly 5 million dog bites that occur yearly, 80% are trivial or minor, and medical care is not required or sought, which demonstrates the importance of knowing first aid. The remainder account for about 1% of all emergency department and physician office visits. Each year, about 19 bite-related deaths occur in the United States **Table 19-1**.

Animal bites represent a major, largely unrecognized public health problem. Two concerns result from an animal bite: immediate tissue damage and later infection from microorganisms. A dog's mouth can carry more than 60 species of bacteria, some of which are dangerous to humans **Table 19-2**. Two examples of infection—tetanus and rabies—have been almost eradicated by medical advances, but they still pose a potential problem.

Although cat bites are less mutilating than dog bites, cat bites have a much higher rate of infection than dog bites. Cats have very sharp teeth, which can create deep puncture wounds and involve muscle, tendon, and bone.

Another pet especially likely to bite children is the ferret. These animals are often unpredictable and can cause severe facial injury to infants. Ferrets sometimes unleash frenzied, rapid-fire, bite-and-slash

Figure 19-1

Dog bite.

Table 19-1	Animal-Related Human Deaths in the United States (1991-2001)
Animal	**Average number of deaths each year**
Venomous animals	
Snake	5.2
Spider	6
Scorpion	0.45
Hornet, bee, wasp	48.5
Centipede	0.45
Other specified venomous arthropod	6
Venomous marine animal	0.18
Other specified venomous animal	2.1
Total venomous	68.88
Nonvenomous animals	
Dog	18.9
Rat	0.27
Nonvenomous snake	0
Other animals except arthropod	4
Other specified animal*	76.9
Unspecified animal	4
Total nonvenomous	104.07
Overall total	172.95

*Note that this category includes bitten or struck by other mammals, contact with marine animal, bitten or stung by nonvenomous insect or other nonvenomous arthropods, bitten or struck by crocodile or alligator, bitten or confronted by other reptiles.
Source: Adapted from Langley RL. 2005. Animal-related fatalities in the United States: An update. *Wilderness Environ Med* 16(2):67-74.

attacks on infants, usually on their heads and throats, and can inflict hundreds of bites.

Besides children, elderly people and people unable to help themselves are especially prone to animal bites because they are sometimes unable to detect or prevent a dangerous situation. Many animal-related deaths occur when the victim is left alone with the offending pet. Contrary to popular belief, wild or stray dogs seldom are involved in fatal attacks.

Damage mostly occurs on the hands, arms, legs, and face. A damaged face presents several problems because the proximity of blood vessels to the skin surface makes it susceptible to copious bleeding. Facial disfigurement and scarring can result in emotional trauma. Complete or partial loss of an eye also is possible.

Wild animal attacks occur most often in rural or wilderness locations (see Chapter 24, *Wilderness First Aid* for more information). Not all injuries are bites. Severe injuries result from victims being thrown in the air, gored by an antler, butted, or trampled on the ground.

Rabies

Rabies is one of the most ancient and feared of diseases **Figure 19-2**. Although human rabies rarely occurs in the United States or in other industrialized nations, it remains a scourge in developing countries. A virus found in warm-blooded animals causes rabies, which spreads from one animal to another in the saliva, usually through a bite or by licking. Bites from cold-blooded animals such as reptiles do not carry the danger of rabies.

A bite or a scratch is considered a significant rabies exposure if it penetrates the skin. Unprovoked attacks are more likely to have been inflicted by a rabid animal than are provoked attacks. Nonbite exposure consists of contamination of wounds, including scratches, abrasions, and weeping skin rashes.

Consider an animal as possibly rabid if any of the following applies:

- The animal made an unprovoked attack.
- The animal acted strangely, that is, out of character (for example, a usually friendly dog is aggressive, or a wild fox seems docile and friendly).
- The animal was a high-risk species (skunk, raccoon, or bat).

Table 19-2 Facts About Dog Bites

- Carefully choose your pet dog. Evaluate your environment and lifestyle and speak with a professional to determine the appropriate type of pet.
- Dogs should be neutered to reduce aggressive tendencies.
- Never leave infants or young children alone with a dog. Be sensitive to cues that a child is fearful or apprehensive about a dog.
- Teach children basic safety around dogs, and review regularly.
- Dogs with histories of aggression are inappropriate for families with children.
- Do not play aggressive games with your dog, for example, wrestling.
- Never approach an unfamiliar dog. Immediately report stray dogs or dogs displaying unusual behavior.
- Remain motionless when approached by an unfamiliar dog—never run or scream.
- Do not disturb a dog that is sleeping, eating, or caring for puppies.
- If knocked down by a dog, lie still and remain in a ball.
- If bitten by a dog, immediately report the bite.

Source: Centers for Disease Control and Prevention: Nonfatal dog bite-related injuries treated in hospital emergency departments—United States 2001. *MMWR Weekly,* 2003;52(26):605-610 accessed at *www.cdc.gov/mmwr/preview/mmwrhtml/mm5226a1.htm.*

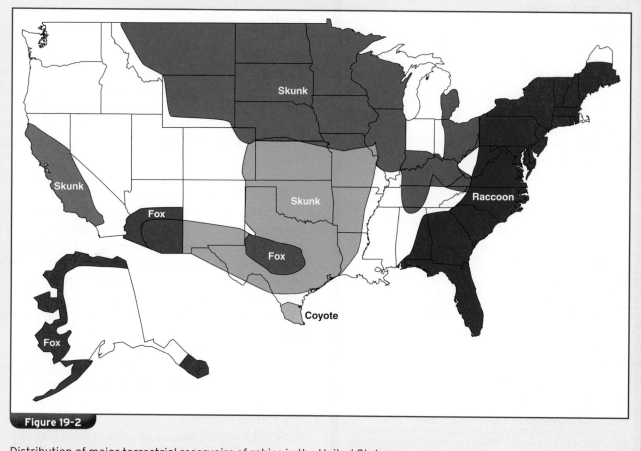

Figure 19-2

Distribution of major terrestrial reservoirs of rabies in the United States.

Source: Centers for Disease Control and Prevention.

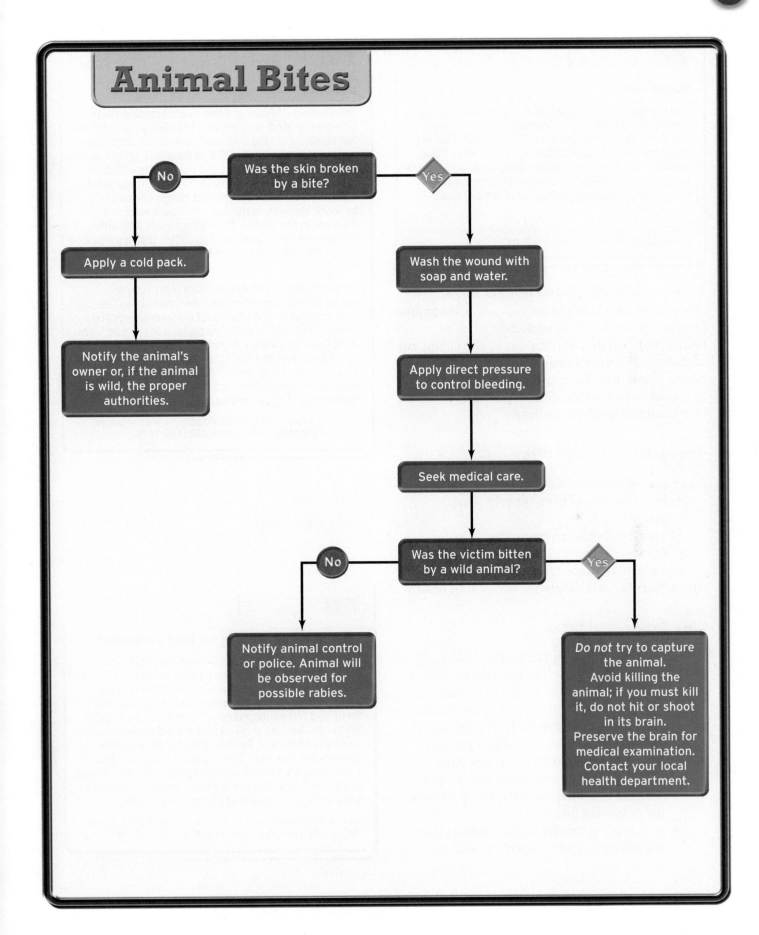

Animal Bites

Was the skin broken by a bite?

No → Apply a cold pack. → Notify the animal's owner or, if the animal is wild, the proper authorities.

Yes → Wash the wound with soap and water. → Apply direct pressure to control bleeding. → Seek medical care. → **Was the victim bitten by a wild animal?**

No → Notify animal control or police. Animal will be observed for possible rabies.

Yes → *Do not* try to capture the animal. Avoid killing the animal; if you must kill it, do not hit or shoot in its brain. Preserve the brain for medical examination. Contact your local health department.

Human Rabies

The number of human deaths in the United States attributed to rabies has declined from 100 or more each year to an average of 1 or 2 each year. Two programs have been responsible for this decline. First, animal control and vaccination programs, which were begun in the 1940s; and second, effective human rabies vaccines and immunoglobulins have been developed.

Sources: Centers for Disease Control and Prevention; United States Rabies Surveillance Data.

Report animal bites to the police or animal control officers; they should be the ones to capture the animal for observation. If a healthy domestic dog or cat up to date with its rabies vaccination bit the victim, the animal should be confined and observed for 10 days for any illness. If a wild animal bit the victim, it should be considered a possible rabies exposure and medical care should be sought immediately.

Recognizing Animal Bites

An animal bite has the following characteristics:
- Puncture wound from animal's sharp, pointed teeth
- Tissue and skin can be crushed
- Open wound on fingers, knuckles, and/or hand

It is important to be cautious when dealing with animal bites because the animal may still be nearby.

Care for Animal Bites

Help an animal bite victim by doing the following:
1. If the wound is not bleeding heavily, wash it with soap and water. Flush the wound with water under pressure from a faucet. Avoid scrubbing, which can bruise the tissues.
2. Control the bleeding with direct pressure.
3. Cover the wound with a sterile or clean dressing. Do not close the wound because doing so could trap bacteria, which increases the chances of infection.
4. Seek medical care for further wound cleaning and closure, and possible tetanus or rabies care.

Dog Bites

The Centers of Disease Control undertook a study of fatalities related to dog bites. The researchers found 157 fatalities during a 10-year period. Pet dogs were responsible for almost 70% of fatalities, strays were involved in 27% of cases, and police or guard dogs in only 2.8% of the deaths. No significant seasonal trends were noted, except that strays seemed to be more involved in the fall, while pets were more involved in the winter. The victims were primarily children under 10 years of age (70%) with a particularly high death rate noted for infants less than one month old.

Pit bulls were implicated in more than 40% of the fatalities, "almost three times more than German shepherds, the next most commonly reported breed." Deaths attributed to pit bulls increased from 20% to 62% during the period. The researchers concluded that dog bite fatalities had been underestimated and suggested "strong animal control laws, public education regarding dog bites, and more responsible dog ownership."

Sources: Sacks JJ et al. 1989. Dog bite-related fatalities from 1979 through 1988. *JAMA* 262:1489-1492.

Dog Bites: Which Breeds Are Most Dangerous?

Researchers who checked Denver records found 178 reports of dog bites for a 1-year period to people outside the dog owners' households (this is more common than bites to family members). They also identified 178 nonbiting dogs from the same neighborhoods. Results showed that male dogs (especially unneutered males), German shepherds, and chow chows were the most likely to bite outsiders, especially children. Children under age 12 were the victims in 51% of cases. Too few pit bulls, Akitas, and collies were involved in this study to rate their risks.

Source: Gershman KA et al. 1993. Which dogs bite? A case-control study of risk factors. *Pediatrics* 93(6):913-917.

Human Bites

After dogs and cats, the animal most likely to bite humans is another human. Human bites can cause severe injury, often more so than other animal bites. The human mouth contains a wide range of bacteria and viruses, so the chance of infection is great from a human bite, especially on the hand **Figure 19-3**.

Most human bites are inflicted by fighting youths, by children at play, by people in mental institutions, or during sexual assaults. Embarrassment sometimes causes a victim not to seek medical care immediately, which greatly increases the risk of infection.

Figure 19-3

Human bites can result in serious, spreading infection.

Although most human bites occur during acts of violence, about one fourth are accidental or sports-related, sustained by hospital workers trying to restrain children or patients having a seizure, or self-inflicted during nail chewing or thumb sucking. Men are more often victims than women, mostly during aggressive altercations, with the peak age being 25 years. The most common injury location is the hand, sustained on a closed fist as the result of a punch.

Recognizing Human Bites

There are two types of human bites. True bites occur when any part of the body's flesh is caught between teeth, usually deliberately. True bites happen during fights and in cases of abuse. Mandatory reporting laws apply if spousal or child abuse is involved. A schoolyard bite, with one child biting another, generally is not reportable.

Much worse than a true bite is the clenched-fist injury, which results from cutting a fist on teeth. It is associated with a high likelihood of infection. The injury is usually a laceration over the knuckles. Although clenched-fist injuries usually result from a fight, unintentional injury can happen during sports and play.

Care for Human Bites

Help someone with a human bite in the following manner:

1. If the wound is not bleeding heavily, wash it with soap and water for 5 to 10 minutes. Avoid scrubbing, which can bruise tissues.
2. Flush the wound thoroughly with running water under pressure from a faucet.
3. Control bleeding with direct pressure.
4. Cover the wound with a sterile dressing. Do *not* close the wound with tape or butterfly bandages. Closing the wound traps bacteria in the wound, increasing the chance of infection.
5. Seek medical care for possible further wound cleaning, a possible tetanus shot, and sutures to close the wound, if needed.

▶ Snake Bites

Throughout the world, about 50,000 people die of snake bites each year. Each year in the United States, 40,000 to 50,000 people are bitten by snakes, 7,000

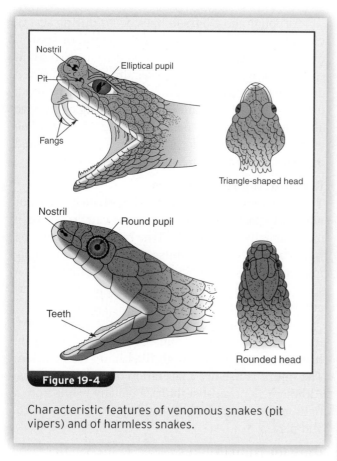

Figure 19-4

Characteristic features of venomous snakes (pit vipers) and of harmless snakes.

Figure 19-5

Rattlesnake.

Figure 19-6

Copperhead snake.

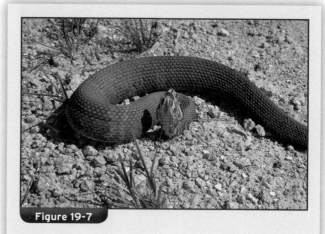

Figure 19-7

Water moccasin (cottonmouth).

to 8,000 of them by venomous snakes Figure 19-4 . Amazingly, fewer than a dozen Americans die each year of snake bites. Victims who die of snake bites in the United States usually do so during the first 48 hours after the bite. Only four snake species in the United States are venomous: rattlesnakes (which account for about 65% of all venomous snake bites and nearly all the snake bite deaths in the United States), copperheads, water moccasins (also known as cottonmouths), and coral snakes Figure 19-5 , Figure 19-6 , Figure 19-7 , and Figure 19-8 . Although uncommon, snake bites can be painful, costly, and potentially deadly. Other than death, disabilities such as partial or complete loss of an extremity or finger or loss of movement in a joint can occur. Most victims fully recover.

The first three are pit vipers, which have three characteristics in common:

- Triangular, flat heads wider than their necks
- Elliptical pupils (cat-like eyes)
- A heat-sensitive pit between the eye and the nostril on each side of the head

The coral snake is small and colorful, with a series of bright red, yellow, and black bands around its body

Figure 19-8

Coral snake; the United States' most venomous snake.

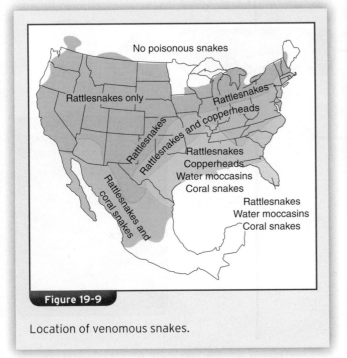

Figure 19-9

Location of venomous snakes.

Map labels:
No poisonous snakes
Rattlesnakes only
Rattlesnakes and copperheads
Rattlesnakes
Rattlesnakes
Copperheads
Water moccasins
Coral snakes
Rattlesnakes and coral snakes
Rattlesnakes
Water moccasins
Coral snakes

Table 19-3 How to Avoid a Snake Bite

Snakebites are best avoided, not treated. These suggestions, when followed, can help you avoid being bitten:

- Do not handle venomous snakes—keep away. They usually do not have to be killed for identification purposes.
- Avoid hiking and camping in snake-infested areas; avoid caves, rock crevices, dens, stone-walls, and wood piles.
- Watch where you sit and step; do not sit on or step over logs until closely checked. Do not reach into holes or hidden ledges.
- Wear protective gear such as boots, gloves, long pants, and long-sleeved shirts when in snake habitats.
- Do not handle a dead venomous snake. The reflex action of the jaws can still inflict a bite up to 90 minutes after the snake has been killed, even if decapitated.
- Do not surprise or corner a snake. Use a walking stick to prod in front of you while walking, and make noise so that a snake can sense you coming.
- Do not keep venomous snakes as pets.
- When unintentionally encountering a snake, remain silent and motionless. If the snake has not fled, step away slowly and cautiously.

(every other band is yellow). Coral snakes are found in Arizona, the southeastern United States, and Texas.

At least one species of venomous snakes is found in every state except Alaska, Hawaii, and Maine **Figure 19-9**. Exotic snakes, whether imported legally or smuggled into the United States, can be found in zoos, schools, snake farms, and amateur and professional collections, and account for at least 15 bites a year. Some of the exotic snakes can be poisonous.

A legitimate snake bite is one in which the victim was bitten before the encounter with a snake was recognized or while trying to move away from the snake. They most often involve the lower extremities and are accidental **Table 19-3**.

An illegitimate snake bite is one in which, before being bitten, the victim recognized the encounter with a snake but did not attempt to move away from the snake. Most illegitimate bites occur on the upper extremities. Most bites of this type occur when the victim tries to kill, capture, play with, or move a snake. Adult snakes deliver more serious bites because they inject more venom than do young snakes, even though a young snake's venom is two to three times more toxic than an adult's.

Pit Vipers

Pit vipers are found in every state but Alaska, Maine, and Hawaii. Rattlesnakes are the most widespread of the pit vipers. Copperheads are found in the central southeastern United States and westward into the Big Bend of Texas. Cottonmouth water moccasins are found in the southeast from Virginia to Florida and into Texas. Snakes benefit us by keeping the rodent

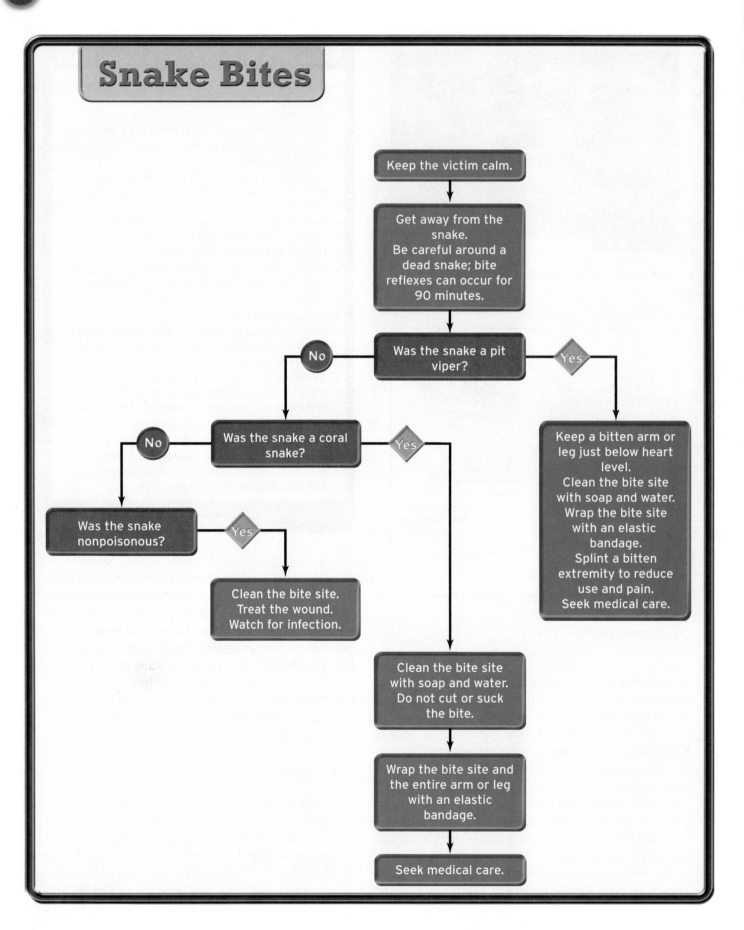

Snake Bites

Keep the victim calm.

Get away from the snake.
Be careful around a dead snake; bite reflexes can occur for 90 minutes.

Was the snake a pit viper? — **Yes** → Keep a bitten arm or leg just below heart level.
Clean the bite site with soap and water.
Wrap the bite site with an elastic bandage.
Splint a bitten extremity to reduce use and pain.
Seek medical care.

No ↓

Was the snake a coral snake? — **Yes** → Clean the bite site with soap and water. Do not cut or suck the bite.
↓
Wrap the bite site and the entire arm or leg with an elastic bandage.
↓
Seek medical care.

No ↓

Was the snake nonpoisonous? — **Yes** → Clean the bite site. Treat the wound. Watch for infection.

Blue Jeans and Snake Bites

Researchers studied whether ordinary clothing (denim material from blue jeans) reduces the amount of venom injected by a rattlesnake.

The investigators used saline solution-filled gloves to simulate human limbs and elicited bites from small and large southern Pacific rattlesnakes. Each snake was videotaped biting a bare glove and a denim-covered glove. The results were that the snakes injected significantly less venom into the denim-covered gloves than into the bare gloves, up to 60% reduction for the small snakes and 66% reduction for the large snakes. The investigators felt that denim interfered with venom delivery and induced a high proportion of "dry" bites (no venom released), as well as harmless spillage of venom from the fangs of the snakes onto the surface of the denim cover. It was interesting to note that larger rattlesnakes struck more readily, maintained longer fang contact during their bites, and delivered 26 to 41 times more venom into the gloves than did the small snakes. This adds to the body of evidence that indicates large venomous snakes are much more dangerous to humans than small ones.

Wearing long denim pants can be an inexpensive and effective way to reduce the severity of snake bites. Other forms of clothing (eg, high leather boots or other types of long pants) may be equally or more effective at deflecting a bite and preventing a snakebite.

Source: Herbert SS, Hayes WK. 2009. Denim clothing reduces venom expenditure by rattlesnakes striking defensively at model human limbs. *Annals of Emergency Medicine* 54(6):830-836.

population from exploding out of control. They consume hundreds of thousands of mice and rats every year. Few snakes act aggressively toward a human unless provoked. The vast majority of bites are not deadly and can be effectively treated.

Ninety-eight percent of snake bites are on the extremities. Alcohol intoxication of the victim is a factor in many bites. The majority of bites in the United States occur in the southwestern part of the country—partly due to the near-extinction of pit vipers in the eastern United States. The eastern and western diamondback rattlesnakes account for almost 95% of the deaths. These deaths occur most often in children, in the elderly, and in victims to whom **antivenom** is not given or is inappropriately given.

Recognizing Pit Viper Bites

Signs of a pit viper bite include:

- Severe burning pain at the bite site.
- Two small puncture wounds about ½″ apart (some cases have only one fang mark) **Figure 19-10**.
- Swelling (occurs within 10 to 15 minutes and can involve an entire extremity).
- Discoloration after 2–3 hours and blood-filled blisters possibly developing in 6 to 10 hours.
- In severe cases, nausea, vomiting, sweating, and weakness.
- In about 25% of venomous snake bites, there is no venom injection, only fang and tooth wounds (known as a dry bite).

Care for Pit Viper Bites

The Wilderness Medical Society lists these guidelines for dealing with pit viper bites:

1. Get the victim and bystanders away from the snake. Snakes have been known to bite more than once. Pit vipers can strike about one half of their body length. Be careful around a decapitated snake head—head reactions can persist for 90 minutes or more.
2. Do not attempt to capture or kill the snake. It wastes valuable time, there is a risk of additional bites, and identification of the snake is not usually needed because the same antivenom is used for all pit viper bites.
3. Keep the victim quiet. Activity increases venom absorption. If possible, carry the victim or have the victim walk very slowly to help to minimize exertion.
4. Gently wash the bitten area with soap and water. Any ring(s) or jewelry that might reduce blood circulation if swelling occurs should be removed.
5. Stabilize the bitten extremity (arm or leg) with a sling or a splint as you would for a

Figure 19-10

Rattlesnake bite.

fracture. Keep the extremity below heart level despite the fact that swelling might occur.

6. Seek medical care *immediately*. This is the most important thing to do for the victim. Antivenom must be given within 4 hours of the bite (not every venomous snake bite requires antivenom).

CAUTION

DO NOT apply cold or ice to a snake bite. It does not inactivate the venom and poses a danger of frostbite.

DO NOT use the cut-and-suck procedure—you could damage underlying structures (for example, blood vessels, nerves, or tendons). Cutting the skin may cause infection and a poorly healing wound.

DO NOT apply mouth suction. Your mouth is filled with bacteria, increasing the likelihood of wound infection.

DO NOT use any form of suction.

DO NOT apply electric shock. No medical studies support this method.

DO NOT apply a constriction band—their use remains controversial. They may increase tissue damage. If applied too tightly or if swelling occurs, they can act as a tourniquet.

FYI

Dead Snakes Can Still Bite

Data collected at the Good Samaritan Regional Medical Center in Phoenix show that fatal injuries do not prevent rattlesnakes from biting humans. Of the 34 patients admitted to the Phoenix Center for Rattlesnake Bites in a recent 11-month period, five were bitten by snakes that had been fatally injured and were presumed dead. One patient was bitten on the index finger after picking up a snake he had bludgeoned in the head and assumed was dead. Another was bitten after picking up a snake he had shot, then decapitated.

Source: Suchard JR, LoVecchio F. 1999. Envenomations by rattlesnakes thought to be dead. *N Engl J Med* 340(24):1930.

Coral Snake Bites

The coral snake is America's most venomous snake, but it rarely bites people. The coral snake has short

fangs and tends to hang on and chew its venom into the victim rather than to strike and release, like a pit viper. Coral snake venom is a neurotoxin, and symptoms can begin 1 to 5 hours after the bite.

Recognizing Coral Snake Bites

Someone who has been bitten by a coral snake might exhibit the following symptoms:

- Minimal pain
- Sagging or drooping of upper eyelids
- Weakness
- Pricking, tingling of skin (often numb at bite site)
- Double vision (seeing two of a single object)
- Difficulty in swallowing
- Sweating
- Abnormal flow of saliva

Care for Coral Snake Bites

You can help a coral snake bite victim in the following manner:

1. Keep the victim calm.
2. Gently clean the bite site with soap and water.
3. Apply mild pressure by wrapping several elastic bandages over the bite site and the entire arm or leg. Applying mild pressure (as tightly as for a sprained ankle) is recommended for any snake bites. The technique originated in Australia, where it has been very successful. Do not cut the victim's skin, suck on the wound, or use a suction device.

   This technique has two parts: (1) The pressure holds the venom at the bite site and prevents it from moving through the lymphatic system to other parts of the body, and (2) immobilization limits the pumping action of the muscles.

4. Seek medical care. Antivenom for coral snakes is no longer produced in the United States.

Nonpoisonous Snake Bites

Nonvenomous snakes inflict the most snake bites. If you are not positive about a snake, assume it was venomous. Some so-called nonpoisonous North American snakes such as the hognose and garter snakes have venom that can cause painful local reactions but no systemic (whole-body) symptoms.

Recognizing Nonpoisonous Snake Bites

A nonpoisonous snake bite results in the following:

- Feeling of a mild to moderate pinch
- Curved lines (horseshoe shaped) of tiny pin-pricks on the skin that correspond with the rows of sharp, pointy teeth
- Bleeding
- Mild itching

Care for Nonpoisonous Snake Bites

A victim of a nonpoisonous snake bite should be treated as follows:

1. Gently clean the bite site with soap and water.
2. Care for the bite as you would a minor wound.
3. Seek medical care.

▶ Insect Stings

The stinging insects belonging to the order of *Hymenoptera* include honeybees, bumblebees, yellow jackets, hornets, wasps, and fire ants **Figure 19-11**. These insects account for more deaths and illnesses each year than all other venomous animals combined. About 1 in every 200 people is dangerously allergic to *Hymenoptera* venom. Fortunately, localized pain, itching, and swelling—the most common consequences of an insect bite—can be treated with first aid.

Generally, venomous flying insects are aggressive only when threatened or when their hives or nests are disrupted. Under such conditions, they sting, sometimes in swarms. Honeybees and some yellow jackets have barbed stingers that become embedded in the victim's skin during the sting. After injecting its

Figure 19-11A

Figure 19-11B

Figure 19-11C

Figure 19-11D

Bees. **A.** Honeybee, **B.** Yellow jacket, **C.** Hornet, **D.** Wasp.

venom, the bee flies away, tearing and leaving behind the embedded stinger and venom sac, which causes it to die. Honeybees and bumblebees do not release all their venom during the initial injection; some remains in the stinger embedded in the victim's skin. If the stinger and venom sac are not removed properly, additional venom can be released and worsen the victim's reaction.

In contrast, the stingers of wasps, yellow jackets, hornets, and fire ants are not barbed and do not become embedded in the victim. Thus, these insects can sting multiple times, and most species (with a few exceptions, such as some yellow jacket species) do not die as a result of the stinging. There are two types of yellow jackets, one is a wasp and can sting multiple times. The other is a ground-nesting bee that stings once then dies, sometimes leaving an embedded stinger like other bees. These bees are smaller than yellow jacket wasps.

Most stings cause only self-limited, local inflammatory reactions consisting of pain, itching, redness, and swelling. These reactions are usually more a nuisance than a medical emergency. However, local reactions can be extensive, for example, involving the victim's entire arm. In an extensive reaction, the swelling and redness might peak 2 to 3 days after the sting and last a week or longer. Signs and symptoms of life-threatening reactions include nausea, vomiting, wheezing, fever, and drippy nose. A victim might go into anaphylaxis almost immediately or after experiencing a variety of symptoms. Most people who have anaphylactic reactions have no history of them. In a study of 400 fatal bee stings, only 15% of the victims had a known sensitivity.

Reactions generally occur within a few minutes to 1 hour after the sting. Bee sting victims who have anaphylactic reactions develop throat swelling and bronchospasm, which are manifested by difficulty speaking, tightness in the throat or chest, wheezing, shortness of breath, and chest pain. Respiratory tract obstruction accounts for the majority of deaths among victims of flying insect stings.

For the severely allergic person, a single sting could be fatal within minutes. Although there are accounts of people who have survived some 2,000 stings at one time, 500 stings will usually kill even people who are not allergic to stinging insects.

Massive numbers of stings are rare. They might occur if a person stumbled into a hive or a truck carrying a load of hives crashed. With the slow migration of Africanized bees (so-called killer bees) from South and Central America into the United States, the number of cases involving multiple stings is likely to increase. The venom of the Africanized bee is no more potent than that of the European type; it is just that the African type is extremely aggressive and, thus, more likely to be involved in multiple stings. A number of child deaths have resulted from the multiple stings of fire ants, which are common in the southeastern United States.

> ### FYI
>
> **Preventing Insect Stings**
>
> People who know they are allergic to insect stings need to exercise extra care to avoid being stung. They should carry a bee sting kit and follow these guidelines:
>
> - Wear long pants and long-sleeved shirts.
> - Because insects are attracted to bright colors and floral patterns, wear white, green, tan, and khaki—the least attractive colors to insects.
> - Wear shoes outdoors.
> - Avoid yard work and other activities in which insect contact is frequent.
> - Keep garbage cans away from the house.
> - Remove insect-attracting plants from inside as well as the immediate proximity of the house.
> - Do not use scented soaps, lotions, or perfumes.
> - Keep car windows closed.
> - If an insect confronts you, avoid quick movements and do not provoke it. Turn away, lower your face, and walk away slowly. Do not run about wildly or move erratically when bees are nearby.
> - Do not eat when bees are nearby.
> - Have insect nests around the house removed by professional exterminators.

Recognizing Insect Stings

A rule of thumb is that the sooner symptoms develop after a sting, the more serious the reaction will be.

- Usual reactions are instant pain, redness around the sting site, and itching.
- Worrisome reactions include hives, swelling of lips or tongue, a tickle in the throat, and wheezing.
- Life-threatening reactions are bluish or grayish skin color, seizures, unresponsiveness, and an inability to breathe because of swelling and spasm of the airway.

About 60% to 80% of anaphylactic deaths are caused by the victim not being able to breathe because

FYI

Fire Ants

Fire ants are aggressive, will defensively attack anything that disturbs them, and can sting repeatedly **Figure 19-12**. The fire ant bites its victim by securing itself to the skin with its mandibles, causing pain, then, using its head as a pivot, the ant swings its abdomen in an arc, repeatedly stinging the victim with an abdominal stinger. Up to 40% of the people who live in infested urban areas are stung each year, and more than 30 deaths have been attributed to these insect bites.

The fire ant sting usually produces immediate pain and a red, swollen area, which disappears within 45 minutes **Figure 19-13**. A blister then forms, rupturing in 30 to 70 hours, and the area often becomes infected. In some cases, a red, swollen, itchy patch develops instead of a blister. Although the stings are not usually life threatening, they are easily infected and can leave permanent scars.

Some people become sensitive to fire ant stings and should seek the advice of an allergist. Anaphylaxis (a life-threatening allergic reaction) occurs in about 1% to 2% of people stung by fire ants. Therefore, if a sting leads to shortness of breath, tightness and swelling in the throat, tightness in the chest, increased pulse rate, swelling of the tongue and mouth, dizziness, or nausea, the person should be taken to a hospital emergency department immediately. Some people lapse into a coma from even one sting.

First aid for fire ant stings includes placing an ice cube over the sting to reduce the pain and to slow absorption of the venom. A topical corticosteroid cream can help combat local swelling and itching. An antihistamine can prevent some local symptoms if given early, but it works too slowly to counteract a life-threatening allergic reaction. People who are allergic to stings should always carry a kit with antihistamine tablets and a preloaded syringe of epinephrine.

Figure 19-12

Fire ants.

Figure 19-13

Fire ant stings.

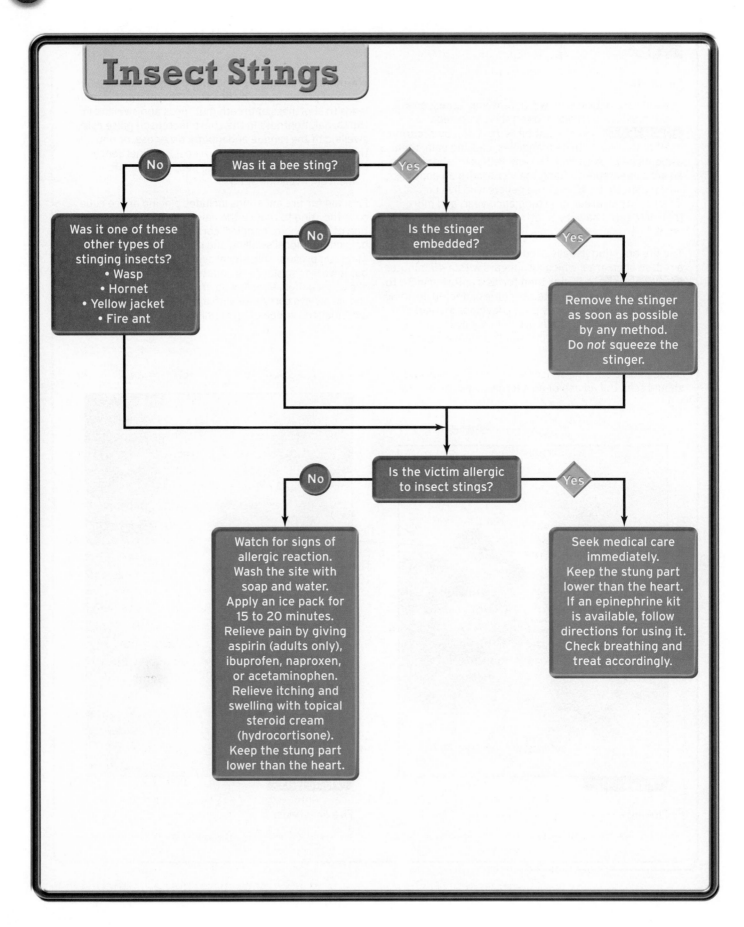

Insect Stings

Was it a bee sting?

No →

Yes →

Was it one of these other types of stinging insects?
- Wasp
- Hornet
- Yellow jacket
- Fire ant

Is the stinger embedded?

No →

Yes →

Remove the stinger as soon as possible by any method. Do *not* squeeze the stinger.

Is the victim allergic to insect stings?

No →

Yes →

Watch for signs of allergic reaction. Wash the site with soap and water. Apply an ice pack for 15 to 20 minutes. Relieve pain by giving aspirin (adults only), ibuprofen, naproxen, or acetaminophen. Relieve itching and swelling with topical steroid cream (hydrocortisone). Keep the stung part lower than the heart.

Seek medical care immediately. Keep the stung part lower than the heart. If an epinephrine kit is available, follow directions for using it. Check breathing and treat accordingly.

swollen airway passages obstruct airflow to the lungs. The second most common cause of death is shock, caused by collapse of blood circulation through the body.

One of the difficulties in dealing with stings is the lack of uniformity in victims' responses. One sting is not necessarily equivalent to another, even within the same species, because the amount of venom injected varies from sting to sting. A person who experiences anaphylactic shock after being stung by a hornet might respond to a bee sting with only a small amount of swelling. One person might have a local reaction involving an entire limb, although the more typical response is a small circle of redness and swelling that disappears without incident in a few days. In beekeepers, for whom stings are an accepted occupational hazard, the response is likely to be even less than in most other people, because they have become tolerant to the toxins in the venom from having been stung many times on different occasions. There seems to be no easy way to predict how a person will react. Most people who are stung, however, have local reactions: redness, swelling, and pain.

Stings to the mouth or eye tend to be more dangerous than stings to other body areas. Also, victims tend to react more severely to multiple stings, especially 10 or more. The most dangerous single stings in nonallergic individuals are those inside the throat, which can result from swallowing an insect that has dropped into a soft drink can or from inhaling one that flies into the victim's open mouth. A sting in the mouth or throat can cause swelling that obstructs the airway even in a person who is not allergic to insect stings. If the sting is not life threatening, have the victim suck on ice or flush his or her mouth with cold water. For a bee sting, dissolve a teaspoon of baking soda in a glass of water. Have the victim rinse his or her mouth and then hold the water in the mouth for several minutes.

Care for Insect Stings

The following outlines how to assist someone who has been bitten or stung by an insect.

1. Most people who have been stung can be treated on site, and everyone should know what to do if a life-threatening allergic reaction (anaphylaxis) occurs. In particular, people who have had a severe reaction to an insect sting should be instructed about what they can do to protect themselves. They also should be advised to wear a medical-alert identification tag identifying them as allergic to insect stings.

2. Look at the sting site for a stinger and venom sac embedded in the skin. Bees are the only stinging insects that leave their stingers and venom sac behind. If the stinger is embedded, remove it or it will continue to inject poison for 2 or 3 minutes. Remove the stinger and venom sac as soon as possible by any method.

3. Wash the sting site with soap and water to prevent infection.

4. Apply an ice pack over the sting site to slow absorption of the venom and relieve pain. Use a commercial sting stick containing a topical anesthetic such as Xylocaine (unless the victim is known to be allergic to the drug). Because bee venom is acidic, a paste made of baking soda and water can help. Sodium bicarbonate is an alkalinizing agent that draws out fluid and reduces itching and swelling. Wasp venom, on the other hand, is alkaline, so apply vinegar or lemon juice. A paste made of unseasoned meat tenderizer can help a bee sting victim if the paste comes in direct contact with the venom. That generally is not possible, however, because the bee will have injected the venom through too small a hole and too deeply into the victim's skin.

5. To further relieve pain and itching, use aspirin (adults only), acetaminophen, or ibuprofen. A topical steroid cream, such as hydrocortisone, can help combat local swelling and itching. An antihistamine can prevent some local symptoms if given early, but it works too slowly to counteract a life-threatening allergic reaction.

6. Observe the victim for at least 30 minutes for signs of an allergic reaction. For a person having a severe allergic reaction, a dose of epinephrine is the only effective treatment. A person with a known allergy to insect stings should have a physician-prescribed emergency kit that includes a prefilled, spring-loaded device that automatically injects epinephrine. The allergic person should take the kit whenever he or she is going someplace where stinging insects are known to

exist. Because epinephrine is short-acting, watch the victim closely for signs of returning anaphylaxis. Another dose of epinephrine as often as every 15 minutes might be needed.

7. Do not use epinephrine to treat a sting unless the victim has a severe allergic reaction. Epinephrine has a shelf life of 1 to 3 years or until it turns brown.

8. Watch for signs and symptoms of a delayed allergic reaction, especially during the first 6 to 24 hours. If the victim develops difficulty breathing, facial swelling, fever, chills, or dizziness, call 9-1-1.

▶ Spider and Insect Bites

Most spiders are venomous, which is how they paralyze and kill their prey. However, most spiders lack an effective delivery system—long fangs and strong jaws—to bite a human. About 60 species of spiders in North America are capable of biting humans, although only a few species have produced significant poisonings **Figure 19-14**.

Most bites are by female spiders. Male spiders are almost always smaller than females and have fangs that are too short and fragile to bite humans. Death rarely occurs and only from bites by brown recluse and black widow spiders.

The number of deaths from spider bites is not accurately known. A spider bite is difficult to diagnose, especially when the spider was not seen or recovered,

because the bites typically cause little immediate pain. In a study of 600 suspected spider bites, 80% were caused by other arthropods (for example, kissing bugs, ticks, fleas, mites, and bedbugs) and 10% by disease states (for example, poison ivy, diabetic ulcer, bedsore, Lyme disease, and gonococcus). Spiders rarely bite more than once, and they do not always release venom.

Black Widow Spiders

Black widow spiders are also commonly known as brown widow spiders and red-legged spiders, depending on the species **Figure 19-15**. The term *black widow* is actually inaccurate, because only three of the five species of widow spider are actually black; the others are brown and gray. Newly hatched spiders are almost entirely red. Males have white stripes along the outside of the abdomen.

The female black widow spider is one of the largest spiders, with a body that ranges up to ½ inch in length and a leg span of up to 2 inches. It is her large size that allows the female black widow's fangs to be large and strong enough to penetrate human skin. The female black widow can live as long as 3 years. Black widow spiders have round abdomens that vary from gray to brown to black, depending on the species. In the female black widow, the abdomen is shiny black with a red or yellow spot (often in the shape of an hourglass) or white spots or bands.

The male is only one third of the size of the female. Contrary to popular myth, the male usually mates safely with the female. Because he is small, his fangs are incapable of penetrating human skin, so bites are

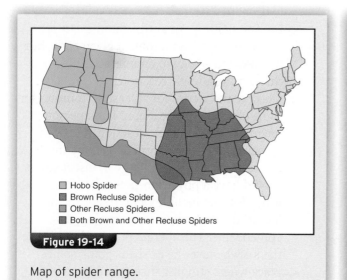

☐ Hobo Spider
☐ Brown Recluse Spider
☐ Other Recluse Spiders
☐ Both Brown and Other Recluse Spiders

Figure 19-14

Map of spider range.

Figure 19-15

Black widow spider.

from the female. Black widow spiders produce one of the most potent venoms known in terms of volume. The venom is chiefly a neurotoxin in humans, with symptoms most often manifested as severe muscle pain and cramping.

Black widow spiders are found throughout the world. In the Western Hemisphere, they are found from southern Canada, throughout every state in the continental United States, to the tip of South America, and in Hawaii.

The web of the black widow spider is an extensive, irregular, shaggy trap for the insects she normally eats. The black widow rarely leaves the web and stays close to her egg mass. She aggressively defends the egg mass and bites if it is disturbed. When she is not guarding eggs, the spider often attempts to escape rather than bite.

Frequent cleaning to remove spiders and their webs from buildings, outbuildings, and outdoor living areas decreases the chance of accidental contact with black widow spiders. Insecticides could decrease the population of the food for the black widows but do not usually affect the spiders themselves.

Recognizing Black Widow Spider Bites

The following could indicate a black widow spider bite:

- If the spider is trapped against the skin or crushed, it will bite. It is difficult to determine if a person has been bitten by a black widow spider or by any spider.
- The victim might feel a sharp pinprick when the spider bites, but some victims are not aware of the bite. Within 15 minutes, a dull, numbing pain develops in the bite area.
- Two small fang marks might be seen as tiny red spots.
- Within 15 minutes to 4 hours, muscle stiffness and cramps occur, usually affecting the abdomen when the bite is on a lower part of the body and the shoulders, back, or chest when the bite is on an upper part. Victims often describe the pain as the most severe they have ever experienced.
- Headache, chills, fever, heavy sweating, dizziness, nausea, and vomiting occur next. Severe pain around the bite site peaks in 2 to 3 hours and can last 12 to 48 hours.

Care for Black Widow Spider Bites

To care for someone who has been bitten by a black widow spider, do the following:

1. If possible, catch the spider to confirm its identity. Even if the body has been crushed, save it for identification (although most spider bite victims never see the spider). The species helps determine the treatment, so the dead spider (if it can be found) should be taken with the victim to the hospital.
2. Clean the bite area with soap and water or rubbing alcohol.
3. Place an ice pack over the bite to relieve pain and delay the effects of the venom.
4. Give aspirin (adults only), ibuprofen, or acetaminophen.
5. Monitor breathing.
6. Seek medical care immediately. For black widow spider bites, an antivenom exists. It is usually reserved for children younger than 6 years, people older than 60 years and with high blood pressure, pregnant women, and victims with severe reactions. The antivenom will give relief within 1 to 3 hours.

Brown Recluse Spiders

Brown recluse spiders are also known in North America as fiddle-back and violin spiders **Figure 19-16**. They have a violin-shaped figure on their backs (several other spider species have a similar configuration on their backs). Color varies from fawn to dark brown, with darker legs. Male and female spiders are

Figure 19-16

Brown recluse spider.

Spider Bites and Scorpion Stings

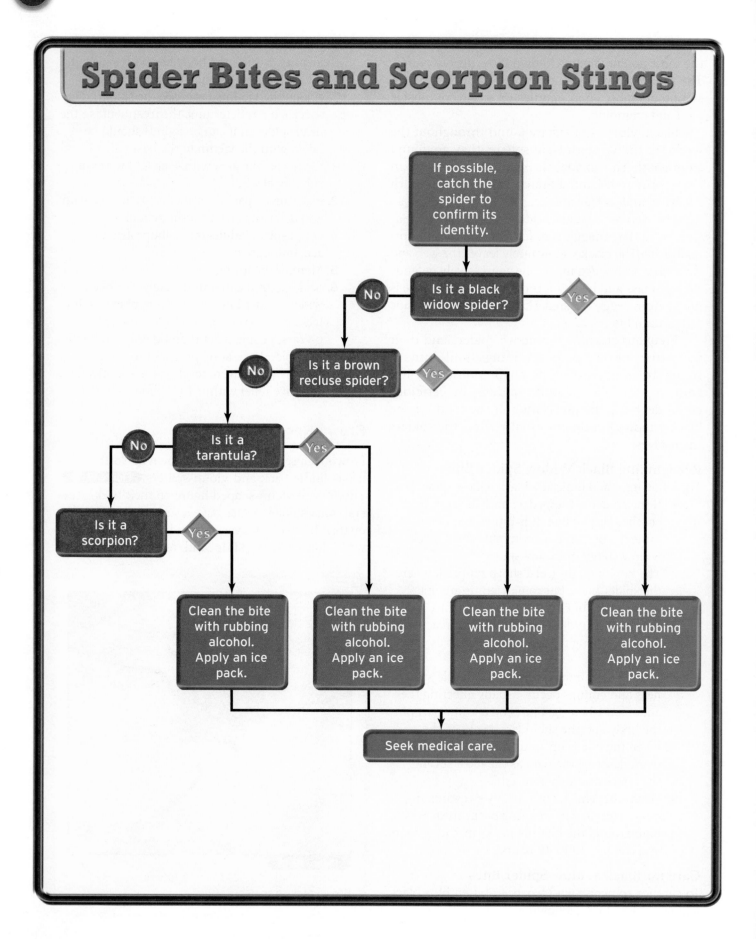

venomous. Brown recluse spiders are found primarily in the southern and midwestern states, with other less toxic but related spiders throughout the rest of the country. They are absent from the Pacific Northwest.

Recognizing Brown Recluse Spider Bites

If you suspect a brown recluse spider bite, remember the following:

- The brown recluse spider bites only when it is trapped against the skin.
- A local reaction usually occurs within 2 to 8 hours with mild to severe pain at the bite site and the development of redness, swelling, and local itching.
- In 48 to 72 hours, a blister develops at the bite site, becomes red, and bursts. During the early stages, the affected area often takes on a bull's-eye appearance, with a central white area surrounded by a reddened area, ringed by a whitish or blue border. A small, red crater remains, over which a scab forms. When the scab falls away in a few days, a larger crater remains. That too scabs over and falls off, leaving a larger crater. The craters are known as *volcano lesions*. This process of slow tissue destruction can continue for weeks or months. The ulcer sometimes requires skin grafting.
- Fever, weakness, vomiting, joint pain, and a rash could occur.
- Stomach cramps, nausea, and vomiting might occur. Death is rare.

Care for Brown Recluse Spider Bites

This is how you can care for someone who has been bitten by a brown recluse spider:

1. If possible, catch the spider to confirm its identity. Even if the body has been crushed, save it for identification (although most spider bite victims never see the spider). The species helps determine the treatment, so the dead spider (if it can be found) should be taken with the victim to the hospital.
2. Clean the bite area with soap and water or rubbing alcohol.
3. Place an ice pack over the bite to relieve pain and delay the effects of the venom.
4. Give aspirin (adults only), ibuprofen, or acetaminophen.
5. Seek medical care immediately.

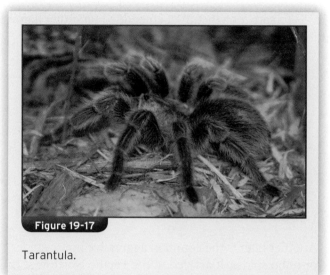

Figure 19-17

Tarantula.

Tarantulas

Tarantulas bite only when vigorously provoked or roughly handled **Figure 19-17**. The bite varies from almost painless to a deep throbbing pain lasting up to 1 hour. The tarantula, when upset, will roughly scratch the lower surface of its abdomen with its legs and flick hairs onto a person's skin.

Recognizing Tarantula Bites and Embedded Hairs

Tarantula bites and embedded hairs have the following characteristics:

- The bite causes pain—aching or stinging.
- The hairs cause itching and inflammation that can last several weeks.

Care for Tarantula Bites and Embedded Hairs

To care for a victim of a tarantula bite:

1. If possible, catch the spider to confirm its identity. Even if the body has been crushed, save it for identification (although most spider bite victims never see the spider). The species helps determine the treatment, so the dead spider (if it can be found) should be taken with the victim to the hospital.
2. Clean the bite area with soap and water or rubbing alcohol.
3. Place an ice pack over the bite to relieve pain and delay the effects of the venom.
4. Give aspirin (adults only), ibuprofen, or acetaminophen.
5. Seek medical care immediately.

To care for a victim of embedded tarantula hairs:

1. Remove the hairs from the skin with sticky tape (repeating as necessary).
2. Wash the area with soap and water.
3. Apply hydrocortisone cream.
4. Give the victim pain medication (aspirin— for adults only—or ibuprofen or acetaminophen)
5. Give the victim an antihistamine.

Common Aggressive House Spider (Hobo Spider)

Another biter is the common aggressive house spider, or hobo spider. It arrived in the Pacific Northwest in 1936 and slowly made its way across Washington State and into surrounding states. In those areas, the hobo spider is the most common large spider.

Recognizing Common Aggressive House Spider Bites

The signs and symptoms of the common aggressive house spider bite are similar to those of the brown recluse spider.

- Redness, blisters, and later, gangrene (dead tissue)
- Headache, visual problems, weakness

Care for Common Aggressive House Spider Bites

If someone has been bitten by a common aggressive house spider, you can help by doing the following:

1. If possible, catch the spider to confirm its identity. Even if the body has been crushed, save it for identification (although most spider bite victims never see the spider). The species helps determine the treatment, so the dead spider (if it can be found) should be taken with the victim to the hospital.
2. Clean the bite area with soap and water or rubbing alcohol.
3. Place an ice pack over the bite to relieve pain and delay the effects of the venom.
4. Give aspirin (adults only), ibuprofen, or acetaminophen.
5. Seek medical care immediately.

Scorpions

Scorpions look like miniature lobsters, with lobsterlike pincers and a long, up-curved taillike appendage with

Figure 19-18

Bark scorpion.

a poisonous stinger **Figure 19-18**. Several species of scorpions inhabit the southwestern United States, but only the bark scorpion poses a threat to humans. Severe cases, which usually appear only in children, could include paralysis, spasms, or breathing difficulties. Death due to scorpion stings in the United States is rare.

The bark scorpion is found primarily in Arizona. Rare stings have been reported in other parts of the United States, after the scorpions traveled from Arizona as stowaways in luggage or in car trunks. The bark scorpion is pale tan and is ¾″ to 1¼″ long, not including the so-called tail.

Stings to adult victims usually are not life threatening. Stings to small children, however, are often dangerous. When a child is stung, every effort should be made to get the victim to medical care as quickly as possible. Pay close attention to make sure the victim's airway is open and that he or she is breathing.

Recognizing Scorpion Stings

The most frequent symptom of a scorpion sting, especially to an adult victim, is local, immediate pain and burning around the sting site. Later, numbness or tingling occurs. There is no swelling or blanching. Tapping a finger over the sting site can cause pain (the tap test) and could serve to indicate a scorpion sting. More severely affected people will experience pain along the stung arm or leg, even paralysis. In more serious stings, uncontrolled jerking movements of the legs or arms and facial twitching might occur.

Victims with a severe reaction will have a fast heart rate, salivate, and experience breathing distress. Symptoms begin from within minutes to half an hour and reach their height within the first few hours. Symptoms usually last from 6 to 24 hours.

Care for Scorpion Stings

Care for a scorpion sting victim by doing the following:
1. Monitor breathing.
2. Gently clean the sting site with soap and water or rubbing alcohol.
3. Apply an ice pack over the sting site to reduce pain and venom absorption.
4. Give aspirin (adults only), ibuprofen, or acetaminophen.
5. Seek medical care. Recently, bark scorpion antivenom production has been discontinued. Its use was controversial. The US Food and Drug Administration has given approval for clinical trials to evaluate a Mexican antivenom for use in the United States.

Centipedes

Centipedes come in various sizes and colors and are found all over the United States and throughout the world. The giant desert centipede, which can be up to 8 inches long, is the only US centipede that is dangerous to humans.

Like spiders, any centipede with fangs that can penetrate human skin can inject venom. These arthropods inject toxic substances into the skin from a pair of hollow jaws that act like fangs. Contrary to popular belief, centipedes do not inject venom with their feet. Exaggerated stories about the deadly effects of their bites and reports that the tip of each leg carries a poisonous spur have caused many people to have an unreasonable fear of centipedes. Their venom is relatively weak.

Recognizing Centipede Bites

Generally, bite indications are burning pain and local inflammation of the wound site, with mild swelling of the lymph nodes. The bite of the giant desert centipede causes inflammation, swelling, and redness that last 4 to 12 hours. Swelling and tenderness can last as long as 3 weeks or can disappear and recur.

Care for Centipede Bites

Centipedes, which have one pair of legs per body segment, are sometimes confused with millipedes, which have two pairs of legs per body segment. Millipedes cannot inject venom, but their secretions can irritate the skin. Treat those who have been exposed to millipede secretions by washing the area of contact with soap and water and applying a cortisone cream or ointment.

Care for a centipede bite victim in the following manner:
1. Clean the wound with soap and water.
2. Apply an ice pack at the bite site.
3. For pain, give aspirin (adults only), acetaminophen, or ibuprofen.
4. Seek medical care for severe reactions.

Mosquitoes

Mosquitoes bite millions of people. Mosquitoes are not only a nuisance, but they also carry many diseases. In developing countries, mosquitoes transmit malaria, yellow fever, and dengue fever; in the United States, they carry encephalitis. There is no evidence that mosquitoes transmit HIV, the virus that causes acquired immunodeficiency syndrome (AIDS).

Female mosquitoes need blood to lay their eggs. Because they breed in water, mosquitoes are most often found in marshes, wetlands, and wooded areas. Mosquitoes usually can be separated into daytime and nighttime biters, but most bite at twilight.

Care for Mosquito Bites

You can care for someone who has mosquito bites in the following manner:
1. Wash the bitten area with soap and water.
2. Apply an ice pack.
3. Apply calamine lotion or hydrocortisone ointment to decrease redness and itching.
4. For a victim with a number of bites or a delayed allergic reaction, an antihistamine every 6 hours or a physician-prescribed cortisone might be useful.

FYI

Preventing Mosquito Bites

To minimize being bitten by mosquitoes, follow these guidelines:

- Wear protective clothing: pants, long-sleeved shirt, and full-brimmed hat. Mosquito netting draped over a hat will protect the face and neck. Mosquito bed nets should be used when sleeping in unscreened rooms.
- Use insect repellents on exposed skin. DEET (diethyltoluamide)-containing repellents are most effective against mosquitoes and, to a lesser extent, helpful in repelling ticks and black flies.
- DEET is considered to have low toxicity. However, it is absorbed through the skin, and hives, skin rashes, and blisters can result when it is used for prolonged periods or in excessive amounts. The long-acting 35% solution has a polymer that prevents evaporation and skin absorption.
- Products that contain 100% DEET are available but unnecessary, especially for children. Long-acting formulations of 35% DEET seem equally effective in protecting against mosquitoes and have far less potential for toxic effects.
- DEET products can be applied over other creams such as sunscreens and moisturizers. Use DEET only on exposed skin, and avoid the hands of young children because they often put their hands in their mouths. Keep DEET out of the reach of small children because ingestion could be fatal. Children younger than 5 years should not be exposed to concentrations greater than 10%, according to the American Academy of Pediatrics. Children younger than 2 months of age should not have DEET applied to their skin. For children ages 5 or older, the DEET concentration should not exceed 30%.
- Other nontoxic insect repellents seem to be less effective than DEET. They might be only 25% as effective as DEET and might need to be reapplied every half hour. Mixed opinions exist about whether 100 mg of vitamin B_1 (thiamine) taken daily for 1 week before being exposed is an effective preventive agent. Some experts believe that a diet high in garlic will make a person undesirable to a mosquito.
- Permethrin is a pesticide, not a repellent. It should be applied to clothing and not the skin.

FYI

Mosquito Bites

In tropical climates, mosquitoes are important carriers of infectious diseases such as malaria and yellow fever. Mosquito bites can also provoke unpleasant skin lesions. In many areas of the world, massive and disturbing mosquito infestations occur. For example, in Alaska it is possible to be bitten by mosquitoes as many as 1,000 times in one hour. Under such conditions, complete avoidance of bites is impossible without use of effective repellents and protective clothing. Topical treatment with over-the-counter sticks, creams, and lotions containing antihistamines, hydrocortisone, or other antipruritic agents is common. However, only a few studies have been made on the effectiveness of these products.

Source: Reunala T, et al. 1993. Treatment of mosquito bites with cetirizine. *Clin Exp Allergy* 23 (1):72-75.

Ticks

Ticks are not insects but are close relatives of mites and spiders. They have eight legs and are classified as hard ticks and soft ticks. Hard ticks are more familiar because of their wide distribution and common occurrence on domestic animals. Soft ticks are found mainly in western states. In the United States, seven kinds of hard ticks and five kinds of soft ticks carry diseases (for example, Lyme disease), are a nuisance (causing itching and swelling), or cause paralysis (toxin injected). Ticks hatch from eggs and grow through three distinct stages: nymph (too small to see), larva (just visible), and adult (ready to lay eggs).

The adult is most likely to be seen. Ticks at any stage of development can use humans for food; at each stage, they need a blood meal before they can grow to the next stage. Ticks are limited in their ability to find their meals. They cannot fly, they crawl very slowly, and, without some help, they cannot travel more than a few yards from where they were hatched. When they are ready for their next meal, they might wait months, years, or even decades for the right host to come along. Bites are nearly painless, so the tick attachment is not noticed until later.

The front part of a tick consists of the head area and the mouthparts. The mouthparts have a central structure, the hypostome, which is shaped like a blunt

Figure 19-19

A. Tick embedded and engorged. **B.** Tick embedded.

Figure 19-20

A bull's-eye rash is a distinctive finding in Lyme disease, but is not always present in victims.

Figure 19-21

Removing a tick with tweezers.

harpoon. A tick makes a hole in the victim's skin with the sharp teeth (barbs) on the front of the hypostome and inserts its hypostome **Figure 19-19**. The barbs anchor the tick to the skin and make it difficult to pull the tick out. Some ticks produce a substance that helps cement them to the host. As they feed, some ticks increase in size 20 to 50 times.

Care for Embedded Ticks

Remove ticks as soon as possible. If a tick is carrying a disease, the longer it stays embedded, the greater the chance of the disease being transmitted. Because its bite is painless, a tick can remain embedded for days before the victim realizes it. Most tick bites are harmless, although ticks can carry Lyme disease, Rocky Mountain spotted fever, and other serious diseases **Figure 19-20**.

To pull off a tick:

1. Use tweezers or a specialized tick removal tool.
2. Grasp the tick as close to the skin as possible, and lift it with enough force to tent the skin surface. Hold it in this position until the tick lets go (about 1 minute). Pull the tick away from the skin. Do not pull hard enough to break the tick apart because this will leave parts of the tick behind, which may cause infection **Figure 19-21**.

After the tick has been removed:

1. Wash the area with soap and water. Apply rubbing alcohol to further disinfect the area.
2. Apply an ice pack to reduce pain.

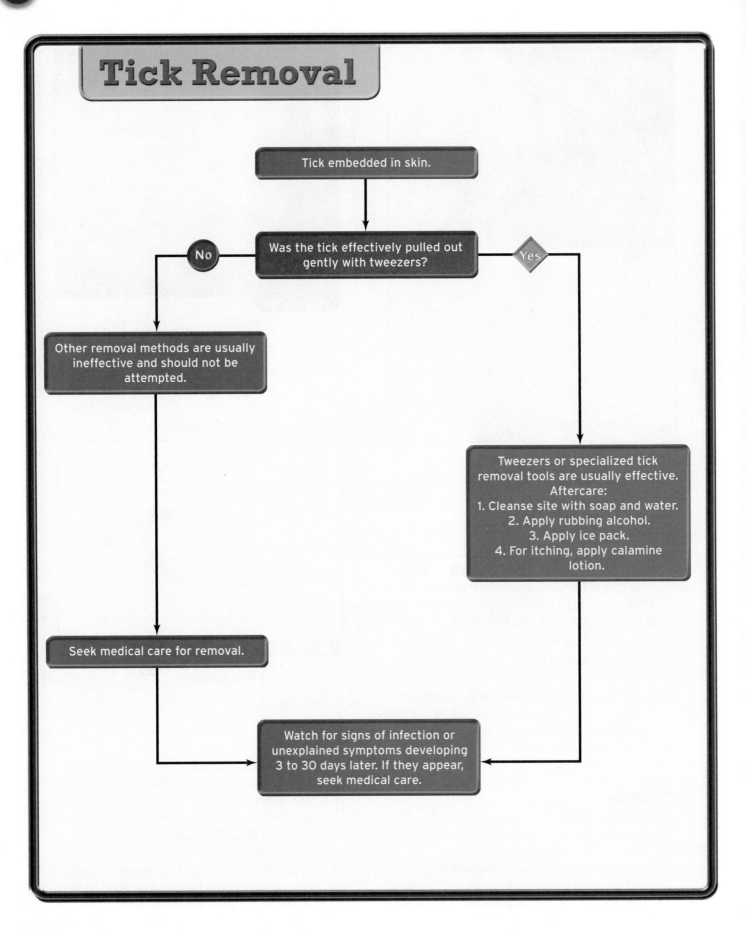

Tick Removal

Tick embedded in skin.

Was the tick effectively pulled out gently with tweezers?

No — Other removal methods are usually ineffective and should not be attempted.

Seek medical care for removal.

Yes — Tweezers or specialized tick removal tools are usually effective.
Aftercare:
1. Cleanse site with soap and water.
2. Apply rubbing alcohol.
3. Apply ice pack.
4. For itching, apply calamine lotion.

Watch for signs of infection or unexplained symptoms developing 3 to 30 days later. If they appear, seek medical care.

FYI

The Knot Method of Tick Removal

An embedded tick should be removed as soon as possible. The longer an infected tick stays embedded, the more likely it is to transmit a disease. An alternative to using tweezers and special commercial tick removal devices, especially when they are not available, is the knot method.

Use cotton thread or dental floss and tie an overhand knot (similar to a shoelace knot without the bows). The open overhand knot is placed over the tick as close as possible to the skin surface and then gently closed to form a loop around the tick. Lift the tick's body over its head in a somersault-type fashion to remove the tick. This method removes the entire tick and is simple and effective.

Source: Celensa A. 2002. The knot method of tick removal. *Wilderness Environ Med* 13(2):181.

CAUTION

DO NOT use the following popular methods of tick removal, which are ineffective:

- Applying petroleum jelly
- Applying fingernail polish
- Applying rubbing alcohol
- Touching a hot match to the tick
- Applying a petroleum product, such as gasoline

DO NOT grab a tick at the rear of its body. The internal organs could rupture, and the contents could be squeezed out, causing infection.

DO NOT twist or jerk the tick, which could result in incomplete removal.

FYI

Preventing Tick Bites

- Wear light-colored clothing so you can see any ticks on your clothes.
- Wear a long-sleeved shirt that fits tightly at the wrists and neck and tuck the shirt into your pants.
- Wear long pants and tuck the pant legs into your boots or socks, or use masking tape to tape the pant legs tightly to your socks, shoes, or boots.
- Check your clothes while you are outdoors and before entering a house. Wash your clothes as soon as possible.
- Inspect your pets for ticks before they come inside.
- After coming indoors, shower or bathe and check your body for ticks, especially in areas that have hair or where clothing was tight. Another person could do the checking.
- Treat your body and clothing with a repellent. The most common, Environmental Protection Agency-approved, and effective tick repellent is DEET.
- You can buy DEET and apply it directly to your skin. Ticks crawling on the treated area are irritated by the repellent and drop off. DEET is most effective against ticks when applied to clothing from a spray can.
- There have been a few reports of adverse toxic reactions to DEET, such as seizures, allergic responses, and skin irritation. To minimize reactions, do the following:
  - Apply DEET sparingly to your skin.
  - Avoid applying high-concentration products (more than 35% DEET) to the skin.
  - Do not inhale or ingest DEET-containing products or get them in your eyes.
  - Do not apply DEET to wounds or irritated skin.
  - Wash your skin after coming indoors.
  - Do not use products with more than 10% DEET on infants and small children (younger than 5 years).
- You can also use 0.5% preparations of permethrin (a pesticide). Permethrin should be applied only to clothing (especially shirt sleeves, pants legs, and collars), never directly on the skin.

Table 19-4 Preventing Shark Attacks

No shark repellents are universally effective. Explosive and electronic devices could threaten diver safety instead of sharks. The following guidelines can help prevent shark attacks:

- Avoid swimming in areas frequented by sharks or where shark attacks have occurred. (In the United States, the greatest concentration of great white shark attacks is off the northern California coast.)
- Do not swim or dive alone.
- Do not swim far offshore, in murky water, or along deep drop-offs.
- People with open wounds and menstruating women should avoid swimming in areas where there is risk of a shark attack.
- Avoid swimming in the vicinity of seal or sea lion colonies or turtle habitats.
- Do not spear fish for an extended period in the same area, and do not attach fish to your body.
- Avoid swimming at dawn, dusk, or night in potentially dangerous waters.

3. Apply calamine lotion to relieve itching. Keep the area clean.
4. For 1 month, continue to watch the bite site for a rash. If a rash appears, seek medical care. Watch for other signs such as fever, muscle aches, sensitivity to bright light, and paralysis that begins with leg weakness.

▶ Marine Animal Injuries

Most marine animals bite or sting in defense, rather than attack. Marine venoms are similar to many venoms found in reptiles and arthropods and can cause anaphylaxis or other types of reactions. The general first aid guidelines are similar to those for any disorder involving trauma, allergy, or cardiopulmonary failure. Serious allergic reactions require primary attention to keeping the airway open.

Sharks

Sharks are the most feared of all marine animals, but the chance of being attacked by a shark along the North American coastline is less than 1 in 5,000,000 Table 19-4 . Although exact figures are unavailable, it is estimated that, worldwide, more than 50 attacks and fewer than a dozen deaths occur each year. The number of unprovoked shark attacks has grown at a steady rate over the past century.

Figure 19-22

Shark.

Most attacks occur within 100 feet of shore, and most victims are attacked by a single shark without warning. In the majority of attacks, the victim does not see the shark before the attack Figure 19-22 . The leg is the most frequently bitten part. Sharks are clearly more attracted to people on the surface than to underwater scuba divers. The greatest attraction for sharks seems to be chemicals found in fish blood—sharks

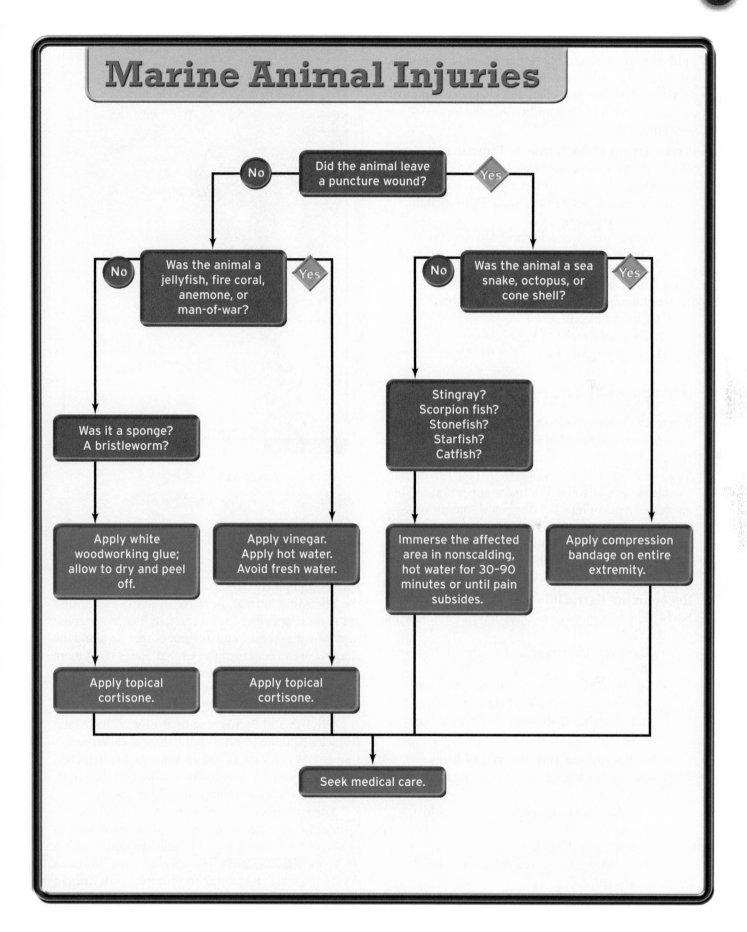

Marine Animal Injuries

Did the animal leave a puncture wound?

No → Was the animal a jellyfish, fire coral, anemone, or man-of-war?

Yes → Was the animal a sea snake, octopus, or cone shell?

Was the animal a jellyfish, fire coral, anemone, or man-of-war?

No → Was it a sponge? A bristleworm?

Yes → Apply vinegar. Apply hot water. Avoid fresh water.

Was the animal a sea snake, octopus, or cone shell?

No → Stingray? Scorpion fish? Stonefish? Starfish? Catfish?

Yes → Apply compression bandage on entire extremity.

Was it a sponge? A bristleworm? → Apply white woodworking glue; allow to dry and peel off.

Stingray? Scorpion fish? Stonefish? Starfish? Catfish? → Immerse the affected area in nonscalding, hot water for 30-90 minutes or until pain subsides.

Apply white woodworking glue; allow to dry and peel off. → Apply topical cortisone.

Apply vinegar. Apply hot water. Avoid fresh water. → Apply topical cortisone.

Seek medical care.

can detect them in quantities as small as one part per million parts of water. Shark bite wounds, among the most devastating of all animal bites, are similar to injuries caused by boat propellers and chainsaws. Immediate control of bleeding and treatment for shock are essential.

Recognizing a Shark Bite or Puncture

Most victims are attacked by single sharks, violently and without warning. In most attacks the victim does not see the shark before the attack. Signs include:

- Severe bleeding
- Large, open wounds, most often on the legs
- Abrasions caused by contact with sharkskin

Care for a Shark Bite or Puncture

To care for a victim of shark bite or puncture:

1. Control bleeding.
2. Treat for shock.
3. Seek medical care.

Barracudas and Moray Eels

Barracudas have a fearsome appearance, but they have an undeserved reputation as attackers of humans. The risk of a barracuda bite is exceedingly small. First aid for a barracuda bite is identical to that for a shark bite.

Moray eels also have a fierce appearance. They are not infrequent biters of divers who handle or tease them, usually in competition for food or in pursuit of lobsters. The multiple puncture wounds created by moray eel bites have a high infection risk. Treat these wounds as you would shark bites.

Recognizing Barracuda and Moray Eel Bites

Barracuda and moray eel bites have the following characteristics:

- Barracuda lacerations are similar to those of a shark.
- Eel bites involve severe puncture wounds with their narrow jaws. Eels will hold onto a victim, rather than strike and release. They leave multiple, small puncture wounds.

Care for Barracuda and Moray Eel Bites

The following list indicates how to care for a barracuda or moray eel bite victim.

- Care for a barracuda bites as you would a shark bite.
- Care for an eel bite by:
  - Flushing the wound with water under pressure.
  - Controlling bleeding.

Figure 19-23

Portuguese man-of-war.

Marine Animals That Sting

Stings from marine animals lead the list of adverse marine animal encounters. It is important to identify the offending animal, because in many cases, first aid is quite specific. Each year, jellyfish, Portuguese man-of-wars, corals, and anemones that lie along the shallow ocean waters of the United States sting more than 1 million people. Reactions to being stung vary from mild dermatitis to severe reactions. Most victims recover without medical attention.

Jellyfish and Portuguese man-of-wars have long tentacles equipped with stinging devices called **nematocysts**. When cast ashore or onto rocks, detached nematocysts retain their ability to sting for a long time, usually until they are completely dried out.

The Portuguese man-of-war sting is usually in the form of well-defined linear welts or scattered patches of welts with redness, which usually disappear within 24 hours **Figure 19-23**. The jellyfish sting produces severe muscle cramping with multiple, thin lines of welts crossing the skin in a zigzag pattern

Figure 19-24

Jellyfish.

Figure 19-25

Anemones.

Figure 19-24. Pain usually is a burning type that lasts 10 to 30 minutes. The welts on the skin usually disappear within an hour.

Anemones are beautiful but potentially dangerous **Figure 19-25**. Many anemone stings result from the improper handling of aquarium animals.

Recognizing Marine Stings

Marine stings cause the following symptoms:

- Stinging
- Severe itching, burning
- Prickling, tingling
- Blisters
- Severe allergic reaction
- Difficulty breathing
- Muscle cramping
- Nausea, vomiting

Care for Marine Stings

Follow these steps to care for a victim of a marine sting:

1. Apply vinegar to the sting area for at least 30 seconds; it deactivates the nematocysts. If vinegar is not available, use a baking soda paste.
2. Use hot water (110° F [43° C]) immersion for at least 20 minutes to reduce pain. If hot water is not available, use hot dry packs.
3. Apply a coating of hydrocortisone (1%) several times a day.

CAUTION

DO NOT try to rub the tentacles off of the victim's skin—rubbing activates the stinging cells.

DO NOT use fresh water for rinsing because it will cause the nematocysts to fire.

DO NOT apply cold packs—they also will cause the nematocysts to fire.

DO NOT touch the tentacles with your bare hands.

Figure 19-26

Stingray.

Stingrays

Stingrays, commonly found in tropical and subtropical waters, are peaceful, reclusive bottom feeders that generally lie buried in the sand or mud **Figure 19-26**. Most wounds inflicted by stingrays are produced on the ankle or foot when the victim steps on a ray. The ray reacts by thrusting its barbed tail upward and forward into the victim's leg or foot. At least 1,500 stingray injuries occur each year in coastal US waters. The stingray's venomous tail barb easily penetrates human skin. The sting usually is more like a laceration because the large tail barb can do significant damage. The venom causes intense burning pain at the site.

Recognizing Stingray Punctures

A stingray puncture results in the following:

- Sudden, intense pain
- An open wound
- Swelling

Care for Stingray Punctures

You can care for stingray puncture victims by doing the following:

1. Relieve pain by immersing the injured body part in hot water (110° F [43° C]) for 30 to 90 minutes. Make sure the water is not hot enough to cause a burn.
2. Wash the wound with soap and water.
3. Irrigate the area with water under pressure to wash out as much of the toxin and foreign material as possible.
4. Treat the wound like any puncture wound.

▶ Emergency Care Wrap-up

Condition	What to Look For	What to Do
Bites and Stings	**Animal and human bites** • Torn tissue • Bleeding	1. Wash wound with soap and water. 2. Flush wound thoroughly with water under pressure. 3. Control bleeding. 4. Seek medical care.
	Venomous snake bites • Severe, burning pain • Small puncture wounds • Swelling • Nausea, vomiting, sweating, weakness • Discoloration and blood-filled blisters developing hours after the bite	1. Get away from the snake. 2. Limit victim's movement and keep bitten extremity below heart level. 3. Call 9-1-1. 4. Gently wash area with soap and water. 5. Apply mild pressure by wrapping the entire affected arm or leg with an elastic bandage.
	Insect stings • Pain • Itching • Swelling • Severe allergic reaction, including breathing problems	1. Remove any stinger. 2. Wash with soap and water. 3. Apply an ice or cold pack. 4. Give pain medication and an antihistamine and apply hydrocortisone cream. 5. Observe for at least 30 minutes for signs of severe allergic reaction. Call 9-1-1 if a severe allergic reaction occurs. If victim has an epinephrine auto-injector, help victim use it.

	Spider bites
	• Black widow
	  • May feel sharp pain
	  • Two small fang marks
	  • Severe abdominal pain
	  • Headache, chills, fever, sweating, dizziness, nausea
	• Brown recluse and hobo
	  • Blister developing several days later
	  • Ulcer in skin
	  • Headache, fever, weakness, nausea
		1. Catch spider for identification.
		2. Wash bitten area with soap and water.
		3. Apply an ice or cold pack.
		4. Seek medical care.

	Scorpion stings • Pain and burning at sting site • Later, numbness or tingling	1. Wash sting site with soap and water. 2. Apply an ice or cold pack. 3. Seek medical care.

Condition	What to Look For	What to Do
Bites and Stings—continued	**Tick bites** • Tick still attached • Rash (especially one shaped like a bull's-eye) • Fever, joint aches, weakness	1. Remove tick. 2. Wash bitten area with soap and water. 3. Apply rubbing alcohol. 4. Apply an ice or cold pack. 5. Watch bitten area for 1 month for rash. Seek medical care if rash or other signs such as fever or muscle joint aches appear.
Marine Animal Injuries	Bites, rips, or punctures from marine animals (for example, sharks, barracudas, moray eels)	1. Control bleeding. 2. Treat for shock. 3. Call 9-1-1.
	Stings from marine animals (for example, jellyfish, Portuguese man-of-war)	1. Apply vinegar (minimum of 30 seconds). 2. Immerse in hot water for 20 minutes to reduce pain.
	Punctures from marine animal spines (for example, stingray)	1. Immerse injured part in hot water for 30 to 90 minutes. 2. Wash with soap and water. 3. Flush with water under pressure. 4. Care for wound.

▶ Ready for Review

- Almost half of all Americans will suffer a bite from either an animal or human.
- Throughout the world, about 50,000 people die each year of snake bites.
- The stinging insects belonging to the order of *Hymenoptera* include honeybees, bumblebees, yellow jackets, hornets, wasps, and fire ants.
- Most spiders are venomous, which is how they paralyze and kill their prey. However, most spiders lack an effective delivery system—long fangs and strong jaws—to bite a human.
- Most marine animals bite or sting in defense, rather than attack.

▶ Vital Vocabulary

<u>antivenom</u> An antiserum containing antibodies against reptile or insect venom.

<u>nematocysts</u> Stinging cells found on certain marine animals.

<u>rabies</u> An acute viral infection of the central nervous system transmitted by the bite of an infected animal.

▶ Assessment in Action

You are enjoying an overnight campout with your family in the springtime. As you get ready for bed, you notice a small lump on your belly and are startled to find an embedded tick.

Directions: Circle Yes if you agree with the statement; circle No if you disagree.

Yes No **1.** You should leave the tick alone because it will cause no harm to humans.

Yes No **2.** Covering the tick with petroleum jelly is very effective for removing the embedded tick.

Yes No **3.** You should touch a hot, blown-out match to the tick.

Yes No **4.** Grabbing the tick as close to the skin as possible with tweezers and pulling upward is usually effective.

Yes No **5.** After removing the tick, clean the wound and use an icepack to reduce pain.

▶ Check Your Knowledge

Directions: Circle Yes if you agree with the statement; circle No if you disagree.

Yes No **1.** Severe abdominal pain is a sign of a black widow spider bite.

Yes No **2.** Apply an ice or cold pack over a snake bite.

Yes No **3.** Use the cut and suck method for a snake bite.

Yes No **4.** Remove a bee's stinger by using tweezers to pull it out.

Yes No **5.** Apply an ice or cold pack over an insect sting or a suspected spider bite.

Yes No **6.** A baking soda paste can help reduce the itching and swelling from an insect sting.

Yes No **7.** A victim's prescribed auto-injector might have to be used if the victim has a life-threatening reaction to an insect sting.

Yes No **8.** Care for stings from marine animals (for example, jellyfish) by pouring hydrogen peroxide on the affected area.

Yes No **9.** Covering an embedded tick with petroleum jelly causes the tick to back out because of the lack of oxygen.

Yes No **10.** Ticks can transmit disease.

Cold-Related Emergencies

Cold-Related Emergencies

Heat flows from an area with a higher temperature to an area with a lower temperature. When a person is surrounded by air or water cooler than body temperature, the body loses heat. If heat escapes faster than the body produces heat, the body temperature falls. Normal body temperature is 98.6° F, and if the body temperature falls much below that, cold injuries can result.

▶ How Cold Affects the Body

Humans protect themselves from cold primarily by avoiding or reducing cold exposure through the use of clothing and shelter. When that protection proves inadequate, the body has biologic defense mechanisms to help maintain correct body temperature. The internal mechanisms to maintain body temperature during cold exposure include vasoconstriction and shivering. Triggering of these responses is a signal that clothing and shelter are inadequate.

<u>Vasoconstriction</u> is the tightening of blood vessels. During cold exposure, vasoconstriction occurs in the exposed skin. The reduced blood flow in the skin conserves body heat but can lead to discomfort, numbness, loss of dexterity in the hands and fingers, and, eventually, cold injuries.

Cold triggers shivering, which increases internal heat production and helps offset the heat lost. Shivering is the body's main involuntary defense against the cold. Shivering produces body heat by forcing muscles to contract and relax rapidly. About 80% of the muscle energy used in shivering is turned into body heat. When the core temperature rises, shivering is no longer needed and is shut down by the brain. When the core temperature falls to about 86° F to 90° F, the shivering reflex stops. Likewise, when there is no further fuel for the body, shivering stops. Several drugs suppress the shivering response, including barbiturates, narcotics, beta-blocking agents, and alcohol.

Internal heat production is also increased by physical activity; the more vigorous the activity, the greater the heat production. In fact, heat production during intense exercise or strenuous work usually is sufficient to compensate completely for heat loss, even when it is extremely cold. However, high-intensity exercise and hard physical work are fatiguing and cannot be sustained indefinitely. If clothes become wet with sweat, heat loss is markedly increased after exertion.

Susceptibility to cold injuries can be minimized by maintaining proper hydration and nutrition; avoiding alcohol, caffeine, and nicotine; and limiting periods of inactivity in cold conditions. Humans do not acclimatize to cold weather nearly as well as they acclimatize to hot weather.

The colder the surrounding temperature, the greater the potential for body heat to escape. When the skin is exposed to cold, the brain signals the blood vessels in the skin to tighten, and blood flow to the skin decreases. This is the body's attempt to prevent heat inside the body from being carried to the skin, where it will be lost. However, because of reduced blood flow to the skin, the skin temperature falls.

When cold exposure lasts more than an hour, cooling of the skin and reduced blood flow to the hands will blunt sensation, touch, and pain, and will cause a loss of dexterity and agility. These changes can impair a person's ability to perform manual tasks and, because symptoms could go unnoticed, can lead to more severe cold injuries.

Heat Loss From the Body

Normal body temperature is maintained by a balance of heat production and heat loss. Heat is produced by food metabolism and muscle activity, and shivering can increase heat production up to 500%. Shivering causes a large increase in heat production, but it rapidly consumes calories stored in the liver and muscles as glycogen. Lack of food limits the body's ability to produce heat; when glycogen stores are depleted, heat output decreases.

Heat loss occurs primarily through the skin. Blood flow to the skin varies in different parts of the body, and some areas lose more heat than others. Thermograms demonstrate high losses from the head and neck (up to 50%), axillary area (armpits), and groin area. The constriction of blood vessels caused by cold conserves heat.

Body heat can be lost by four mechanisms:

- Conduction, or direct contact with a colder object (for example, lying on the snow), normally accounts for only a small fraction of heat loss. The exception is immersion in cold water, in which heat loss can be 25 to 30 times greater than in air and even more in moving water.
- Convection is the loss of heat from the body by air blowing over the skin or through porous clothing. **Windchill** is the combined effect of the ambient temperature and wind speed.
- Evaporation, or conversion of liquid on the skin to a vapor, normally accounts for about 20% of heat loss (two thirds through sweating and one third through respiration).
- Radiation is the primary method of heat loss, accounting for about 65% of the body's heat loss. A warm object gives off (radiates) heat to cooler air. It has been demonstrated that up to 50% of the body's total heat production can be lost by radiation through a person's unprotected head **Figure 20-1** .

Q&A

How is shivering related to the muscular system?

Shivering is the body's natural way of keeping warm and can actually serve as a lifesaver in extreme cold. Shivering produces heat by forcing skeletal muscles to contract and relax rapidly. About 80% of the muscle energy used in this process is turned into body heat. Studies have shown that applying hot water bottles or hot objects can actually be harmful in some cases of hypothermia because the shivering reflex is shut down.

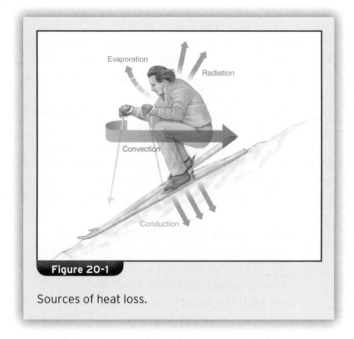

Figure 20-1

Sources of heat loss.

Susceptibility to Cold Injury

A person's susceptibility to cold injury is affected by many factors. Physically unfit people are more susceptible to cold injury. They tire more quickly and are unable to stay active to keep warm as long as people who are physically fit.

Dehydration reduces blood flow in the skin, which increases susceptibility to cold injury. Fat functions as an insulator against heat loss because it has less blood flow than muscle and loses less heat. Therefore, a very lean person may be susceptible to the effects of cold if clothing is inadequate or wet or if the person is relatively inactive. Elderly people are less tolerant of the cold than younger people because of the decline in physical fitness that often occurs with aging.

Alcohol and, to a lesser extent, caffeine cause the blood vessels in the skin to open, which can accelerate body heat loss. Also, alcohol and caffeine both increase urine formation, leading to dehydration, which can further degrade the body's defenses against cold. Most important, alcohol blunts the senses and impairs judgment, so a person may not feel the signs and symptoms of developing cold injury.

Because nicotine decreases blood flow to the skin, smoking and chewing tobacco can increase susceptibility to frostbite. Inadequate nutrition, illness, and injury compromise the body's responses to cold and a person's ability to recognize and react appropriately to the symptoms of developing cold injury. People who have experienced a cold injury are at greater risk of experiencing another cold injury.

Effects of Altitude

Assessing weather conditions in mountainous regions must include altitude considerations, especially if the assessment is based on weather measurements obtained at lower elevations. Temperatures, windchill, and the risk of cold injury at high altitudes can differ considerably from those at lower elevations.

In general, it can be assumed that air temperature drops 3.6° F every 1,000 feet above the original measurement site. Winds usually are more severe at high altitudes, and there is less cover above the tree line. People are more susceptible to frostbite and other cold injuries at altitudes above 8,000 feet than at sea level because of lower temperatures, higher winds, and less oxygen.

Effects of Water

Water can conduct heat away from the body much faster than air of the same temperature. When clothing becomes wet because of snow, rain, splashing water, or accumulated sweat, the body's loss of heat is accelerated, up to 25 times faster. Swimmers and people working or wading in water can lose a great deal of body heat, even when the water temperature is only mildly cool. People working in cold water should be closely watched as they enter the water because sudden plunging into cold water can produce an irregular heartbeat, gasping, and hyperventilation, which can cause inhalation of water, heart failure, and drowning.

Effects of Wind

For any given air temperature, the potential for body heat loss, skin cooling, and decreased internal temperature is increased by wind. Wind increases heat loss from skin exposed to cold air, in effect lowering the temperature. The windchill index integrates wind speed and air temperature to provide an estimate of the cooling power of the environment and the associated risk of cold injury.

Windchill temperatures obtained from weather reports do not take into account artificial wind, which worsens the windchill effect of natural wind. For example, riding in an open vehicle can subject the passengers to dangerous windchill, even when natural winds are low.

Effects of Metals and Liquid Fuels

Metal objects and liquid fuels that have been left outdoors in the cold pose a serious hazard. Both can conduct heat away from the skin rapidly. Fuels and solvents remain liquid at very low temperatures. Skin contact with fuel or metal at below-freezing temperatures can result in nearly instantaneous freezing. Fuel handlers must use great care and not allow exposed skin to come into contact with spilled fuels or metals.

Minimizing Effects of Cold on the Body

When adequately protected, humans can tolerate temperatures as low as −72° F. Adequate clothing maintains the microclimate surrounding the body. Air is an excellent insulator, and the basis for most clothing is to trap a layer of air around the body. Layering, which has been used for centuries, allows the removal or opening of a garment to vent excess heat during times of greater activity or changes in environment, and it accommodates individual needs and preferences. Wearing layered clothing is especially important for people who frequently change environments by going in and out of buildings or who periodically undertake vigorous physical activity **Figure 20-2** .

Three important layers are recommended for most outdoor activities. The first layer (undergarments) removes perspiration from the skin, the middle layers insulate, and the outer layer or outer shell protects against wind. By understanding this principle, people can vary their clothing for protection and comfort.

For the first layer, use underwear that wicks away perspiration; that is, it stays dry by drawing moisture away from the skin to the next layer of clothing. Wet clothing transfers heat away from the body. Cotton holds moisture next to the skin, so the person feels cold and clammy. Silk feels warm and soft, but it also retains moisture. Fabrics such as polypropylene or one of the new types of polyesters such as Capilene or Thermax should be considered.

The middle layer can be a synthetic pile or fleece jacket that is warm and dries quickly or a wool or synthetic sweater. Synthetic insulating materials, unlike down or wool, provide warmth without bulk or heavy weight. Insulation should be effective even when wet. In that respect, synthetics are clearly superior to natural fibers and natural products. Duck or goose down, for example, is virtually useless when wet, and it dries slowly. One exception, however, is the insulating ability of wool, even when wet.

Physically active people can sweat even in extremely cold weather. Therefore, the best choice for an outside layer is a jacket that is waterproof, wind resistant, and "breathable." Materials such as Gore-Tex allow perspiration to evaporate. A zipper is preferable, so the clothing can be opened easily to increase ventilation. Nylon and vinyl are poor choices because they produce a sauna effect by holding in perspiration. Because the head loses more body heat than any other part (up to 50%), heed the admonition, "If the feet are cold, cover the head." A wool or synthetic cap serves well.

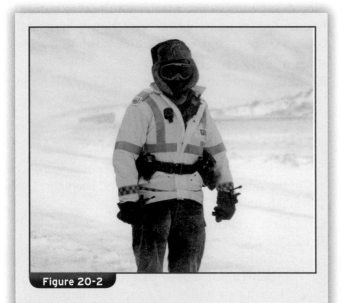

Figure 20-2

Wearing layered clothing can help your body adapt to changing conditions.

▶ Nonfreezing Cold Injuries

Nonfreezing cold injuries can occur when conditions are cold and wet (air temperatures between 32° F and 55° F) and the hands and feet cannot be kept warm and dry. The most prominent nonfreezing cold injuries are chilblain and trench foot.

Chilblain

Chilblain is a nonfreezing cold injury that, while painful, causes little or no permanent damage. Chilblain can develop in 3 to 6 hours in skin exposed to cold and moisture.

Recognizing Chilblain

The signs of chilblain include:

- Skin is swollen.
- Skin is tender, hot to the touch, and possibly itchy.
- Blisters might form.
- Condition can worsen to an aching, prickly (pins and needles) sensation and then numbness.

Care for a Victim of Chilblain

To care for a victim of chilblain, get the victim out of the cold.

Trench Foot/Immersion Foot

Trench foot (also called immersion foot) is a serious non-freezing cold injury that develops when the skin on the feet is exposed to moisture and cold for prolonged periods (12 hours or longer). Wearing wet boots or shoes and socks causes trench foot; prolonged immersion of the feet in cold water causes immersion foot. The combination of cold and moisture softens the skin, causing tissue loss and, often, infection. The risk of this potentially crippling injury is high during wet weather. People who wear rubberized or tight-fitting boots are at risk for trench foot regardless of weather conditions because sweat accumulates inside the boots and keeps the feet wet.

Recognizing Trench Foot/Immersion Foot

Signs of trench foot include:

- Itching, numbness, or tingling pain
- Swollen feet and pale skin that feels cold when touched

Q&A

What is the origin of the term *trench* or *immersion* foot?

The term *immersion foot* was coined during World War I as a description of those victims who were shipwrecked and isolated in a lifeboat for a prolonged period of time.

The term *trench foot* was applied to a similar situation during World War I when the infantry would be pinned down in trenches filled with cold mud and water.

Both conditions occur after prolonged exposure to wet and cold. The temperature usually ranges from just above freezing to about 50° F. The duration of exposure to the wet and cold usually exceeds 10 to 12 hours.

- Red or bluish blotches on the skin, sometimes with open weeping or bleeding

Care for a Trench Foot/Immersion Foot Victim

Care for someone with trench foot includes these guidelines:

1. Dry the skin.
2. Rewarm the foot gradually.
3. Care for open weeping areas by cleansing with mild soap and water and applying breathable dressings.

▶ Freezing Cold Injuries

Freezing cold injuries can occur whenever the air temperature is below freezing (32° F). Freezing limited to the skin surface is <u>frostnip</u>. Freezing that extends deeper through the skin and into the flesh is <u>frostbite</u>.

Frostbite is prevalent during military campaigns and is a known hazard for outdoor workers, the homeless, mountain climbers, and explorers. As more people pursue cross-country skiing, snowmobiling, and other outdoor winter sports, the number of frostbite cases probably will increase. However, it is still thought to be rare in nonmilitary situations.

Frostnip

Frostnip is caused when water on the skin surface freezes. Frostnip should be taken seriously because it could be the first sign of impending frostbite.

Recognizing Frostnip

It is difficult to tell the difference between frostnip and frostbite. Signs of frostnip include:

- Skin appears red and sometimes swollen.
- Painful, but usually no further damage after rewarming.
- Repeated frostnip in the same spot can dry the skin, causing it to crack and become sensitive.

Care for a Frostnip Victim

To care for a frostnip victim:

1. Gently warm the affected area by placing it against a warm body part (for example, put bare hands under the armpits or on the stomach) or by blowing warm air on the area. After rewarming, the affected area can be red and tingling.
2. Do not rub the affected area.

Frostbite

Frostbite happens only in below-freezing temperatures. Tissue is not composed of water alone, so it will not freeze until it has been cooled to about 28° F. Tissue is damaged in two ways: (1) actual tissue freezing, which results in the formation of ice crystals within the tissue (the ice crystals expand as they freeze, damaging cells), and (2) the obstruction of the blood supply to the tissue, which causes sludged blood clots and further prevents blood from flowing to the tissues. The second type of tissue damage is more extensive than the first. In severely cold temperatures, flesh can freeze in less than a minute **Figure 20-3** .

Frostbite affects mainly the feet, hands, ears, and nose. These areas do not contain large heat-producing muscles and are some distance from the body's heat-generation sources. The most severe consequences of frostbite occur when tissue dies (gangrene), and the affected part might have to be amputated. The longer the tissue stays frozen, the worse the injury. Check for hypothermia in any frostbitten victim.

Recognizing Frostbite

The severity and extent of frostbite are difficult to judge until hours after thawing. Frostbite can be classified as superficial or deep before thawing.

The signs and symptoms of superficial frostbite are as follows:

- The skin is white, waxy, or grayish yellow.
- The affected part feels very cold and numb. There might be tingling, stinging, or an aching sensation.
- The skin surface feels stiff or crusty and the underlying tissue soft when depressed gently and firmly.

The following signs and symptoms indicate deep frostbite:

- The affected part feels cold, hard, and solid and cannot be depressed—it feels like a piece of wood or frozen meat.
- Blisters might appear after rewarming.
- The affected part is cold, with pale, waxy skin.
- A painfully cold part suddenly stops hurting.

After a part has thawed, frostbite can be categorized by degrees, similar to the classification of burns. First-degree frostbite is superficial, and second-, third-, and fourth-degree frostbite are deeper.

- First-degree frostbite: The affected part is warm, swollen, and tender.
- Second-degree frostbite: Blisters form minutes to hours after thawing and enlarge over several days **Figure 20-4** and **Figure 20-5** .
- Third-degree frostbite: Blisters are small and contain reddish blue or purplish fluid. The surrounding skin can be red or blue and might not blanch when pressure is applied.
- Fourth-degree frostbite: No blisters or swelling occur. The part remains numb, cold, and white to dark purple.

Care for a Frostbite Victim

All frostbite injuries require the same first aid treatment. Seek medical care immediately. Rewarming of frostbite should seldom be attempted outside a medical facility.

Figure 20-3

Frostbitten fingers 6 hours after rewarming in 108°F water.

Figure 20-4

Second-degree frostbite.

CAUTION

DO NOT use water hotter than 104° F—burns can result.

DO NOT use water cooler than 100° F—it will not thaw frostbite rapidly enough.

DO NOT break any blisters.

DO NOT rub or massage the affected part—ice crystals can be pushed into body cells, rupturing them.

DO NOT rub the affected part with ice or snow.

DO NOT rewarm the part with a heating pad, hot-water bottle, stove, sunlamp, radiator, or exhaust pipe or over a fire. Excessive temperatures cannot be controlled, and burns can result.

DO NOT allow the victim to drink alcoholic beverages. Alcohol dilates blood vessels and causes loss of body heat.

DO NOT allow the victim to smoke. Smoking constricts blood vessels, thus impairing circulation.

DO NOT rewarm if there is any possibility of refreezing.

DO NOT allow the thawed part to refreeze because the ice crystals formed will be larger and more damaging. If refreezing is likely or even possible, it is better to leave the affected part frozen.

DO NOT use the dry rewarming technique (putting the victim's hands in your armpits) because that takes three to four times longer than the wet, rapid method to thaw frozen tissue. Slow rewarming results in greater tissue damage than rapid rewarming.

DO NOT rewarm if close to a medical facility.

Figure 20-5

Frostbitten ear.

1. Get the victim out of the cold and to a warm place.
2. Remove any wet clothing or constricting items, such as rings, that could impair blood circulation.
3. Seek immediate medical care.

4. If the affected part is partially thawed, and you have warm water, use the following wet, rapid rewarming method. If there is risk of refreezing, do not rewarm. Place the frostbitten part in warm (100° F to 104° F) water. If you do not have a thermometer, pour some of the water over the inside of your arm or put your elbow into it to test that it is warm, not hot. Maintain water temperature by adding warm water as needed. Rewarming usually takes 20 to 40 minutes or until the tissues are soft. To help control the severe pain during rewarming, give the victim aspirin (adults only) or ibuprofen. For ear or facial injuries, it is best but may be difficult to apply warm, moist cloths, changing them frequently.
5. After thawing:
   - If the feet are affected, treat the victim as a stretcher case—the feet will be impossible to use after they are rewarmed.
   - Protect the affected area from contact with clothing and bedding.
   - Place dry, sterile gauze between the toes and the fingers to absorb moisture and keep them from sticking together.
   - Slightly elevate the affected part to reduce pain and swelling.

Frostbite

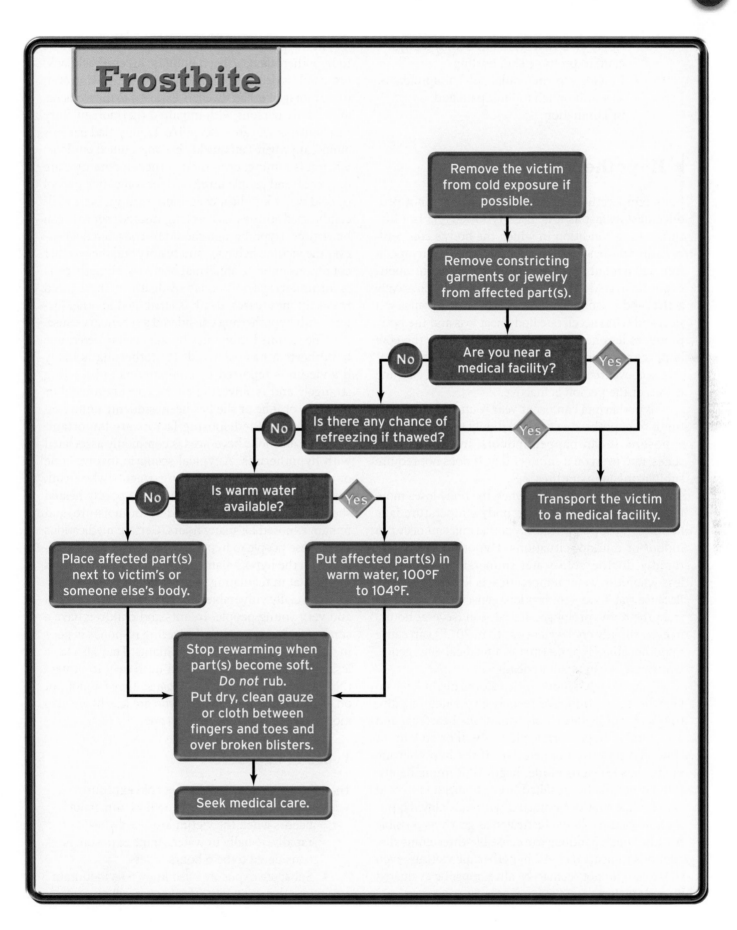

Remove the victim from cold exposure if possible.

↓

Remove constricting garments or jewelry from affected part(s).

↓

Are you near a medical facility?

No →

Yes →

Is there any chance of refreezing if thawed?

No →

Yes →

Transport the victim to a medical facility.

Is warm water available?

No →

Yes →

Place affected part(s) next to victim's or someone else's body.

Put affected part(s) in warm water, 100°F to 104°F.

Stop rewarming when part(s) become soft. *Do not* rub. Put dry, clean gauze or cloth between fingers and toes and over broken blisters.

↓

Seek medical care.

- Apply aloe vera gel, if advised by a physician, to promote skin healing.
- Provide aspirin (adults only), ibuprofen, or acetaminophen to limit pain and inflammation.

▶ Hypothermia

Body temperature falls when the body cannot produce heat as fast as it is lost. **Hypothermia** is a life-threatening condition in which the body's core temperature falls below 95° F. Generally, the core temperature will not fall until after many hours of continuous exposure to cold air, if the person is healthy, physically active, and reasonably dressed. However, because wet skin and wind accelerate body heat loss and the body produces less heat during inactive periods, the core body temperature can fall even when the air temperature is above freezing if conditions are windy, clothing is wet, or the person is inactive.

Hypothermia can occur year round. Most people think of hypothermia as related only to cold outdoor exposure. It can happen indoors, in the southern states, and even on a summer day. It does not require subfreezing temperatures.

Hypothermia happens when the body loses more heat than it produces. If the body temperature falls to 80° F, most people die. Hypothermia can occur in indoor or outdoor situations. Hypothermia occurs rapidly during cold-water immersion (1 hour or less when the water temperature is less than 45° F). Because water has a tremendous capacity to drain heat from the body, prolonged immersion (several hours) in even slightly cool water (less than 70° F) can cause hypothermia. Hypothermia is a medical emergency. Untreated, it can result in death.

Even though hypothermic victims might have no heartbeat, breathing, or response to touch or pain, they may not be dead. Sometimes, the heartbeat and breathing of hypothermic victims will be so faint or slow that they are not detected. If the hypothermic victim has no signs of life, begin CPR immediately. If hypothermia has resulted from submersion in cold water, CPR should be started without delay. Hypothermic victims should be treated as gently as possible because rough handling can cause life-threatening disruptions in heart rate. All hypothermic victims, even those who do not seem to be alive, must be evaluated by a physician.

In the past, the people believed most vulnerable to hypothermia have been hunters, hikers, backpackers, careless drinkers, and accident victims. However, disadvantaged urban dwellers exposed to the elements and elderly persons with impaired thermoregulatory mechanisms also are susceptible. Lightly clad persons almost anywhere can quickly become chilled outdoors when it is raining, even though the temperatures are only cool, and people immersed for some time in cool or cold water lose heat even more readily. Even well-conditioned athletes such as long-distance runners can be victims. Hypothermia should be considered whenever the victim's behavior and history and the weather conditions indicate abnormal heat loss. Hypothermia is an underreported cause of death in the United States. In most cases, death is attributed to other factors, with hypothermia considered a secondary cause.

The victim's history may be sufficient to determine hypothermia has occurred. Hypothermia is likely if a victim is reported by companions to be acting strangely and is shivering after exposure to cold or moisture or if he or she has been suddenly immersed in cold water. Predisposing factors are important: drinking alcoholic beverages is commonly associated with hypothermia. A typical scenario involves one or more people in lightweight garments who drink too much, fall asleep outdoors or in a poorly heated shelter, become chilled by cold air or moisture, and remain exposed for many hours. Certain medications predispose people to hypothermia because they interfere with the hypothalamus, which acts as the brain's thermostat in regulating body heat.

Especially vulnerable to hypothermia are very old and very young people. Infants and children have a small muscle mass, so the shivering response is poor in children and nonexistent in infants. They also have less body fat. Younger children need help to protect themselves against the cold because they cannot put on or take off clothes. People who are less fit are also more likely to become hypothermic.

Types of Exposure

There are three classifications of cold exposure:
- Acute exposure (also known as immersion) occurs when the victim loses body heat very rapidly, usually in water. Acute exposure is considered to be 6 hours or less.
- Subacute exposure (also known as mountain or exhaustion exposure) occurs when

exposure is 6 to 24 hours and can be land or water based.

- Chronic exposure (also known as urban exposure) involves long-term cooling. It generally occurs on land and exceeds 24 hours.

Recognizing Hypothermia

Consider hypothermia in all victims who have been exposed to cold and who have an altered mental status. Suspect hypothermia in any person who has a temperature of less than 95° F. (Keep in mind that some thermometers do not measure below 95° F.) Shivering is a good clue, but it could be suppressed when energy stores (glycogen) are depleted. Suspect hypothermia in people with frostbite and those injured in a cold environment.

Some people die of hypothermia because they or those around them do not recognize the symptoms, which are difficult to recognize in the early stages. Here are some signs to watch for:

- *Change in mental status.* This is one of the first symptoms of developing hypothermia. Examples are disorientation, apathy, and changes in personality, such as unusual aggressiveness.
- *Shivering.* Shivering is the first, and most important, body defense against a falling body temperature. Shivering starts when the body temperature drops 1° F and can produce more heat than many rewarming methods. As the core temperature continues to fall, shivering decreases and usually stops at about 86° F. Shivering also stops as body temperature rises. If shivering stops as responsiveness decreases, assume that the core temperature is falling. If, on the other hand, shivering stops while the victim is becoming more coordinated and feeling better, assume that the core temperature is rising.
- *Cool abdomen.* Place the back of your hand between the clothing and the victim's abdomen to assess the victim's temperature. When the victim's abdominal skin under clothing is cooler than your hand, consider the victim hypothermic until proven otherwise.
- *Low core body temperature.* The best indicator of hypothermia is a thermometer reading of the core body temperature. The ability to reliably measure core temperature depends on the

availability of an appropriate thermometer and access to the victim's rectum. Normal thermometers do not register below 94° F and so do not indicate whether the hypothermia is mild or severe. Because first aid for mild hypothermia is different from that for severe hypothermia, it is helpful to have a rectal thermometer that registers below 90° F. Oral and axillary (armpit) temperatures are influenced by too many external factors to make them reliable.

Measuring rectal temperatures in wilderness or remote locations is seldom done, mainly because low-reading rectal thermometers usually are not readily available. Also, taking a rectal temperature can be difficult, inconvenient, and embarrassing to the victim and rescuer. If done outdoors, such a procedure can further expose the already cold victim.

Types of Hypothermia

The difference between mild and severe hypothermia is based on the core body temperature, but taking a rectal temperature often is not possible. The second most significant difference is that with severe hypothermia, the victim becomes so cold that shivering stops, which means the victim's body cannot rewarm itself internally and requires external heat for recovery. In fact, 50% to 80% of all victims of severe hypothermia die.

The National Association of Emergency Medical Service Physicians recommends that CPR not be started on a severe hypothermic victim if one of the following applies:

- The victim's core body temperature is less than 60° F.
- The victim's chest is frozen (cannot be compressed).
- The victim was submerged in water for more than 60 minutes.
- The victim has a lethal injury.
- Transport for controlled rewarming will be delayed.
- Rescuers are endangered.

For CPR to be effective, heart activity must be restored within a short time, which requires defibrillation, oxygen, and medications. Do not start CPR until you have checked the victim's circulation for 30 to 45 seconds. A hypothermic victim will have an extremely slow pulse rate. CPR can cause cardiac arrest in an already beating heart.

Recognizing Mild Hypothermia

Signs of mild hypothermia include the following:

- Vigorous, uncontrollable shivering
- Victim has the "umbles"
  - Grumbles—decreased mental skills
  - Mumbles—slurred speech
  - Fumbles—difficulty using fingers or hands
  - Stumbles—staggers while walking
- Has cool or cold skin on the abdomen, chest, or back
- Victims have a core body temperature above 90° F

Care for a Mild Hypothermia Victim

Do the following to care for victims of mild hypothermia:

1. Stop further heat loss:
   - Get the victim out of the cold.
   - Handle the victim gently.
   - Prevent heat loss by replacing wet clothing with dry clothing and placing insulation (blankets, towels, pillows, wadded-up newspapers) beneath and over the victim. Cover the victim's head (50% to 80% of the body's heat loss is through the head).
   - Cover the victim with a vapor barrier (such as a tarp, sheet of plastic, or trash bags). If you are unable to remove wet clothing, place a vapor barrier between clothing and insulation. For a dry victim, the vapor barrier can be placed outside of the insulation.
   - Keep the victim in a horizontal (flat) position. Do not raise the legs.
   - Do not let the victim walk or exercise. Do not massage the victim's body. Either activity could drive cold blood from the extremities to the torso and produce what is known as temperature after drop.
2. Call 9-1-1 for immediate medical transportation. Remember that hypothermia is more common in urban settings than in victims found in the wilderness.
3. Allow the victim to shiver—do not stop the shivering by adding heat to the victim. Shivering that generates heat will rewarm mildly hypothermic victims.
4. Give warm, sugary drinks, which can provide energy (calories) for the shivering to continue. They may also provide a

psychological boost. These drinks will not provide enough warmth to rewarm the victim.

Recognizing Severe Hypothermia

The following signs indicate severe hypothermia:

- No shivering.
- Skin feels ice cold and appears blue.
- Muscles can be stiff and rigid, similar to rigor mortis.
- Altered mental status—not alert.
- Breathing and pulse slow.
- Victim might appear to be dead.
- Victim has a core body temperature below 90° F.

Care for a Severe Hypothermia Victim

Care for someone with severe hypothermia by doing the following:

1. Stop further heat loss:
   - Get the victim out of the cold.
   - Handle the victim gently. Rough handling can cause cardiac arrest.
   - Prevent heat loss by replacing wet clothing with dry clothing and placing insulation (blankets, towels, pillows, wadded-up newspapers) beneath and over the victim. Cover the victim's head (50% to 80% of the body's heat loss is through the head).
   - Cover the victim with a vapor barrier (such as a tarp, plastic sheets, or trash bags). If you are unable to remove wet clothing, place a vapor barrier between clothing and insulation. For a dry victim, the vapor barrier can be placed outside of the insulation.
   - Keep the victim in a horizontal (flat) position. Do not raise the legs.
   - Do not let the victim walk or exercise. Do not massage the victim's body. Either activity could drive cold blood from the extremities to the torso and produce what is known as temperature after drop.
2. Call 9-1-1 for immediate medical transportation. Remember that hypothermia is more common in urban settings than in victims found in the wilderness.
3. When the victim is in a remote location and far from medical care, warm the victim by any available external heat source (such as body-to-body contact).

Adding Heat

Adding heat to a victim is extremely difficult. The longer the victim has been exposed to the cold, the longer it will take to raise the core temperature to normal. Trying to rewarm a hypothermic victim could cause cardiac arrest.

Although surface rewarming suppresses shivering, it might be the only option when the victim is far from medical care. In that case, the victim must be warmed by any available external heat source.

There are problems with the commonly recommended rewarming methods:*

*Paton BC: Field treatment of hypothermia. Second World Congress on Wilderness Medicine, Wilderness Medical Society. 1995.

Warm water immersion requires a lot of warm water (no hotter than 106° F) and a bathtub—both rarely found in remote locations. Hot baths can produce rapid changes in the blood that can produce cardiac arrest.

Recent studies show that body-to-body contact in an insulated sleeping bag is no better than shivering for rewarming. Reasons include the following:

- All the heat produced by the rescuer's body is not enough to rewarm a victim. For example, heat loss of adults cooled to 91° F exceeds 300 kcal (kilocalories); heat production of a rescuer is only 100 kcal per hour.
- There usually is only a small amount (less than 50%) of direct skin contact, which is

---

FYI

How Cold Is It?

In addition to cold, two other factors account for body heat loss: moisture and wind. Moisture—whether from rain, snow, or perspiration—speeds the conduction of heat away from the body.

Wind causes sizable amounts of body heat loss. If the thermometer reads 20° F and the wind speed is 20 mph, the exposure is comparable to 4° F. This is called the windchill factor. Use the following rough measures of wind speed: if you feel the wind on your face, wind speed is at least 10 mph; if small branches move or if dust or snow is raised, it is 20 mph; if large branches are moving, it is 30 mph; and if a whole tree bends, it is about 40 mph.

To determine the windchill factor:

1. Estimate the wind speed by checking for the aforementioned signs.
2. Look at an outdoor thermometer reading (in degrees Fahrenheit).
3. Match the estimated wind speed with the actual thermometer reading in the following table.

Wind Chill Chart

Effective 11/01/01

Calm	40	35	30	25	20	15	10	5	0	-5	-10	-15	-20	-25	-30	-35	-40	-45
5	36	31	25	19	13	7	1	-5	-11	-16	-22	-28	-34	-40	-46	-52	-57	-63
10	34	27	21	15	9	3	-4	-10	-16	-22	-28	-35	-41	-47	-53	-59	-66	-72
15	32	25	19	13	6	0	-7	-13	-19	-26	-32	-39	-45	-51	-58	-64	-71	-77
20	30	24	17	11	4	-2	-9	-15	-22	-29	-35	-42	-48	-55	-61	-68	-74	-81
25	29	23	16	9	3	-4	-11	-17	-24	-31	-37	-44	-51	-58	-64	-71	-78	-84
30	28	22	15	8	1	-5	-12	-19	-26	-33	-39	-46	-53	-60	-67	-73	-80	-87
35	28	21	14	7	0	-7	-14	-21	-27	-34	-41	-48	-55	-62	-69	-76	-82	-89
40	27	20	13	6	-1	-8	-15	-22	-29	-36	-43	-50	-57	-64	-71	-78	-84	-91
45	26	19	12	5	-2	-9	-16	-23	-30	-37	-44	-51	-58	-65	-72	-79	-86	-93
50	26	19	12	4	-3	-10	-17	-24	-31	-38	-45	-52	-60	-67	-74	-81	-88	-95
55	25	18	11	4	-3	-11	-18	-25	-32	-39	-46	-54	-61	-68	-75	-82	-89	-97
60	25	17	10	3	-4	-11	-19	-26	-33	-40	-48	-55	-62	-69	-76	-84	-91	-98

Wind (mph) — left axis

Frostbite Times: ■ 30 minutes ■ 10 minutes ■ 5 minutes

Wind Chill (°F) = 35.74 + 0.6215T - 35.75 (V^{0.16}) + 0.4275T (V^{0.16})

$$\text{Wind Chill (°F)} = 35.74 + 0.6215T - 35.75\,(V^{0.16}) + 0.4275T\,(V^{0.16})$$

Where, T=Air Temperature (°F) V=Wind Speed (mph)

Source: Courtesy of the National Weather Service/NOAA.

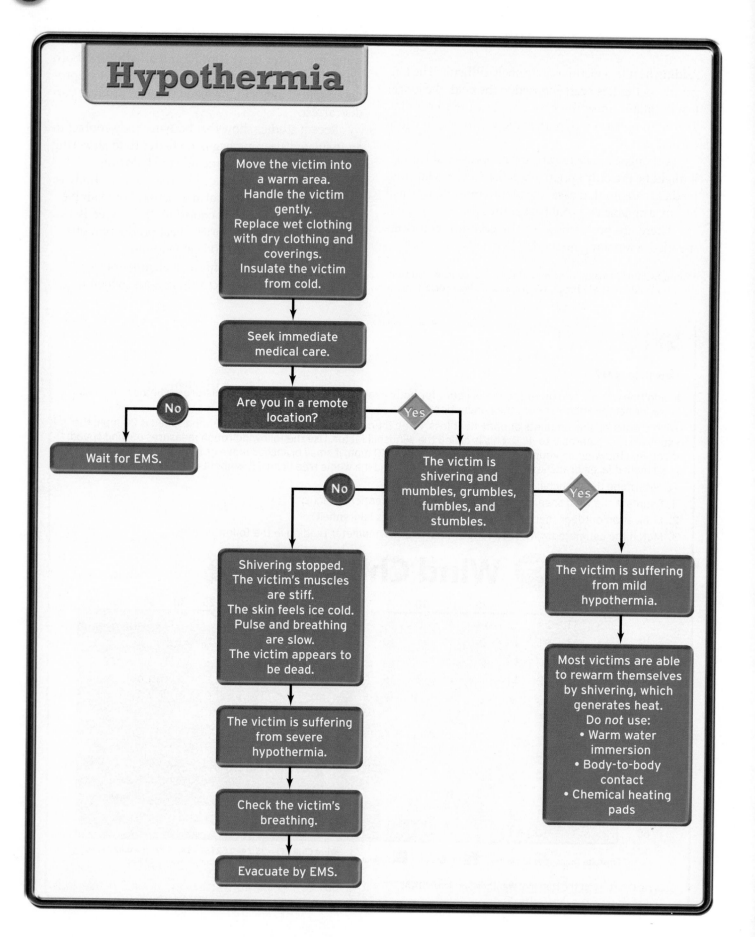

Hypothermia

Move the victim into a warm area.
Handle the victim gently.
Replace wet clothing with dry clothing and coverings.
Insulate the victim from cold.

↓

Seek immediate medical care.

↓

Are you in a remote location?

No →

Wait for EMS.

Yes →

The victim is shivering and mumbles, grumbles, fumbles, and stumbles.

No →

Shivering stopped.
The victim's muscles are stiff.
The skin feels ice cold.
Pulse and breathing are slow.
The victim appears to be dead.

↓

The victim is suffering from severe hypothermia.

↓

Check the victim's breathing.

↓

Evacuate by EMS.

Yes →

The victim is suffering from mild hypothermia.

↓

Most victims are able to rewarm themselves by shivering, which generates heat.
Do *not* use:
• Warm water immersion
• Body-to-body contact
• Chemical heating pads

CAUTION

DO NOT allow the victim to exert himself or herself (no walking, no climbing).

DO NOT try to rewarm a hypothermic victim outside a medical facility. External measures to rewarm should not be used, especially on the extremities, because surface rewarming leads to vasodilation (wider blood vessels), which can lead to a drop in blood pressure and temperature after drop.

DO NOT try to rewarm a hypothermic victim outside a medical facility because rewarming the skin will stop shivering, which is the most effective way to rewarm.

DO NOT put an unconscious victim in a bathtub.

DO NOT give the victim alcohol. Alcohol interferes with shivering and accelerates heat loss by dilating the blood vessels in the skin. The victim might feel warmer temporarily, but there is a greater risk of hypothermia.

DO NOT give the victim a caffeine drink. Caffeine has a diuretic effect, and the victim probably is already dehydrated.

DO NOT rub or massage the victim's arms or legs. Rubbing the skin suppresses shivering, dilates the blood vessels in the skin (resulting in more heat loss), and produces temperature after drop.

DO NOT raise the victim's legs, which allows cold blood from the legs to flow into the body core and adversely affect the heart. Keep the victim in a flat position.

essential for effective heat transfer, between the victim and the rescuer.

- The victim's peripheral blood vessel constriction can impair heat transfer to the body's core.
- Skin warming can slow the victim's shivering response, which effectively rewarms the body.

Because skin rewarming suppresses shivering, which slows the rate of core rewarming, body-to-body rewarming should be used only when there will be a long delay in getting the victim to medical care and when more appropriate methods of adding heat are unavailable. Several types of chemical heating pads are available. Although they might be effective for warming hands and feet, there is no evidence that they are capable of rewarming a hypothermic victim. For example, one type of heating pad is 7″ × 9″ and provides 14.5 kcal of total heat, with a maximum temperature of about 125° F. A minimum of 20 pads

would be needed to provide enough heat to rewarm a victim with a temperature of 91° F, even if heat transfer were 100% efficient. This method can stop the desirable effects of shivering, leaving the victim hypothermic.

▶ Dehydration

Dehydration occurs because of unperceived fluid loss combined with inadequate fluid intake. In very cold weather, the humidity approaches zero, and large quantities of fluid are lost through exhaled breath.

People in a cold environment must drink even when they are not thirsty. Inactive people in comfortable climates need two quarts of water a day to prevent dehydration.

A person's hydration status can be monitored by noting the color and the volume of the urine. The lighter the color, the better hydrated; dark yellow urine is a definite indication that fluid consumption should be increased.

Unmelted snow and ice should not be consumed for water. Eating snow and ice irritates the mouth, wastes body heat, and, if enough is consumed, lowers body temperature. When snow and ice are the only available sources of water, they should be melted before being consumed. Melted snow or ice should not be considered drinkable until it has been appropriately disinfected (by boiling, filtering, or using chemicals).

Q&A

What is the coldest body temperature?

The lowest recorded body temperature with a full recovery was 56.6° F (13.7° C). This was the temperature of D. Anna Bagenholm, age 29, who was trapped under ice for 80 minutes in May 2000, while skiing with friends near Narvik, Norway.

▶ Emergency Care Wrap-up

Condition	What to Look For	What to Do
Frostbite	• White, waxy-looking skin • Skin feels cold and numb (pain at first, followed by numbness) • Blisters, which may appear after rewarming	1. Move victim to a warm place. 2. Remove tight clothing or jewelry from injured part(s). 3. Place dry dressings between toes and/or fingers. 4. Seek medical care.

Hypothermia	• Mild
	  • Uncontrollable shivering
	  • Confusion, sluggishness
	  • Cold skin even under clothing
	• Severe
	  • No shivering
	  • Muscles stiff and rigid
	  • Skin ice cold
	  • Appears to be dead
		All victims:
		1. Move victim to a warm place.
		2. Prevent heat loss by
		  • Replacing wet clothing with dry clothing
		  • Covering victim's head
		Mild
		1. Give warm, sugary beverages.
		2. Do not add anything warm to the skin—let the shivering rewarm the body.
		Severe
		1. Do not rewarm unless in a very remote location.
		2. Call 9-1-1.

▶ Ready for Review

- When a person is surrounded by air or water cooler than body temperature, the body loses heat.
- Humans protect themselves from cold primarily by avoiding or reducing cold exposure through the use of clothing and shelter.
- Nonfreezing cold injuries can occur when conditions are cold and wet and the hands and feet cannot be kept warm and dry.
- Freezing cold injuries can occur whenever the air temperature is below freezing.
- Hypothermia is a life-threatening condition in which the body's core temperature falls below 95° F.
- Dehydration occurs because of unperceived fluid loss combined with inadequate fluid intake.

▶ Vital Vocabulary

<u>frostbite</u> The damage to tissues as a result of prolonged exposure to extreme cold.

<u>frostnip</u> The superficial local tissue destruction caused by freezing; it is limited in scope and does not destroy the full thickness of skin.

<u>hypothermia</u> Decreased body temperature.

<u>vasoconstriction</u> The narrowing of the diameter of a blood vessel.

<u>windchill</u> The relationship of wind velocity and temperature in determining the effect of cold on living organisms.

prep kit

▶ Assessment in Action

You are on a winter hike with five friends high in the mountains. The snowshoeing has been great but it is very cold. At the trailhead, the temperature was 15° F (–9° C) and it has not warmed up much during your hike. One of your friends wore only tennis shoes but has not been complaining. When you return to the trailhead and begin to warm up in your car, your friend begins to complain of tingling and aching in his toes.

Directions: Circle Yes if you agree with the statement; circle No if you disagree.

Yes No **1.** It is difficult to determine if your friend has frostnip or frostbite.

Yes No **2.** Frostbite requires freezing temperatures (below 32° F [0° C]).

Yes No **3.** The skin and underlying tissue affected by superficial frostbite feel hard and solid.

Yes No **4.** As long as there is no danger of refreezing, you could begin warming his toes in warm water.

Yes No **5.** If you do not have warm water, you could rub his toes to increase circulation.

▶ Check Your Knowledge

Directions: Circle Yes if you agree with the statement; circle No if you disagree.

Yes No **1.** Shivering is a signal that clothing and shelter are inadequate to protect the body from the cold.

Yes No **2.** Up to 100% of the body's total heat production can be lost by radiation through a person's unprotected head.

Yes No **3.** Physically unfit people are more susceptible to cold injury.

Yes No **4.** Frostnip is caused when water on the skin surface freezes.

Yes No **5.** Shivering produces body heat.

Yes No **6.** Rub a frostbitten part to rewarm it.

Yes No **7.** Rewarm a hypothermic victim quickly in a hot shower or with chemical heat packs.

Yes No **8.** Replace any wet clothing with dry clothing for a hypothermic victim.

Yes No **9.** Seek medical care for a severe hypothermic victim.

Yes No **10.** Below-freezing temperatures are required for hypothermia to occur.

21 Heat-Related Emergencies

Heat-Related Emergencies

When the temperature goes up, a multitude of problems can—and do—arise. Given the right (or wrong) conditions, anyone can develop heat illness. Some victims are lucky enough to have only **heat cramps**, but less fortunate people could be laid low by heat exhaustion or devastated by heatstroke.

▶ How the Body Stays Cool

The human body is constantly engaged in a life-and-death struggle to disperse the heat that it produces. If allowed to accumulate, the heat would quickly increase your body temperature beyond its comfortable 98.6° F. That does not normally happen, because your body is able to lose enough heat to maintain a steady temperature. Usually, you are aware of this struggle only during hard labor or exercise in a hot environment, when your body produces heat faster than it can lose it. In certain circumstances, your body can build up too much heat, your temperature might rise to life-threatening levels, and you can become delirious or lose consciousness. This condition is called **heatstroke** and is a serious medical emergency. If you do not rid your body of excess heat fast enough, it cooks the brain and other vital organs. It is often fatal, and people who survive might have permanent damage to their vital organs. Before your temperature reaches heatstroke level, however, you might experience heat exhaustion with its flulike symptoms. By treating the symptoms of **heat exhaustion**, you avoid heatstroke.

How does the body dispose of excess heat? Humans lose heat largely through their skin, much as a car loses heat through its radiator. Exercising muscles warms the blood, just as the car's hot engine warms its radiator fluid. Warm blood travels through the skin's dilated blood vessels, losing heat by evaporating sweat to the surrounding air, just as the car loses engine heat through the radiator.

When blood delivers heat to the skin, the body loses heat primarily in two ways: radiation and evaporation (vaporization of sweat). When the air temperature is 70° F or less, the body releases heat into its surroundings by radiation. As the environmental temperature approaches the body's temperature, however, heat loss through radiation is greatly reduced. In fact, people working or exercising on a hot summer day actually gain heat through radiation from the sun, leaving evaporation as the only way to control body temperature effectively.

FYI

World Record: Highest Body Temperature

The person with the highest body temperature who lived to tell about it is Willie Jones. On July 10, 1980, a day when the temperature reached 90° F (32.2° C) with 44% humidity, Mr. Jones was admitted to Grady Memorial Hospital, Atlanta, Georgia, with heatstroke. His temperature was 115.7° F (46.5° C). The record temperature was taken after he had been immersed for 25 minutes in cold water. The attending physician said that his body temperature may have exceeded 120° F when he first arrived at the hospital. After 24 days in the hospital, he was discharged. Body temperatures of 109° F can be fatal.

Source: Guinness Book of World Records. Bantam. 2008, page 112.

Water Loss

Water makes up about 50% to 60% of an adult's body weight. You lose about 2 quarts every day through breathing, urinating, bowel movements, and sweat. The lost fluid must be replaced. Although the amount of water used each day varies from person to person, an adult requires about 2 quarts a day from water, other beverages, and food (about 70% of most food

is water). A working adult can produce 2 to 3 quarts of sweat an hour for short periods and up to 10 to 15 quarts a day. When the body's water absorption rate of 1.5 quarts per hour is pitted against a sweat loss of 2 quarts per hour, dehydration results—drinking water cannot keep up with sweat losses.

When you are thirsty, you are already dehydrated. Thirst is not a good guide for when to drink water. In fact, in hot and humid conditions, people could be so dehydrated by the time they become thirsty that they have trouble catching up with their fluid losses. One guideline regarding water intake is to monitor urine output. You are getting enough water if you are producing clear urine at least five times a day. Cloudy or dark urine or urinating fewer than five times a day probably means you should drink more.

If possible while working, especially in hot weather, drink 1 cup (8 ounces) of water every 20 minutes. Usually, 1 pint (16 ounces) is the most a person can comfortably drink at once. It takes time for water to pass from the stomach into the blood, so you cannot catch up by drinking extra water later; about 1 quart of water per hour can pass out of the stomach.

Cool water (50° F) is easier for the stomach to absorb than warm water, and a little flavoring can make the water more tasty. The best fluids are those that leave the stomach fast and contain little sodium and less than 8% sugar. Coffee and tea should be avoided because they contain caffeine, a diuretic that increases water loss through urination. Alcoholic beverages also dehydrate by increasing urination. Soda pop contains about 10% sugar and, therefore, is not absorbed as well as water or commercial sports drinks (which contain about 5% to 8% sugar). Fruit juices range from 11% to 18% sugar and have an even longer absorption time.

Electrolyte Loss

Sweat and urine contain potassium and sodium, essential electrolytes that control the movement of water in and out of the cells. These electrolytes can be found in many everyday foods. Bananas and nuts are rich in potassium, and most American diets have up to 10 times as much sodium as the body needs. Acclimatizing to heat can reduce sodium loss tenfold. Getting enough salt (sodium chloride) is rarely a problem in the typical American diet. In fact, most Americans consume an excessive amount of sodium, averaging 5 to 10 grams of sodium per day, although

FYI

Water Intoxication in Recreational Hikers

Water intoxication (hyponatremia), often seen in endurance athletes, has been reported in recreational hikers. Water intoxication results when people replace sweat loss with plain water instead of an enhanced product that more nearly resembles sweat. Differentiating water intoxication from heat exhaustion is difficult. Recreational wilderness hikers performing sustained exercise in the heat might require electrolyte replacement similar to endurance athletes.

Source: Backer H, et al. 1993. Hyponatremia in recreational hikers in Grand Canyon National Park. *J Wilderness Med* 4(4):391–406.

humans probably require only 1 to 3 grams. Sodium loss, therefore, is seldom a problem, unless a person is sweating profusely for long periods and drinking large amounts of water (more than 1 quart an hour).

Most people require only water most of the time. Commercial sports drinks can be useful for participants in vigorous physical activity lasting for longer than 1 hour. The human body needs water more than it needs salt. Whenever extra sodium is added to a diet, more water should be consumed. Otherwise, excessive sodium can draw water out of the cells, accelerating dehydration.

Drinking large amounts of water (more than 1 quart an hour) and profuse sweating for long periods can lead to a condition called water intoxication, in which electrolytes are flushed from the body. Symptoms of water intoxication include frequent urination and behavior changes (irrationality, combativeness, seizures, and coma).

Effects of Humidity

Sweat can cool the body only if it evaporates (vaporizes). In dry air, you will not notice sweat evaporating. In high humidity, no sweat can evaporate. It drips off the skin without cooling the body. At about 75% humidity, sweating is ineffective in cooling the body.

Because humidity can significantly reduce evaporative cooling, a very humid but mildly warm day can be more stressful than a very hot, dry day. The higher the humidity, the lower the temperature at which heat risk begins, especially for people generating heat with vigorous work.

Who Is at Risk?

Everyone is susceptible to heat illness if environmental conditions overwhelm the body's temperature-regulating mechanisms. Heat waves can set the stage for a rash of heatstroke victims. For example, in the 1995 Chicago heat wave, the death toll reached 591 in 5 days. Several groups are at particular risk, including people who are obese, people with a chronic illness, and people with alcoholism.

Elderly people are at higher risk because of impaired cardiac output and decreased ability to sweat. Infants and young children are also susceptible to heatstroke. Children (and pets) are especially vulnerable when they are left in automobiles. The temperature in a parked car can soar to 150° F, even when a window is open. The fluid loss and dehydration resulting from physical activity put outdoor laborers and athletes at particular risk.

Certain medications predispose to heatstroke. They include drugs that alter sweat production (for example, antihistamines, antipsychotics, and antidepressants) and those that interfere with **thermoregulation**.

FYI

Heat-Related Deaths of Young Children in Parked Cars

Each year, many young children in the United States die of heatstroke caused by being enclosed in parked motor vehicles. Researchers located and analyzed 171 heat-related deaths in children under 5 years:

- 39% involved a child "forgotten by a caregiver"
- 27% involved a child playing in an unattended vehicle
- 20% involved a child intentionally left in a vehicle by an adult
- 14% involved unclear circumstances

Source: Guard, A and SS Gallagher. 2005. "Heat-Related Deaths to Young Children in Parked Cars: An Analysis of 171 Fatalities in the United States" *Injury Prevention* 11 (1):33–37.

▶ Heat Illnesses

Heat illnesses include a range of disorders Table 21-1 . Some of them are common, but only heatstroke is life threatening. Untreated heatstroke victims always die.

Table 21-1 Heat Illnesses

Condition	Symptoms	What to do
Heat cramps	Painful muscle spasms Sweaty skin Normal body temperature	1. Sit or lie down in the shade. 2. Drink cool, lightly salted water or a sports drink. 3. Stretch affected muscles.
Heat exhaustion	Profuse sweating Flulike symptoms Clammy or pale skin Dizziness Nausea, vomiting Rapid pulse Thirst Normal or slightly above normal body temperature	1. Treat mild cases the same way as heat cramps (but do not stretch the muscles). 2. If persistent, gently apply wet towels and call 9-1-1.
Heatstroke	Unresponsiveness (if responsive, victim will be confused, stagger, be agitated) Hot skin, which can be dry or wet	1. Move person to a half-sitting position in the shade. 2. Call 9-1-1. 3. If humidity is below 75%, spray victim with water and vigorously fan. If humidity is above 75%, apply ice packs on neck, armpits, and groin.

Heat Cramps

Heat cramps are painful muscle spasms that occur suddenly during or after vigorous exercise or activity. They usually involve the muscles in the back of the leg (calf and hamstring muscles) or the abdominal muscles. Some experts state they are caused by water and electrolyte losses during times of excessive sweating. Victims might be drinking fluids without adequate salt content. However, other experts disagree because the typical American diet is heavy with salt.

Recognizing Heat Cramps
Heat cramps have the following characteristics:
- Painful muscle spasms that happen suddenly
- Affect the muscles in the back of the leg or abdomen
- Occur during or after physical exertion

Care for Someone With Heat Cramps
To relieve heat cramps (it could take several hours), follow these steps:
1. Have the victim rest in a cool place.
2. Have the victim drink lightly salted, cool water (dissolve ¼ teaspoon salt in 1 quart of water) or a commercial sports drink. (A commercial sports drink is easier to absorb if diluted to half strength to reduce the sugar content.)

3. Stretch the cramped calf muscle. Place an ice bag (over a towel or cloth, to protect the skin) on the painful muscle. Also, try an acupressure method: pinch the upper lip just below the nose.

Heat Exhaustion

Heat exhaustion is characterized by heavy perspiration with a normal or slightly above-normal body temperature. Heavy sweating causes water and electrolyte losses. Some experts believe that a better term would be *severe dehydration*. Heat exhaustion affects workers and athletes who do not drink enough fluids while working or exercising in hot environments. Symptoms include severe thirst, heavy sweating, fatigue, headache, nausea, vomiting, and sometimes diarrhea. The affected person often mistakenly believes he or she has the flu. Uncontrolled heat exhaustion can evolve into heatstroke.

Recognizing Heat Exhaustion
Heat exhaustion differs from heatstroke by having (1) no altered mental status and (2) skin that is not hot, but clammy. Heat exhaustion causes the following symptoms:
- Sweating
- Thirst

- Fatigue
- Flulike symptoms (headache and nausea)
- Shortness of breath
- Fast heart rate

Care for Heat Exhaustion Victims

Use the following guidelines to care for a victim of heat exhaustion:

1. Move the victim immediately out of the heat to a cool place.
2. Give cool liquids, adding electrolytes (lightly salted water or a commercial sports drink) if plain water does not improve the victim's condition in 20 minutes. Do not give salt tablets; they can irritate the stomach and cause nausea and vomiting.
3. Consider raising the victim's legs 6 to 12 inches (keep the knees slightly bent).
4. Remove excess clothing.
5. Sponge the victim with cool water and fan him or her; or, place ice bags on the sides of the chest, neck, and armpits.
6. If no improvement is seen within 30 minutes, seek medical care.

Heatstroke

Two types of heatstroke exist: classic and exertional Table 21-2 . Classic heatstroke, also known as the slow cooker, can take days to develop. It is often seen during summer heat waves and typically affects poor, elderly, chronically ill, alcoholic, and obese people. Because elderly people, who often have medical problems, are frequently afflicted, this type of heatstroke has a 50% death rate, even with medical care. It results from a combination of a hot environment and dehydration. Under normal conditions, temperature and humidity are the most important elements influencing body comfort. The heat index compiled by the National Weather Service lists apparent temperatures (how hot it feels) at various combinations of temperature and humidity Table 21-3 .

Q&A

What is the difference between fever and hyperthermia?

Fever and hyperthermia have different causes. Fever is an elevation of body temperature and involves a change in the hypothalamic "set point." In other words, in a fever the body is trying to raise the temperature above normal to fight a disease (eg, a virus).

Hyperthermia is related to environmental heat exposure. It occurs when the body absorbs more heat than it can handle. It is caused by an inability to cool the body. Hyperthermia is more commonly known as heatstroke.

Table 21-2 Classic or Exertional Heatstroke?

Characteristics	Classic	Exertional
Age group usually affected	Elderly	Males 15-45 years
Claims many victims at the same time	During heat waves	During athletic competition
Health status of victims	Chronically ill	Healthy and physically fit
Activity at the time of incident	Sedentary	Strenuous exercise
Medication use	Common	Usually none
Sweating	Absent	Often present (50% of victims)

Table 21-3 Heat Index

Relative Humidity (%)	Temperature (°F)															
	80	82	84	86	88	90	92	94	96	98	100	102	104	106	108	110
40	80	81	83	85	88	91	94	97	101	105	109	114	119	124	130	136
45	80	82	84	87	89	93	96	100	104	109	114	119	124	130	137	
50	81	83	85	88	91	95	99	103	108	113	118	124	131	137		
55	81	84	86	89	93	97	101	106	112	117	124	130	137			
60	82	84	88	91	95	100	105	110	116	123	129	137				
65	82	85	89	93	98	103	108	114	121	128	136					
70	83	86	90	95	100	105	112	119	126	134						
75	84	88	92	97	103	109	116	124	132							
80	84	89	94	100	106	113	121	129								
85	85	90	96	102	110	117	126	135								
90	86	91	98	105	113	122	131									
95	86	93	100	108	117	127										
100	87	95	103	112	121	132										

Likelihood of Heat Disorders with Prolonged Exposure or Strenuous Activity
■ Caution ■ Extreme Caution ■ Danger ■ Extreme Danger

Exertional heatstroke is also more common in the summer. It is frequently seen in athletes, laborers, and military personnel, all of whom often sweat profusely. This type of heatstroke is known as the fast cooker. It affects healthy, active people who are strenuously working or playing in a warm environment. Because its rapid onset does not allow enough time for severe dehydration to occur, 50% of exertional heatstroke victims usually are sweating. (Classic heatstroke victims are not sweating.)

FYI

Heat Illness Among High School Athletes

Heat illness during practice or competition is a leading cause of death and disability among high school athletes in the United States. The 100 schools sampled by CDC reported a total of 118 heat illnesses among high school athletes resulting in at least 1 day of time lost from athletic activity (ie, time-loss heat illness). The highest rate of time-loss heat illness was among football players at a rate 10 times higher than the average rate for the eight other sports surveyed. Time-loss heat illnesses occurred most frequently during August and while practicing or playing football.

Consistent with guidelines from the National Athletic Trainers' Association (NATA), to reduce the risk for heat illness, high school athletic programs should implement heat-acclimatization guidelines (eg, set limits on summer practice duration and intensity). All athletes, coaches, athletic trainers, and parents/guardians should be aware of the risk factors for heat illness, follow recommended strategies, and be prepared to respond quickly to symptoms of illness. Coaches also should continue to stress to their athletes the importance of maintaining proper hydration before, during, and after sports activities.

Source: Centers for Disease Control and Prevention. Heat Illness Among High School Athletes—United States, 2005-2009. *Morbidity and Mortality Weekly Report (MMWR).* 59(32):1009-1013.

There are several ways to tell the difference between heat exhaustion and heatstroke.

- If the victim's body feels extremely hot when touched, suspect heatstroke.
- Altered mental status (behavior) occurs with heatstroke, ranging from slight confusion and disorientation to coma. Between those extreme conditions, victims usually become irrational, agitated, or even aggressive, and they might have seizures.

- In severe heatstroke, a coma can occur in less than an hour. The longer a coma lasts, the lower the chance for survival.
- Rectal temperature can also distinguish heatstroke from heat exhaustion, although obtaining a rectal temperature is usually not practical. A responsive heatstroke victim might not cooperate, taking a rectal temperature can be embarrassing to the victim and the rescuer, and rectal thermometers are seldom available.

Recognizing Heatstroke

Signs of heatstroke include:

- Extremely hot skin when touched—usually dry, but can be wet from sweating related to strenuous work or exercise.
- Altered mental status ranging from slight confusion, agitation, and disorientation to unresponsiveness.

Care for Heatstroke Victims

Heatstroke is a medical emergency and must be treated rapidly! Every minute delayed increases the likelihood of serious complications or death. Do the following:

1. Move the victim immediately to a cool place.
2. Remove clothing down to the victim's underwear.
3. Keep the victim's head and shoulders slightly elevated.
4. Call 9-1-1 immediately even if the victim seems to be recovering.
5. The only way to prevent damage is to cool the victim quickly and by any means possible. Cooling methods include the following:
   - Spraying the victim with water and then fanning **Figure 21-1**. This method is *not* as effective in high humidity (more than 75%) conditions.
   - Applying cool, wet sheets or cloths.
   - Placing ice bags against the large veins on the groin, armpits, and sides of the neck; this cools the body, regardless of humidity.
   - Placing the victim in an ice bath; this cools a victim quickly, but it requires a great deal of ice—at least 80 pounds—to be effective. The need for a big enough tub also limits this method.
   - Placing the victim in a cool water bath (less than 60° F) can be successful if the water is stirred to prevent a warm layer

from forming around the body. This is the most effective method in high humidity (greater than 75%) conditions.

Vigorously fan the victim to keep the person cool.

Keep the sheet wet by continually sprinkling it with water.

Figure 21-1

Spraying with water and fanning are effective in low humidity conditions.

Other Heat Illnesses

Less serious heat illnesses include heat syncope, heat edema, and prickly heat.

- **Heat syncope**, in which a person becomes dizzy or faints after exposure to high temperatures, is a self-resolving condition. Victims should lie down in a cool place and, if not nauseated, drink water. Syncope may be associated with heat exhaustion.
- **Heat edema**, which is also a self-resolving condition, causes the ankles and feet to swell from heat exposure. It is more common in women who are not acclimatized to a hot climate. It is related to salt and water retention and tends to disappear after acclimatization. Wearing support stockings and elevating the legs could help reduce the swelling.
- **Prickly heat**, also known as a heat rash, is an itchy rash that develops because of unevaporated moisture on skin wet from sweating. Treat by drying and cooling the skin.

FYI

Hot Weather Precautions

These simple preventive measures can reduce heat stress:

1. Keep as cool as possible.
   - Avoid direct sunlight.
   - Stay in the coolest available location (usually indoors).
   - Use air conditioning, if available.
   - Use electric fans to promote cooling.
   - Place wet towels or ice bags on the body or dampen clothing.
   - Take cool baths or showers.
2. Wear lightweight, loose-fitting clothing.
3. Avoid strenuous physical activity, particularly in the sun and during the hottest part of the day.
4. Increase intake of fluids, such as water and fruit or vegetable juices. Thirst is not always a good indicator of adequate fluid intake. Fluid intake in hot weather should be one and a half times the amount that quenches thirst. People who are overweight or have a large build or who engage in strenuous activities, such as sports, can require more than a gallon of fluid intake daily in very hot weather. People for whom salt or fluid is restricted should consult their physicians for instructions on appropriate fluid and salt intake.
5. Do not take salt tablets unless instructed to do so by a physician.
6. Avoid alcoholic beverages (beer, wine, and liquor).
7. Stay in contact with other people.

CAUTION

DO NOT delay initiating cooling while waiting for an ambulance. The longer the delay, the greater the risk of tissue damage and prolonged hospitalization.

DO NOT continue cooling after the victim's mental status has improved. Unnecessary cooling could lead to hypothermia.

DO NOT use rubbing alcohol to cool the skin. It can be absorbed into the blood and cause alcohol poisoning. Also, the vapors are a potential fire hazard.

DO NOT give the victim aspirin or acetaminophen. The brain's control center is not elevated, as it is with fever caused by diseases, so these products are not effective for lowering body temperature.

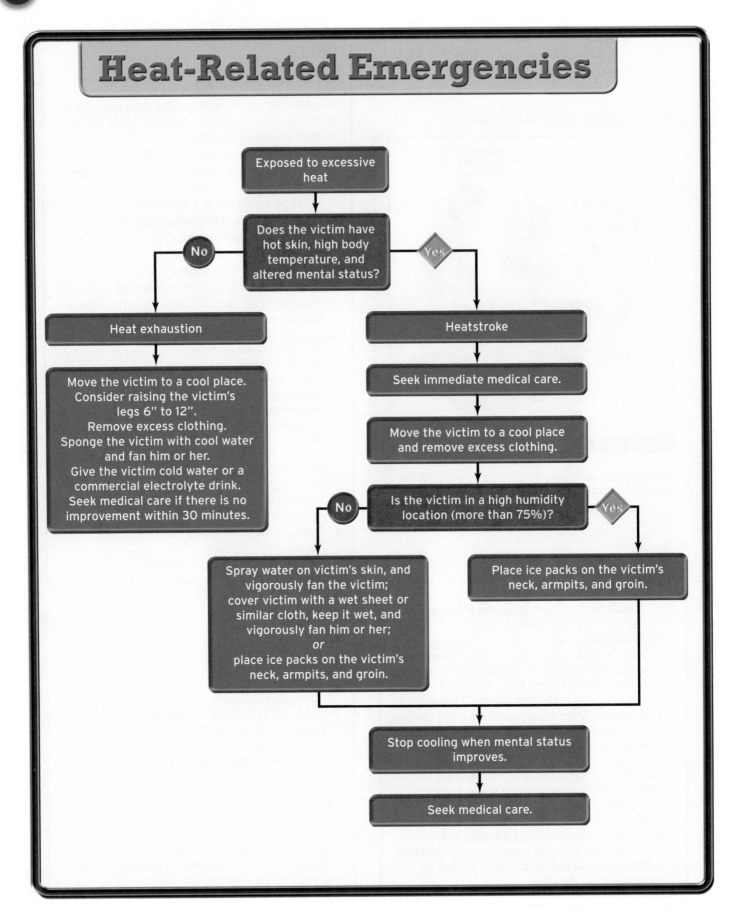

Heat-Related Emergencies

Exposed to excessive heat

Does the victim have hot skin, high body temperature, and altered mental status?

No → Heat exhaustion

Move the victim to a cool place.
Consider raising the victim's legs 6" to 12".
Remove excess clothing.
Sponge the victim with cool water and fan him or her.
Give the victim cold water or a commercial electrolyte drink.
Seek medical care if there is no improvement within 30 minutes.

Yes → Heatstroke

Seek immediate medical care.

Move the victim to a cool place and remove excess clothing.

Is the victim in a high humidity location (more than 75%)?

No → Spray water on victim's skin, and vigorously fan the victim;
cover victim with a wet sheet or similar cloth, keep it wet, and vigorously fan him or her;
or
place ice packs on the victim's neck, armpits, and groin.

Yes → Place ice packs on the victim's neck, armpits, and groin.

Stop cooling when mental status improves.

Seek medical care.

FYI

Heat-Related Deaths in Cars

Case 1

Hawaii, March 2007: A 3-year-old girl from Honolulu died from hyperthermia. The child's father told police that he left her in a child seat in the back seat of the car for an hour and a half late that morning while he visited friends in a Makiki apartment building. The outside temperature was only 81 degrees.

Case 2

South Carolina, April 2006: A mother left her 15-month-old son locked in a car. He was left in the car for 9 hours while his mother went to work. She is currently serving a 20-year prison sentence.

Case 3

Colorado, August 2008: Two children who died in an overheated car may have been on their own for more than 3 hours as their mother slept after working a night shift. The children died in a closed but unlocked car; investigators believe the temperature where the children were found may have reached 123 degrees.

Case 4

Mississippi, July 2001: A man died of heatstroke after falling asleep in his car with the windows rolled up in a supermarket parking lot.

Source: National Weather Service.

▶ Emergency Care Wrap-up

Condition	What to Look For	What to Do
Heat Cramps	• Painful muscle spasm during or after physical activity • Usually lower leg affected	1. Move victim to cool place. 2. Stretch the cramped muscle. 3. Remove excess or tight clothing. 4. If the victim is responsive, give water or sports drink.
Heat Exhaustion	• Heavy sweating • Severe thirst • Weakness • Headache • Nausea and vomiting	1. Move victim to cool place. 2. Have victim lie down. 3. Apply cool, wet towels to head and body. 4. If victim is responsive, give water or sports drink. 5. Seek medical care if no improvement within 30 minutes.
Heatstroke	• Extremely hot skin • Dry skin (may be wet at first) • Confusion • Seizures • Unresponsiveness	1. Move victim to cool place. 2. Call 9-1-1. 3. If unresponsive, open airway, check breathing, and provide appropriate care. 4. Rapidly cool victim by whatever means possible (cool, wet sheets; ice or cold packs against armpits, side of neck, and groin).

▶ Ready for Review

- Given the right conditions, anyone can develop a heat illness.
- The human body is constantly dispersing the heat that it produces.
- Heat illnesses include a range of disorders from heat cramps to heatstroke. Heatstroke is life threatening.

▶ Vital Vocabulary

heat cramps A painful muscle cramp resulting from excessive loss of salt and water through sweating.

heat exhaustion A prostration caused by excessive loss of water and salt through sweating; characterized by clammy skin and a weak, rapid pulse.

heatstroke A life-threatening condition of severe hyperthermia caused by exposure to excessive natural or artificial heat.

thermoregulation The body's ability to maintain a normal body temperature despite the weather.

▶ Assessment in Action

You decide to watch your local high school football team practice before its first game in late August. The coach has the defense running sprints for the last 30 minutes without rest breaks. At the end of the sprints, all but one player walk over to the water station. That player falls to the ground and you are the first to respond. The victim is responsive and his skin is moist and clammy.

Directions: Circle Yes if you agree with the statement; circle No if you disagree.

Yes   No   **1.** The victim is most likely suffering from heatstroke.

Yes   No   **2.** The first thing you should do is to help the coach and athletic trainer move the victim out of the heat and to a cool place.

Yes   No   **3.** The victim should drink cool water or a sports drink.

Yes   No   **4.** Giving several salt tablets, if available, should always be considered.

Yes   No   **5.** Removing the player's jersey, shoulder pads, and helmet and sponging him with cool water is recommended.

Yes   No   **6.** The coach and/or athletic trainer should seek medical care if there is no improvement within 30 minutes.

▶ Check Your Knowledge

Directions: Circle Yes if you agree with the statement; circle No if you disagree.

Yes   No   **1.** For heat cramps in the legs, stretch the cramped muscle.

Yes   No   **2.** Commercial sports drinks can be given to victims of heat-related emergencies.

Yes   No   **3.** Move victims of heat-related illness to a cool place.

Yes   No   **4.** Victims of heatstroke need immediate medical care—it is a life-threatening condition.

Yes   No   **5.** Cool heatstroke victims rapidly, including the use of ice packs applied to the neck, armpits, and groin.

Yes   No   **6.** Fruit juices are digested quickly and rehydrate the body most rapidly.

Yes   No   **7.** You can drink too much water and cause water intoxication.

Yes   No   **8.** Humidity cannot significantly reduce evaporative cooling.

Yes   No   **9.** Certain medications predispose to heatstroke.

Yes   No   **10.** Heat exhaustion can feel like the flu.

Childbirth and Gynecologic Emergencies

Childbirth and Gynecologic Emergencies of Pregnancy

Handling childbirth and gynecologic situations of pregnancy requires that a first aider be familiar with the terminology used to describe female reproductive anatomy and physiology.

- The <u>birth canal</u> includes the vagina and the lower part of the uterus.
- The <u>cervix</u> is the small opening at the lower end of the uterus through which the baby passes.
- The <u>placenta</u> (afterbirth) is the organ through which the mother and the fetus exchange nourishment and waste products during pregnancy. It is expelled after the baby's birth.
- The <u>umbilical cord</u> is the extension of the placenta through which the fetus receives nourishment while in the uterus.
- The <u>amniotic sac</u> (bag of waters) surrounds the fetus inside the uterus. Amniotic fluid in the sac cushions the fetus and helps protect it from injury.
- <u>Crowning</u> occurs when the fetus's head presses against the vaginal opening and begins to bulge out.
- <u>Bloody show</u> is the mucus and blood that might be discharged from the vagina as labor begins.
- <u>Labor</u> is the process of childbirth (defined in three stages), from the first regular uterine muscle contractions until delivery of the placenta.

- A <u>miscarriage</u> (medical term is *spontaneous abortion*) is the delivery of a fetus before it can live independent of the mother.

Predelivery Emergencies

▶ Miscarriage

Miscarriages usually occur during the first 3 months (first trimester) of pregnancy. Most occur because the fetus was not developing properly and was not able to survive. The woman will be emotionally upset. She might be hesitant about confiding in a stranger, especially a man; help from a woman, if possible, might be wise.

Recognizing Miscarriage

Signs of a miscarriage include the following:
- Cramping pain in lower abdomen resembling menstrual cramps
- Aching in the lower back
- Vaginal bleeding, which could be sudden and heavy
- Passage of tissue from the vagina

Care for a Woman Having a Miscarriage

Follow these guidelines to care for a woman having a miscarriage:
1. Reassure the woman.
2. Help her into a comfortable position with legs bent.
3. Have the woman place a sanitary pad over the outside of the vagina. Do not place pads in the vagina. Replace blood-soaked pads or dressings.
4. Any tissue that passes through the vagina should be transported with the woman to the hospital. Do not try to pull tissue out of the vagina; instead, cover it with a sterile pad.
5. Seek medical care.
6. Call 9-1-1 if bleeding is heavy or there are signs of shock.

Vaginal Bleeding

▶ Vaginal Bleeding During Pregnancy

A woman experiencing vaginal bleeding late in her pregnancy (third trimester, or last 3 months) usually constitutes an emergency. Find out how long she has been bleeding and how many sanitary pads she has used so that you can report the information to medical personnel. An increase in pulse rate of more than 20 beats per minute when the victim goes from a lying-down to a sitting position suggests blood loss of more than 1 pint. The woman might feel embarrassed. She might be hesitant about confiding in a stranger, especially a man; and therefore, help from a woman might be wise.

Recognizing Vaginal Bleeding During Pregnancy

Signs of vaginal bleeding during pregnancy include the following:
- Bleeding may be mild spotting but can indicate a severe problem.
- Bleeding may be heavy.
- Signs of shock may be present.

Care for a Woman With Vaginal Bleeding During Late Pregnancy

To care for someone with vaginal bleeding during late pregnancy, do the following:
1. Place the woman on her left side to relieve pressure from the fetus on the inferior vena cava (large vein between the spine and the abdominal organs).
2. Have the woman place a sanitary pad over the outside of the vagina.
3. Call 9-1-1 immediately.
4. Treat for shock (eg, maintain body temperature, avoid giving fluids).

▶ Vaginal Bleeding Caused by Injury

It is difficult to determine the source of the bleeding. Vaginal bleeding can be difficult to care for because of the woman's modesty and pain.

Recognizing Vaginal Bleeding Caused by Injury

The following signs could indicate vaginal bleeding caused by injury:
- Injuries of the external female genitalia, including all types of soft-tissue injuries (such as wounds or contusions)
- Severe pain
- Blood in the vaginal area
- Massive internal vaginal bleeding

Care for a Woman With Vaginal Bleeding Caused by Injury

To assist a woman with injury-related vaginal bleeding, follow these guidelines:

1. Use direct pressure over a bulky dressing or sanitary pad to control external bleeding from a laceration or other injury.
2. Apply an ice pack to reduce swelling and pain.
3. Never place or pack dressings into the vagina. It is useless and dangerous to introduce packs blindly into the vagina in an attempt to control bleeding.
4. Place the victim on her left side to help prevent vomiting, to prevent aspiration of vomitus, and, if the woman is pregnant, to relieve pressure on the vena cava from the fetus.
5. Seek medical care.

Q&A

Are pregnant women more susceptible to injury?

More injuries are seen in pregnant women because many of them are active and often work and travel throughout all stages of pregnancy. In addition, there is a significant incidence of violence and battering of pregnant women.

Factors predisposing a woman to injury in early pregnancy are fainting episodes, hyperventilation, and becoming easily fatigued. In the last trimester, an enlarged abdomen changes the woman's center of gravity, making her more susceptible to falls, and pelvic pressure causing leg pain.

Motor vehicle crashes in which the seat belt is not used or is used in an improper position is also a common cause of injury.

▶ Non–Injury-Related Vaginal Bleeding

Bleeding from the vagina is most likely to be menstrual bleeding. However, such bleeding can indicate more serious conditions (such as miscarriage, childbirth, infection).

Recognizing Non-Injury-Related Vaginal Bleeding

Abdominal cramps can be a sign of non–injury-related vaginal bleeding.

Care for Victims of Non-Injury-Related Vaginal Bleeding

Non–injury-related vaginal bleeding can result from various causes, but treatment is similar. Here is what you can do:

1. Reassure the woman.
2. Help her into a comfortable position with legs bent.
3. Have the woman place a sanitary pad over the outside of the vagina.
4. Seek medical care.

Delivery

Emergency childbirth occurs when a baby is born at an unplanned time or at an unplanned place. Most babies in the United States are delivered in a hospital. Occasionally, the birth process moves along faster than expected. Because of the infrequency, taking care of an anxious mother and her newborn infant is a stressful event for a first aider. On the other hand, assisting in the birth of a baby is one of the few situations in which first aiders have the opportunity to participate in a happy event rather than an unpleasant one.

▶ Imminent Delivery

Consider transporting the woman to a hospital only if she is not straining or crowning and this is her first pregnancy. Making a hasty decision to transport the woman means that the delivery could take place under the worst possible circumstances. When there is enough time to transport the woman to a hospital the woman should wear seat belts. Neither the lap belt nor the shoulder harness should be worn alone—both should be worn at the same time to avoid rupturing the uterus if a crash occurs. If she needs to lie down, place her on her left side. This position prevents a possible drop in blood pressure caused by pressure on the inferior vena cava, which reduces venous blood returning to the heart.

If the woman is straining or crowning, has had previous pregnancies, and there is not enough time to get to the hospital, you must prepare to assist in the delivery. First, call (or have a bystander call) 9-1-1. Then, if the woman is in a crowded or public place, try to find a private, clean area. The mother might find it reassuring to have a companion, such as her husband, a friend, or a relative, present. Follow these guidelines:

- Wear exam gloves. If available, wear a mask, a gown, and eye protection.
- Do not touch the vaginal area except during delivery and, if possible, with a witness present.
- Do not let the mother use the toilet.
- Do not hold the mother's legs together.

If the baby's head is not the presenting part (the first part to come out of the birth canal), the delivery will be complicated. Tell the mother not to push and attempt to calm and reassure her. Call 9-1-1 if you have not already done so.

CAUTION

DO NOT allow the mother to go to the toilet if delivery seems imminent.

DO NOT attempt to delay or restrain delivery in any way (for example, holding the mother's legs together).

Stages of Labor

Labor is a three-stage process that begins with the first regular uterine contractions, includes delivery of the baby, and ends with delivery of the placenta. The first stage usually lasts several hours (possibly 12 hours or more for a first baby), from the first contraction until the cervix is fully open (dilated). The cervix gradually stretches until it is large enough to let the baby pass through. (Outside a hospital setting, rescuers cannot safely check for dilation of the cervix.) The contractions usually begin as acutely aching sensations in the small of the back; in a short time, they turn into cramplike pains recurring regularly in the lower abdomen. At first, the contractions are 10 to 15 minutes apart, are not very severe, and last less than 1 minute. Gradually, the intervals between contractions grow shorter, and the contractions increase in intensity. A slight, watery, bloodstained discharge (bloody show) from the vagina might accompany contractions or might occur before labor begins.

At the end of the first stage of labor, the amniotic sac breaks, and a pint or more of watery fluid, the amniotic fluid, discharges. Sometimes the amniotic sac breaks during the first stage of labor, but this is no cause for concern because it usually does not affect labor. If the amniotic sac breaks prematurely and labor

does not begin within 12 hours, the risk of infection to mother and baby is great, and medical care should be sought.

The second stage usually lasts from 30 minutes to 2 hours. It begins when the neck of the cervix is fully open and ends with the actual birth of the baby. The baby is normally head down; once the head gets through the pelvis, the rest of the body should follow easily. During the third stage, which lasts about 15 minutes or more, the afterbirth (placenta) is expelled **Figure 22-1**.

Recognizing Signs of Impending Delivery

At the scene of a woman in labor, you will need to determine whether delivery is imminent or whether there is time to transport the woman to the hospital. To make that decision, answer the following questions:

- *Has the woman had a baby before?* Labor during a first pregnancy is usually longer than in subsequent pregnancies. If this is her first pregnancy, there might be more time for transport to a hospital.
- *How frequent are the contractions?* Contractions more than 5 minutes apart are a good indication that there will be enough time to get the mother to a nearby hospital. Contractions less than 2 minutes apart that last 45 to 60 seconds, especially in a woman who has had more than one pregnancy, signal imminent delivery.
- *Has the amniotic sac ruptured? If so, when?* Labor usually proceeds more rapidly after rupture. If the sac ruptures more than 18 hours before birth occurs, the likelihood of fetal infection increases, and the hospital staff should be alerted. Delivery might be more difficult when the amniotic sac ruptures prematurely because amniotic fluid serves as a lubricant.
- *Does the mother feel as though she has to move her bowels?* That sensation is caused by the fetal head in the vagina pressing against the rectum and indicates that delivery is imminent.

Only if the answers to these questions seem to indicate an imminent birth should you examine the mother for crowning. Look to see if there is bulging at the vaginal opening or if part of the baby is visible. Crowning indicates that the baby is about to be born and that there is no time to get to a hospital before delivery. Because this step might be embarrassing to the mother,

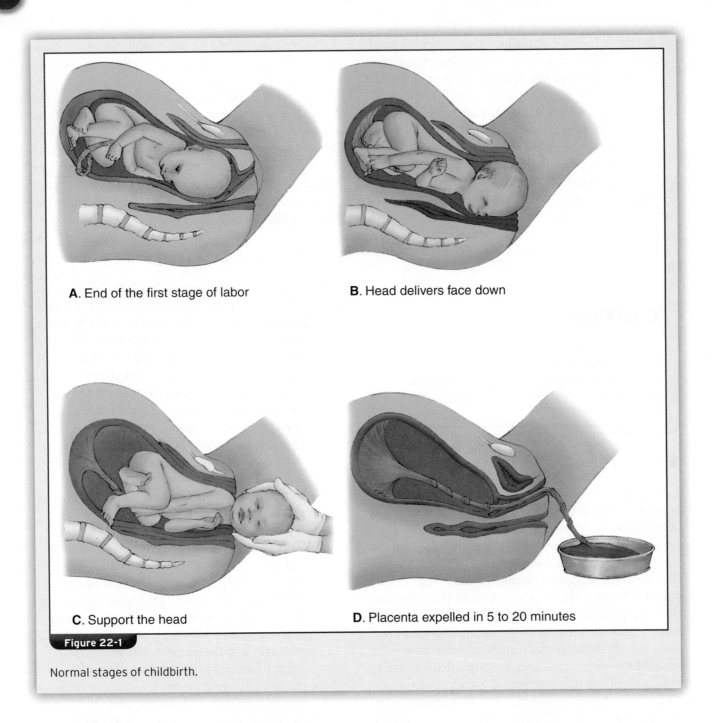

A. End of the first stage of labor

B. Head delivers face down

C. Support the head

D. Placenta expelled in 5 to 20 minutes

Figure 22-1

Normal stages of childbirth.

the father, bystanders, or even you, it is important that you explain fully what you are doing and why. Make every effort to protect the woman from embarrassment during such an examination by removing only enough clothing to expose the vaginal area. Use something to shield the woman from prying eyes—for example, a blanket used to make a tent, or even a human shield, with people standing with their backs toward her.

Delivery Procedures

Ideally, you should have the following supplies for delivery:

- Clean sheets, towels, and blankets to cover the mother and baby
- A plastic bag or towel to wrap the placenta for delivery to the hospital

- Clean, unused, exam gloves to reduce the likelihood of infection
- Sanitary pads
- Newspapers, plastic, or a cloth sheet to place under the woman to provide a clean delivery area
- Rubber bulb syringe for suctioning the baby's mouth and nostrils
- Sterile gauze pads for wiping blood and mucus from the baby's mouth and nose
- Strips of gauze, new or clean shoelaces, or similar materials to tie the cord. (Do not use thread, wire, or string because they might cut through the cord.) Gauze bandages or pads opened into strips can be used.

Care for a Woman During Delivery

If you are faced with an imminent delivery, follow the steps in **Skill Drill 22-1**:

1. Take standard precautions by washing your hands thoroughly and wearing exam gloves. If possible, wear a mask, a gown, and eye protection.
2. Have the mother lie on her back with her head slightly elevated, knees drawn up, and legs spread apart. The mother might want to be in a different position. Other safe positions for childbirth include the following:
   - Sitting up or squatting, with someone behind supporting her. These two positions place less tension on the vaginal tissues, reducing the likelihood of a tear, and allow the force of gravity to help.
   - Lying on her left side, which improves blood return to her heart and prevents aspiration should she vomit. Have someone hold the woman's right leg up out of the way.
   - Kneeling in a knee-chest position, which is used in many countries and in cases of breech presentations.

   Remind the woman to take short, quick breaths during each contraction. Between contractions, she should rest and breathe deeply through her mouth.
3. Place absorbent, clean materials (such as sheets or towels) under the mother's buttocks.
4. Elevate her buttocks with blankets or a pillow.
5. When the baby's head appears, place the palm of your hand on top of the head and exert very gentle pressure to prevent an explosive delivery. Have the woman stop pushing. Do not push on the fontanelles (soft spots on the top and back of the infant's head).
6. If the amniotic sac does not break or has not broken, tear it with your fingers and push it away from the baby's head and mouth as they appear. The baby could suffocate if the sac is not removed.
7. As the baby's head emerges from the vagina, determine whether the umbilical cord is wrapped around the baby's neck. If it is, gently slip the cord over the baby's head. If you cannot do that, attempt to alleviate pressure on the cord. (See Step 17 for instructions on how to cut the cord).
8. Support the baby's head as it emerges.
9. Suction the baby's mouth and then the nostrils two or three times with the bulb syringe. Use caution to avoid contact with the back of the baby's mouth. If a bulb syringe is not available, wipe the baby's mouth and then the nose with gauze (**Step ❶**).
10. As the torso and full body emerge, support the baby with both hands—he or she will be slippery (**Steps ❷ and ❸**).
11. Do not pull on the baby, which could cause cervical spine damage. Do not put your fingers in the baby's armpits; pressure on the nerve centers there could cause paralysis.
12. Keep the baby level with the vagina, slightly head down, to improve drainage from the mouth and nose.
13. Wipe blood and mucus from the baby's mouth and nose with sterile gauze; suction the mouth, and then suction the nose again.
14. Dry the infant to reduce heat loss and help stimulate breathing. Rub the baby's back or flick the soles of its feet to stimulate breathing. The baby should breathe within 30 seconds, especially after the cord stops pulsating (**Step ❹**). (Do not hold the baby up by the feet and slap its buttocks, which could cause an increase in intracranial pressure.) If

breathing does not start within 30 seconds, begin cardiopulmonary resuscitation (CPR).

15. Wrap the infant in a warm blanket and place on his or her side, head slightly lower than the trunk. Keep the infant level with the mother's vagina until the cord is cut. Raising the baby above the mother's abdomen (location of the placenta) while the umbilical cord is intact will allow the baby's blood to drain out and might result in shock in the baby. Holding the baby below the mother's abdomen allows her blood to flow into the baby, and the extra blood cells can cause serious problems such as jaundice.

16. When the umbilical cord stops pulsating, tie it with gauze (or similar material) or a clean shoelace between the mother and the infant.

17. If the mother is going to the hospital soon after the birth, and it was a normal delivery, there is no need to cut the cord. Keep the infant warm and wait for EMS personnel, who will have the proper equipment to clamp and cut the cord. If you are in a remote location, you might have to cut the cord yourself. In such a situation and after cord pulsations stop, tie the cord about 4″ away from the baby and make a second tie 2″ from the first tie. Cut the cord between the two ties.

18. Watch for delivery of the placenta, which usually takes a few minutes, but could take as long as 30 minutes. Do not pull on the end of the umbilical cord to speed the placenta's delivery (**Step ❺**).

19. When the placenta is delivered, wrap it in a towel with three quarters of the umbilical cord and place the towel in a plastic bag. Keep the bag at the level of the infant. Take the placenta to the hospital, where it will be examined for completeness. This procedure is necessary because pieces of placenta retained in the uterus can cause persistent bleeding or infection.

20. Place a sterile pad over the vaginal opening, lower the mother's legs, and help her hold them together.

21. Gently massage the woman's abdomen, just below the navel, to help control bleeding.

Delivery Aftercare

After delivery, monitor the mother's breathing and pulse. Replace any blood-soaked sheets and blankets while awaiting transport. A woman can be expected to lose from 1 to 2 cups (300 to 500 mL) of blood after delivery. You should be aware of this amount of blood loss so it does not cause undue psychological stress to the new mother or to you. If blood loss continues, massage the uterus. Uterine massage stimulates the uterus to contract, thus constricting blood vessels within its walls and decreasing bleeding.

1. Use your hand with your fingers fully extended.
2. Place the palm of your hand on the lower abdomen, where you should be able to feel a grapefruit-sized mass.
3. Gently massage over the area with a firm, circular motion.
4. If bleeding continues, check your massage technique.
5. The mother can also breast-feed the baby following delivery of the placenta to stimulate uterine contractions and, thus, help control bleeding.

Initial Care of the Newborn

Normal findings in a newborn are a pulse rate of more than 100 beats per minute (feel the brachial artery) and a respiratory rate of more than 40 breaths per minute. The baby often will be crying. The most important care is positioning, drying, keeping warm, and stimulating the newborn to breathe. Wrap the newborn in a blanket, making sure the head is covered. Repeat suctioning if necessary, and continue to stimulate the newborn if he or she is not breathing (flick the soles of the feet and rub the infant's back).

If the newborn is motionless, tap the infant on the bottom of a foot or a shoulder for a response. If the infant does not respond and is not breathing, or is only gasping, begin CPR starting with 30 chest compressions followed by two breaths. Initially, give a total of five sets of 30 chest compressions and two breaths before calling 9-1-1 unless a bystander has already done so. Continue sets of 30 chest compressions and two breaths until EMS personnel take over or an automated external defibrillator (AED) arrives.

22-1 **Childbirth**

1 Support the baby's head and suction its mouth and nose.

2 Once the head delivers, the upper shoulders will be visible.

3 Support the baby's head and body as the shoulders deliver.

4 Clean and dry the infant to reduce heat loss and stimulate breathing.

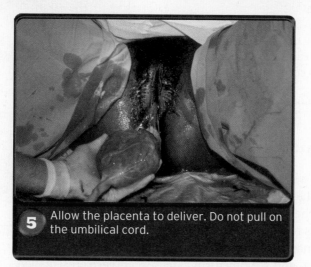

5 Allow the placenta to deliver. Do not pull on the umbilical cord.

▶ Abnormal Deliveries

Most childbirths are normal and natural. Sometimes, however, complications arise. It is essential that you be calm, deliberate, and gentle in a situation that becomes even more stressful because of complications. Call 9-1-1 for all of these situations.

Prolapsed Cord

A prolapsed cord is a condition in which the umbilical cord comes through the birth canal before delivery of the head. The cord is squeezed between the baby's head and the mother's body (vaginal wall), and oxygen supply to the baby could be stopped. This puts the baby in danger of suffocation **Figure 22-2**. This situation is rare and very dangerous.

Recognizing a Prolapsed Cord
If the umbilical cord can be seen before the baby's head, the cord is prolapsed.

Care for an Infant With a Prolapsed Cord
1. Position the woman with her head down or buttocks raised to use gravity to lessen pressure in the birth canal.
2. Insert fingers of your gloved hand into the vagina, placing fingers on either side of the cord to hold pressure from the presenting part (most often the head) of the fetus away from the pulsating cord. Continue until EMS arrives. Do *not* push the cord back into the vagina. This is one of only two circumstances for putting your fingers into the vagina.
3. Call 9-1-1 immediately.

CAUTION

DO NOT attempt to push the cord back into the vagina.

Breech Birth Presentation

A breech presentation occurs when the baby's buttocks or lower extremities emerge before the head or shoulders. Breech presentation is the most common type of abnormal delivery and occurs in 3% to 4% of all deliveries. Place the mother in a kneeling, head-down position, with her pelvis elevated, and seek medical care immediately **Figure 22-3**.

Figure 22-2

Prolapsed cord.

Figure 22-3

Breech presentation.

In a breech presentation, if the baby's head is not delivered within 3 minutes of the body, you must act to prevent suffocation of the baby. Suffocation can occur when the baby's face is pressed against the vaginal wall or when the umbilical cord is compressed by the baby's head in the vagina.

Recognizing Breech Birth Presentation
In a breech birth, the baby's buttocks come out first (most babies are born head first).

Care for an Infant With Breech Birth Presentation
To establish an airway, do the following:

1. Place one hand in the vagina, positioning the palm toward the baby's face. This is one of only two circumstances for putting your fingers into the vagina.
2. Form a V with your fingers on either side of the baby's nose.
3. Push the vaginal wall away from the baby's face until the head is delivered.
4. Have someone call 9-1-1 immediately.
5. Have the woman continue to push with contractions and attempt to deliver the baby.

CAUTION

DO NOT pull out the baby's head during a breech delivery.

Figure 22-4

Limb presentation.

Limb Presentation

Limb presentation occurs when an arm, leg, or foot of the infant protrudes from the birth canal. A foot more commonly presents when the infant is in a breech presentation **Figure 22-4**.

FYI

Emergencies During Pregnancy

What Medical Specialties Take Care of Women?

A gynecologist specializes in treating conditions related to the female reproductive tract. An obstetrician specializes in treating pregnant women. A pediatrician specializes in treating newborn babies, toddlers, and young teens.

How Is Emergency Care for a Pregnant Woman Different?

There are two people involved—the mother and fetus. Even minor trauma to the mother's abdomen can result in life-threatening consequences. All pregnant women with trauma to the abdomen need a medical examination in a hospital emergency department and often need fetal monitoring. Fetal viability is determined by maternal viability. Position the mother on her left side to help venous blood return to the heart. Care for the pregnant woman the same way you would treat a non-pregnant woman.

What Are Some Indications of Pregnancy Problems?

• The big three warning signs of a serious problem are bleeding, abdominal cramps, and weakness.
• Morning sickness, swollen ankles, and urinary tract infections are not usually dangerous, but call the physician anyway.
• If a pregnant woman is spotting (small amount of vaginal bleeding), have her lie down immediately. Call for medical attention. Spotting can signal the onset of a miscarriage.

Recognizing Limb Presentation

In a case of limb presentation, an arm, leg, or foot appears first.

Care for an Infant With Limb Presentation

1. Place the mother in a head-down position with the pelvis elevated. Do *not* pull on the baby or attempt to push the limb back into the vagina.
2. Call 9-1-1 immediately. The baby cannot be delivered in this position by a first aider.

Meconium

Meconium is the baby's first feces (bowel movement) and can be present in the amniotic fluid. Its presence is associated with fetal distress during labor and a greater risk for infant death. The danger to the baby is the possibility of breathing the meconium into the lungs, where it can cause severe respiratory problems.

Recognizing Meconium

Amniotic fluid containing meconium is greenish or brownish-yellow in color rather than clear. It is tarry and almost odorless.

Care for an Infant in Danger of Inhaling Meconium

Follow these steps to prevent a newborn infant from inhaling meconium:

1. Keep the infant in a moderately head-down position to aid with drainage.
2. Suction the mouth and nostrils thoroughly, or the baby will inhale meconium with its first breath into the lungs. Clear amniotic fluid, however, is harmlessly absorbed through the baby's lungs. Try not to stimulate the infant to breathe before suctioning.
3. Maintain the baby's open airway.
4. Call 9-1-1 immediately.

Premature Birth

Any baby born prior to 37 completed weeks of pregnancy is defined as premature and will require special care. Premature babies develop problems because they are smaller and less developed than full-term infants. For example, their cardiovascular and respiratory systems are often immature.

Recognizing Premature Birth

It is difficult without scales to weigh an infant. Signs of premature birth include:

- Premature infant will be smaller and thinner than a full-term infant.
- Premature infant has a head proportionately larger in comparison with the rest of the body.
- The cheesy, white coating on the skin (*vernix caseosa*) of a full-term infant will be minimal or absent on the premature infant.

Care for a Premature Infant

Care for a premature baby in the following manner:

1. Keep the baby warm. Premature babies are always at risk for hypothermia.
2. Keep the mouth and nose clear of mucus.
3. Monitor breathing and perform CPR, if necessary.

Gynecologic Emergencies

Gynecologic emergencies are reproductive system problems that occur in nonpregnant females.

Q&A

What is pelvic inflammatory disease (PID)?

PID is caused by the spread of microorganisms from the vagina and cervix to reproductive organs. The organisms (the most common being *Chlamydia* and gonorrhea) are typically sexually transmitted. A victim with PID can have more than one sexually transmitted disease (STD) at the same time. Other important conditions may cause confusion about the problem (eg, ectopic pregnancy, acute appendicitis). The inflammatory response can range from mild to severe. No reliable signs or symptoms exist, but may involve vaginal discharge and abdominal tenderness. Because the consequences of unrecognized and untreated PID can be severe, medical care should be sought.

Q&A

What are the signs and symptoms of an ectopic pregnancy?

Pelvic pain and vaginal bleeding or spotting in a woman of childbearing age should be treated as an ectopic pregnancy until the condition is ruled out by a physician. Predisposing factors for ectopic pregnancy are previous ectopic pregnancies, surgeries, pelvic infections, and presence of an intrauterine device (IUD). Common signs and symptoms are vaginal bleeding and abdominal tenderness.

Emergency Childbirth

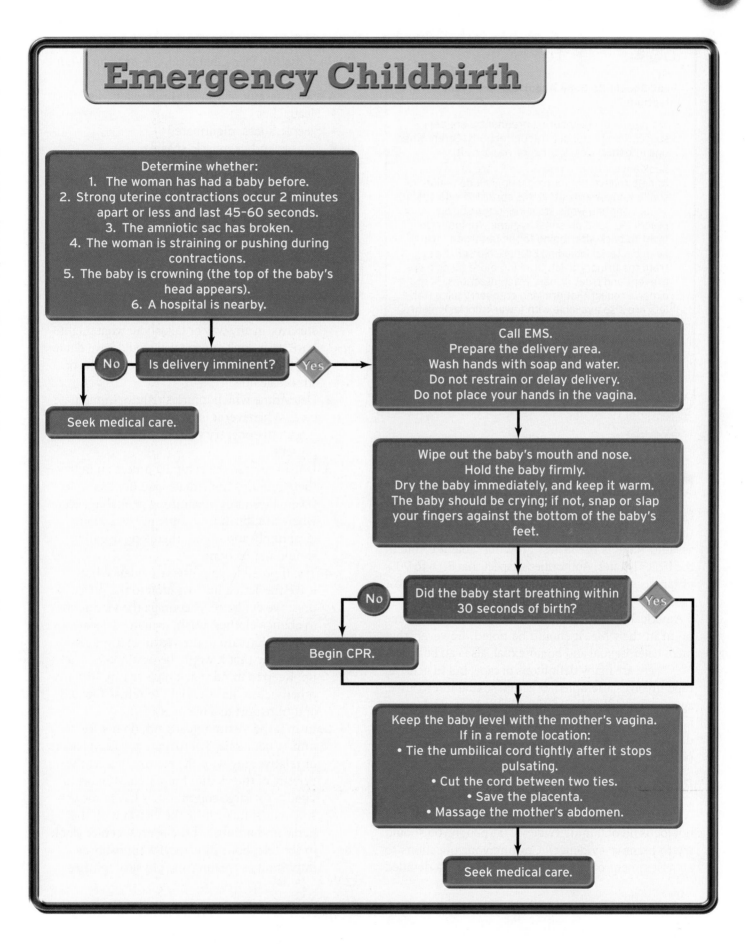

Determine whether:
1. The woman has had a baby before.
2. Strong uterine contractions occur 2 minutes apart or less and last 45–60 seconds.
3. The amniotic sac has broken.
4. The woman is straining or pushing during contractions.
5. The baby is crowning (the top of the baby's head appears).
6. A hospital is nearby.

Is delivery imminent?

No → Seek medical care.

Yes → Call EMS.
Prepare the delivery area.
Wash hands with soap and water.
Do not restrain or delay delivery.
Do not place your hands in the vagina.

Wipe out the baby's mouth and nose.
Hold the baby firmly.
Dry the baby immediately, and keep it warm.
The baby should be crying; if not, snap or slap your fingers against the bottom of the baby's feet.

Did the baby start breathing within 30 seconds of birth?

No → Begin CPR.

Yes →

Keep the baby level with the mother's vagina.
If in a remote location:
• Tie the umbilical cord tightly after it stops pulsating.
• Cut the cord between two ties.
• Save the placenta.
• Massage the mother's abdomen.

Seek medical care.

Q&A

What Should Be Done About Urinary Tract Infections?

- Women, especially during pregnancy, are very susceptible to urinary tract infections. Often, when one infection clears, another replaces it.
- Seek advice from a doctor. Self-care measures to help relieve the burning pain include taking shallow, lukewarm sitz baths sprinkled with baking soda; urinating while standing in the shower; and practicing good personal hygiene. Wiping from front to back after going to the bathroom helps keep bacteria, including *Escherichia coli*, away from the urinary tract. Drinking more fluids helps prevent and treat urinary tract infections. Some experts report that drinking cranberry juice (tablets are also available with fewer calories) might help inhibit urinary tract infections.
- A urinary tract (bladder) infection can lead to the more serious kidney infection. Signs of a kidney infection include, pain in the lower back or flank, fever, and nausea or vomiting.

▶ Sexual Assault and Rape

Perhaps one of the most difficult emergency situations that a first aider might have to deal with is sexual assault. Rape is the fastest growing violent crime in the United States. Authorities suspect that 80% to 90% of rape cases are not reported to authorities. In most cases, the rape victim is a woman. An estimated 1 in 3 American women will be sexually assaulted at some point in their life. It should be noted, however, that men, heterosexual and homosexual, also can be raped.

There are many definitions of rape, but in general, rape involves attempted or actual sexual intercourse, against the will of the victim. Related physical injury is common, but the psychological trauma may be more damaging. It is essential that you be calm and sympathetic when dealing with a victim of sexual assault.

Recognizing Sexual Assault and Rape

A first aider should provide care for the victim and not focus on obtaining evidence (although you should try to *preserve* evidence). Confine your questions to an assessment of the victim's injuries, not a detailed description of the events. Ask questions based on the SAMPLE history (see Chapter 4, *Finding Out What's Wrong*).

A sexual assault victim might display:
- Headaches
- Sleeplessness, nightmares
- Nausea and/or muscle spasms
- Confusion
- Depression
- Anxiety, jumpiness

Care for a Victim of Sexual Assault and Rape

The following list outlines what you should do and not do for a victim of sexual assault and rape.

1. Don't ask a lot of questions. Don't blame the survivor in any way or talk about what might have been done or what you would have done. Be supportive. Remind him or her that he or she is safe now.
2. Determine which injuries require immediate care. Whenever it is necessary that a female victim disrobe, try to have another woman present.
3. Do not expose the genitalia unless an injury there requires immediate care (for example, severe bleeding). Examining genitalia, except when childbirth is imminent, has serious legal implications and, therefore, usually should not be done.
4. Try, if possible, to preserve evidence but leave the actual investigation to the police. To preserve evidence, encourage the victim not to change clothes, wash, urinate, defecate, or douche. Explain to the victim in a sympathetic way that it would be best not to clean up. Keep in mind that a rape victim, like any other victim, has the right to refuse first aid and transport to a hospital.
5. Even if the victim refuses aid, do not leave him or her alone. Try to have a trusted friend or relative stay with the victim. Protect the privacy of the victim. Emotional support is vital. Most large communities have rape crisis centers; furnishing the victim with the name and number of the nearest center (look in the telephone directory) is probably as important as treating any physical injuries.

Trained volunteers can talk to the victim and give you and the victim information about what to do next.

6. Get the victim medical care. The victim could be in shock and unaware of the severity of her or his injuries. Strongly encourage a rape victim to receive medical care, even if the person does not show any signs of injury and does not want medical care. However, be aware that the medical exam following a rape is intrusive and includes a full gynecologic exam. Victims will need information about what is going to happen before receiving medical care.

prep kit

▶ Ready for Review

- Miscarriages usually occur during the first trimester of pregnancy.
- If a woman experiences vaginal bleeding late in her pregnancy, it usually constitutes an emergency.
- Emergency childbirth occurs when a baby is born at an unplanned time or at an unplanned place.
- In most cases, childbirth is normal and natural. Sometimes complications can arise.
- Perhaps one of the most difficult emergency situations that a first aider might have to deal with is sexual assault.

▶ Vital Vocabulary

<u>amniotic sac</u> A thick, transparent sac that holds the fetus suspended in the amniotic fluid.

<u>birth canal</u> The vagina and the lower part of the uterus.

<u>bloody show</u> The bloody mucus plug that is discharged from the vagina when labor begins.

<u>cervix</u> The small opening at the lower end of the uterus through which the baby passes.

<u>crowning</u> The stage of birth when the presenting part of the baby is visible at the vaginal orifice.

<u>labor</u> The process or period of childbirth; especially, the muscular contraction of the uterus designed to expel the fetus from the mother.

<u>miscarriage</u> Delivery of the fetus before it is mature enough to survive outside the womb (about 20 weeks), from either natural (spontaneous abortion) or induced causes.

<u>placenta</u> The vascular organ attached to the uterine wall that supplies oxygen and nutrients to the fetus; also called afterbirth.

<u>umbilical cord</u> The flexible structure that connects the fetus to the placenta.

▶ Assessment in Action

You are visiting a local museum when you respond to calls for help in the exhibit hall. A young woman has gone into labor. When you arrive on scene, she tells you this is her third child and that her due date is next week. She says she thought she would have time to get to the hospital when the contractions started. However, the contractions intensified and got closer together very quickly. Contractions are now less than 2 minutes apart and last up to 60 seconds. A hospital is 10 minutes away.

Directions: Circle Yes if you agree with the statement; circle No if you disagree.

Yes   No   **1.** Labor during a third pregnancy is usually longer than in previous pregnancies.

Yes   No   **2.** If the amniotic sac ruptures, you should assume that delivery may be imminent.

Yes   No   **3.** With contractions less than 2 minutes apart, you should have time to get her to the hospital.

Yes   No   **4.** Call 9-1-1 and immediately prepare a delivery area.

Yes   No   **5.** If the baby is crowning, you should not restrain or delay delivery.

▶ Check Your Knowledge

Directions: Circle Yes if you agree with the statement; circle No if you disagree.

Yes   No   **1.** An aching in the lower back is a sign of a miscarriage.

Yes   No   **2.** It is normal for a woman to experience vaginal bleeding in her last trimester.

Yes   No   **3.** Most babies in the United States are delivered at home.

Yes   No   **4.** Place a pregnant woman on her left side when transporting her to the hospital.

Yes   No   **5.** Labor is a four-stage process.

Yes   No   **6.** The second stage of labor lasts from 30 minutes to 2 hours.

Yes   No   **7.** New or clean shoelaces can be used to tie the umbilical cord.

Yes   No   **8.** A prolapsed umbilical cord is a normal occurrence.

Yes   No   **9.** The placenta is also called the afterbirth.

Yes   No   **10.** Whether or not the woman has given birth before will usually affect the length of the labor.

23

Behavioral Emergencies

Behavioral Emergencies

Behavior is how a person acts. Although each person acts or behaves differently, sometimes a person exhibits unacceptable or intolerable behavior. The abnormal behavior may be due to a psychological condition (such as a mental illness) or a physical condition. For example, a person with diabetes who has an uncorrected low blood glucose level can display aggressiveness, restlessness, or anxiety. Because the brain lacks energy in the form of blood glucose, altered mental status results. Likewise, lack of oxygen and inadequate blood flow to the brain also cause altered mental status, resulting in similar behavior. Behavior that leads to violence or other inappropriate activities is known as a <u>behavioral emergency</u>.

Several factors can change a person's behavior, including situational stresses, medical illnesses, psychiatric problems, alcohol, and drugs. The following are common reasons for behavioral changes:

- Low blood glucose level in a person with diabetes
- Lack of oxygen (known as *hypoxia*)
- Inadequate blood flow to the brain
- Head trauma
- Excessive cold
- Excessive heat
- Mind-altering substances, such as alcohol, depressants, stimulants, hallucinogens, and narcotics
- Psychogenic or psychiatric illness that leads to psychotic thinking, depression, or panic

▶ Depression

Depression is more than the sad feeling that everyone experiences at times. Depression is one of the most common and treatable of all mental illnesses. There are several types of depression: *reactive depression* (following tragic events), *major* or *clinical depression* (with no apparent cause, lasts more than 2 weeks, and prevents functioning in top form at work or socially), and *bipolar depression*, a type that includes episodes of euphoria. *Depression* is believed to be due to a chemical imbalance in the brain, which causes the nerves in the brain not to work properly. This is why it is often treated using medications that act on the brain. Depression can lead to suicide; in fact, untreated depression is the main cause of suicide.

Recognizing Depression

Not everyone who is depressed experiences every symptom. Some people experience a few symptoms, others many. Severity of symptoms varies with individuals and also varies over time.

- Persistent sad, anxious, or "empty" moods
- Feelings of hopelessness, pessimism
- Feelings of guilt, worthlessness, helplessness
- Loss of interest or pleasure in hobbies and activities that were once enjoyed, including sex
- Decreased energy, fatigue, feeling "slowed down"
- Difficulty concentrating, remembering, making decisions
- Insomnia, early-morning awakening, or oversleeping
- Appetite and/or weight loss or overeating and weight gain
- Thoughts of death or suicide; suicide attempts
- Restlessness, irritability
- Persistent physical symptoms that do not respond to treatment such as headaches, digestive disorders, and chronic pain

Care for Depression

Some depressed people do not feel like talking. In such cases, saying, "You look very sad," often allows the person to talk about the depressed feelings. The person might burst into tears. Do not discourage the crying. Maintain a sympathetic silence and let the person "cry it out."

A depressed person needs empathetic attention and reassurance and needs to know that the first aider is concerned. It is usually best to interview a depressed person in private because the presence of several people may make the person uncomfortable. Ask open-ended questions such as, "Tell me how you feel." Tell the depressed person that many people have periods of unhappiness, but they can be helped to feel better. Mention community resources where such help can be found.

▶ Suicide

Suicide is defined as any willful act that ends one's own life. Each year, about 30,000 Americans commit suicide; it is the eleventh reported leading cause of death in the United States. Many experts, however, believe that suicide is vastly underreported. Suicide in the United States is increasingly a problem of adolescents, college-age students, and the very old.

The rate for suicide in men is more than three times that for women. It is most common in men who are single, widowed, or divorced. Slightly more than half of all suicides—both men and women—use firearms. The next most common method is hanging. Poisoning by solids or liquids is the most common method used by people who attempt but do not complete suicide. Jumping from high places, carbon monoxide poisoning by auto exhaust, drowning, and self-inflicted (non-firearm) wounds are less common methods.

The number of suicides peaks during spring months and is lowest in the winter. Suicide rates are lowest in the Northeast and highest in the mountain states.

Suicide attempts are eight times more common than completed suicides. In addition, although males complete suicide three times more often than females, females are reported to attempt suicide three times more often. It is not known if males are more reluctant to seek help and, thus, less likely to report their attempts. It also is not known if the lower rate of suicide among females results from their choice of less-lethal methods.

Despite its ranking as a major cause of death, suicide is rare. Except in the case of suicide clusters (three or more completed suicides closely related in time and place), no community is likely to experience many suicides.

Suicide is often attempted by people who are depressed or have alcoholism. About 60% of all suicide victims previously attempted suicide, and about 75% gave clear warning that they intended to kill themselves. Typically, a suicide attempt occurs when a person's close emotional attachments are in danger or when he or she physically loses a significant family member or friend. Suicidal people often feel unable to manage their lives. Frequently, they lack self-esteem.

Many suicidal people make last-minute attempts to communicate their intentions. When a person phones to threaten suicide, try to keep the suicidal person on the line until EMS reaches the scene.

If you encounter a person who is attempting or threatening suicide, discreetly remove any dangerous articles. Talk quietly with the person and encourage the person to discuss the situation. Ask the following: Have you attempted suicide before? Have you made any concrete plans for a method of suicide? Has any family member committed suicide? People who have made a previous suicide attempt, who have detailed suicide plans, or who have a close relative who committed suicide are more likely to try to kill themselves **Table 23-1** . They must be reassured and taken to medical help, usually at a hospital. Do not leave them alone under any circumstances.

When a person attempts suicide, first aid care has priority. Drug overdoses must be managed. Bleeding from slashed wrists must be controlled. As you give first aid, try to encourage the person to talk about the situation. If a drug overdose is involved, collect any medication containers, pills, or other drugs found on the scene and take the items to the hospital emergency department with the victim. In many cases, law enforcement authorities should be contacted.

Recognizing a Potential Suicide Victim

If you observe someone:
- Getting their affairs in order (paying off debts, making or changing a will)
- Giving away articles of either personal or monetary value
- Exhibiting signs of planning a suicide such as obtaining a weapon or writing a suicide note

If someone says:
- Life isn't worth living.
- My family would be better off without me.
- Next time I'll take enough pills to do the job right.

Table 23-1 Suicide Risk Factors

The SAD PERSONS scale is a mnemonic list of known suicide high-risk characteristics. A score of nine or greater indicates the probable need for psychiatric consultation.

Mnemonic	Characteristics	Score
S Sex	Male	1
A Age	Younger than 19 or older than 45 years	1
D Depression or hopelessness	Admits to depression or decreased concentration, appetite, sleep, libido	2
P Previous attempts or psychiatric care	Previous inpatient or outpatient psychiatric care	1
E Excessive alcohol or drug use	Chronic addiction or recent frequent drug use	1
R Rational thinking loss	Brain dysfunction (unknown or nonspecific cause) or psychosis	2
S Separated, widowed, or divorced		1
O Organized or serious attempt	Well-thought-out plan or life-threatening display	2
N No social support	No close family, friends, job, or active religious affiliation	1
S Stated future intent	Determined to repeat attempt	2

Determining whether high-risk factors are involved will help first aiders maintain objectivity. It is important to maintain a nonjudgmental approach. Using the SAD PERSONS mnemonic acknowledges the seriousness of the situation and reminds first aiders that ridiculing, making demeaning comments, or ignoring the person are not helpful or proper.

Take precautions by keeping the person under close observation, removing any potentially dangerous items (for example, glass, razors, and medicines) from the immediate area, and not allowing the person to go *anywhere*, even to the bathroom, unaccompanied.

Source: Hockberger RS, Rothstein RJ. 1988. Assessment of suicide potential by non-psychiatrists using the SAD PERSONS score. *J Emerg Med* 6(2):99-107.

- Take my (prized collection, valuables); I don't need this stuff anymore.
- I won't be around to deal with that.
- You'll be sorry when I'm gone.
- I won't be around much longer.
- I just can't deal with everything—life's too hard.
- Nobody understands me; nobody feels the way I do.
- There's nothing I can do to make it better.
- I'd be better off dead.
- I feel like there is no way out.

CAUTION

DO NOT ignore a suicide threat. Every suicidal act or gesture should be taken seriously and the person referred to a professional counselor.

Care for a Potential Suicide Victim

If someone tells you they are thinking about suicide, you should take their distress seriously. Here are some ways to be helpful to someone who is threatening suicide:

- Be direct. Talk openly and matter-of-factly about suicide.
- Be willing to listen. Allow expressions of feelings. Accept the feelings.
- Be nonjudgmental. Don't debate whether suicide is right or wrong.
- Get involved. Become available. Show interest and support.
- Do not dare him or her to do it.
- Do not act shocked. This will put distance between the two of you.
- Do not be sworn to secrecy. Seek support.

FYI

Common Myths About Suicide

Myth	Fact
People who talk about suicide do not commit suicide.	Of every 10 people who kill themselves, 8 have given definite warnings of their suicidal intentions. Suicide threats and attempts must be taken seriously.
Suicide happens without warning.	Studies reveal that the suicidal person gives many clues and warnings about suicidal intentions. Being alert to these cries for help may prevent suicidal behavior.
Suicidal people are fully intent on dying.	Most suicidal people are undecided about living or dying, and they gamble with death, leaving it to others to save them. Almost no one commits suicide without letting others know how he or she is feeling. Often this cry for help is given in code. Decoding these distress signals can save lives.
Once a person is suicidal, he or she is suicidal forever.	Fortunately, people who want to kill themselves are suicidal only for a limited time. If they are saved from self-destruction, they can lead useful lives.
Improvement following a suicidal crisis means that the suicidal risk is over.	Most suicides occur within 3 months after the beginning of improvement, when the individual has the energy to put morbid thoughts and feelings into effect. Relatives and physicians should be especially vigilant during this period.
Suicide strikes more often among the rich—or, conversely, it occurs more frequently among the poor.	Suicide is neither the rich man's disease nor the poor man's curse. Suicide is democratic and is represented proportionately at all levels of society.
Suicide is inherited or runs in a family (that is, is genetically determined).	Suicide does not run in families. It is an individual matter and can be prevented.
All suicidal people are mentally ill, and suicide is always the act of a psychotic person.	Studies of hundreds of genuine suicide notes indicate that although a suicidal person is extremely unhappy, he or she is not necessarily mentally ill. The overpowering unhappiness may result from a temporary emotional upset, a long and painful illness, or a complete loss of hope.

Source: US Department of Health and Human Resources.

- Offer hope that alternatives are available but do not offer glib reassurance.
- Take action. Remove means of suicide, such as guns or stockpiled pills.
- Get help from persons or agencies specializing in crisis intervention and suicide prevention.

▶ Emotional Injury

First aid for an emotional "injury" means being supportive of people with emotional injuries, whether the injuries are from physical injury or excessive or unbearable strain on the victim's emotions.

Emotional first aid often goes hand in hand with physical first aid because a physical injury and the circumstances surrounding it may actually cause emotional injury. On the other hand, emotional injury may occur when there is no physical injury. Emotional injuries usually are not as obvious as physical injuries, but both can be severe and require "first aid."

Although most emotional reactions are temporary, lasting only minutes, hours, or, at the most, a few days, they are seriously disabling and may upset others. It is important to know that first aid can be applied to emotional as well as to physical injuries.

Typical Reactions

With few exceptions, all people experience fear in the face of an emergency. Feeling shaky, perspiring profusely, and becoming nauseated are common. Such reactions are normal and no cause for concern. Most people are able to regain their composure reasonably quickly.

Extensive training is not needed to recognize severe, abnormal reactions. To determine whether a person needs help, find out whether he or she is doing something that makes sense and is able to take care of him- or herself. For the most part, emotional first aid measures are simple and easy to understand Table 23-2 .

However, improvisation is often needed, just as it is in splinting a fracture. Whatever the situation, you will have your own emotional reactions toward the victim. These reactions are important; they can enhance or hinder your ability to help the person. Especially when you are tired or worried, you may easily become impatient with the victim who seems to be "making a mountain out of a molehill." You may feel resentful toward the victim for being a burden. Be on guard against becoming impatient, intolerant, or resentful. Victims who can see the first aider's calmness, confidence, and competence will be reassured.

On the other hand, do not be overly sympathetic or overly solicitous. Excessive sympathy for an incapacitated person can be as harmful as negative feelings. The victim needs solid help but does not need to be overwhelmed with pity.

Recognizing Aggressive, Hostile, and Violent Behavior

When you are faced with aggressive, hostile, or violent behavior, size up the situation before you do anything. It may be unsafe for you and for others. The person may be standing or sitting in a threatening position. For example, does the person have clenched fists? Is he or she holding a lethal object? Is the person yelling or verbally threatening harm to anyone? If the scene appears unsafe, do not enter. If necessary, contact law enforcement officers.

An angry, violent person is ready to fight with anyone who approaches and may be difficult to control. Remember that anger may be a response to illness or that aggressive behavior may be a person's way of coping with feelings of helplessness. Avoid responding with anger. Many angry or violent persons can be calmed by someone who is trained and who appears confident that the person will behave well. Encourage the person to speak directly about the cause of his or her anger. A statement like "I'm not sure I understand why you are angry" often brings results. Reassure the person that you are there to help.

A person who is violent and out of control presents a special problem. Notify the police if you are unable to communicate with a person who is dangerous to him- or herself or to others.

Care for Aggressive, Hostile, and Violent Behavior

Confronting a person who is experiencing a behavioral emergency can be a trying and frustrating experience. Use these guidelines if you must try to calm a person who is upset:

- Acknowledge that the person seems upset, and reiterate that you are there to help.
- Maintain a comfortable distance.

Table 23-2 Psychological First Aid for Reactions to Emergency Situations

Reaction	Symptoms	Do...	Do Not...
Normal	Trembling Muscle tension Perspiration Nausea Mild diarrhea Urinary frequency Pounding heart Rapid breathing Anxiety	Give reassurance. Provide group identification. Motivate. Talk with the person. Observe to see that the person is gaining composure, not losing it.	Show resentment. Overdo sympathy.
Individual panic (flight reaction)	Unreasoning attempt to flee Loss of judgment Uncontrolled weeping Wildly running about	Try kind firmness. Give the person something warm to eat or drink. Get help to isolate the person from others, if necessary. Be empathetic. Encourage the person to talk. Be aware of your own limitations.	Use brutal restraint. Strike the person physically. Douse the person with water. Give sedatives.
Depression (underactive reactions)	Stands or sits without moving or talking Vacant expression Lack of emotional display	Make contact gently. Secure a rapport. Get the person to tell you what happened. Be empathetic. Recognize feelings of resentment in the person and yourself. Give the person a simple, routine task to complete. Offer warm food or drink.	Tell the person to "snap out of it." Overdo sympathy. Give sedatives. Argue with the person.
Overactive	Argumentative Talks rapidly Jokes inappropriately Makes endless suggestions Jumps from one activity to another	Let the person talk about the situation. Find the person a job that requires physical effort. Offer warm food or drink. Supervision is necessary. Be aware of your own feelings.	Suggest that the person is acting abnormally. Give sedatives. Argue with the person.
Physical (conversion disorder)	Severe nausea and vomiting Cannot use some part of the body	Show interest in the person. Find a small job for the person to distract and occupy his or her thoughts. Make the person comfortable. Get medical care as soon as possible.	Tell the person that there's nothing wrong with him or her. Place blame. Ridicule the person. Ignore the disability.

Source: Modified from M51-400-603-1, Department of Nonresident Instruction, Medical Field Service School, Brooke Army Medical Center, Fort Sam Houston, Texas.

- Encourage the person to state what is troubling him or her.
- Do not make quick moves.
- Respond honestly to the person's questions.
- Do not threaten, challenge, or argue with a disturbed person.
- Tell the truth—do not lie.
- Do not "play along" with any of a disturbed person's visual or auditory disturbances.
- Involve trusted family members or friends.
- Be prepared to stay with the person for an extended period of time.

- Never leave the person alone.
- Avoid unnecessary physical contact.
- Maintain eye contact.

▶ Sexual Assault and Rape

The definitions of rape and sexual assault vary widely. *Rape* is generally defined as forcible sexual intercourse without the consent of one participant. Categories of rape include the following:

- *Acquaintance rape,* which involves people who knew each other before the rape; includes relatives, neighbors, or friends.
- *Date rape,* which takes place within a relationship but without the consent of one person and may involve harm or the threat of harm by the other person.
- *Marital rape,* which occurs when the victim and the offender are married to each other.
- *Stranger rape,* which occurs when the victim and the offender have no relation to each other.

The victim may hesitate to report a rape for various reasons, such as shame, guilt, fear of retaliation, or reluctance to deal with law enforcement officials or the judicial system. The victim may even begin to doubt whether a "real" rape occurred. Rape is a traumatic crisis that disrupts the physical, psychological, social, and sexual aspects of the victim's life. The most common physical injuries are bruises, black eyes, and cuts.

As a first aider, you must be tactful and sensitive with the victim. The victim may find it extremely difficult to discuss what happened and may feel fear or hostility toward a first aider of the opposite sex. Every effort should be made to understand the victim's feelings and to respond with kindness and reassurance. The emotional trauma of rape is usually more prolonged and severe than the physical trauma. The attitude shown toward the victim during the initial care can have a substantial influence—for good or ill—on future psychological and physical recovery. Convince the victim to seek counseling through community resources such as a rape crisis center and to report the crime to the police. Ask the victim not to change clothes or to bathe because doing so can alter legal evidence. For the same reason, suggest that the victim not urinate, douche, defecate, or wash before being examined by a physician. Care for any injuries incurred during the attack. For more information, see Chapter 22, *Childbirth and Gynecologic Emergencies.*

▶ Child Abuse and Neglect

Because child abuse and neglect usually occur in the privacy of the home, no one knows exactly how many children are affected. More than 2.5 million cases of child abuse and neglect cases are reported each year. Of these, 35% involve physical abuse, 15% involve sexual abuse, and 50% involve neglect. Child abuse and neglect can cause permanent damage to a child's physical, emotional, and mental development. The physical effects can include damage to the brain, vital organs, eyes, ears, arms, and legs, which, in turn, can result in mental retardation, blindness, deafness, or loss of a limb. At its most serious, abuse or neglect can result in a child's death.

Child abuse and neglect are usually divided into four major categories: physical abuse, neglect, sexual abuse, and emotional maltreatment. Each has recognizable characteristics, and all may be encountered by a first aider.

The National Center on Child Abuse and Neglect has set forth physical and behavioral indicators of child abuse and neglect. The list is not intended to be exhaustive; many more indicators exist than can be included. The presence of a single indicator does not necessarily prove that child abuse or neglect has occurred Table 23-3.

However, the repeated occurrence of an indicator, the presence of several indicators in combination, or the appearance of serious injury should alert the first aider to the possibility of child abuse Figure 23-1.

Recognizing Child Abuse and Neglect

It is not always easy to recognize when a child has been abused. Children who have been mistreated are often afraid to tell anyone because they think they will be blamed or that no one will believe them. Other parents or teachers also tend to overlook symptoms because they do not want to face the truth. The longer a child continues to be abused or is left to deal with the situation on his or her own, the less likely he or she is to make a full recovery.

The best way to check for signs of abuse is to be alert to any unexplainable changes in a child's body or behavior.

- Physical abuse: any injury (bruise, burn, fracture, abdominal or head injury) that cannot be explained.
- Sexual abuse:

Table 23-3 Physical and Behavioral Indicators of Child Abuse and Neglect

Type of Child Abuse or Neglect	Physical Indicators	Behavioral Indicators
Physical Abuse	Unexplained bruises and welts on face, lips, mouth, torso, back, buttocks, and/or thighs in various stages of healing Clustered injuries on several different surface areas; formed by regular patterns reflecting the shape of the articles used to inflict the injury (electric cord, belt buckle) Regularly appearing injuries after an absence, weekend, or vacation, especially about the trunk and buttocks Old bruises in addition to fresh ones Unexplained burns (such as those from a cigar or cigarette) especially on soles, palms, back, or buttocks Immersion burns (socklike, glovelike, doughnut shaped on buttocks or genitalia) Pattern burns as from an electric burner or iron, for example Rope burns on arms, legs, neck, or torso Unexplained fractures (particularly if multiple) to skull, nose, and/or facial structures in various stages of healing Multiple or spiral fractures Unexplained lacerations or abrasions to mouth, lips, gums, eyes, and/or external genitalia	Wary of adult contacts Apprehensive when other children cry Behavioral extremes: aggressiveness or withdrawal Frightened of parents Afraid to go home Reports injury by parents Acts apathetic and does not cry despite injuries Has been seen by emergency personnel for related complaints Was injured several days before medical attention was sought
Physical Neglect	Consistent hunger, poor hygiene, inappropriate dress Consistent lack of supervision, especially in dangerous activities or for extended periods of time Unattended physical problems or medical needs Abandonment	Begs, steals food Extended stays at school (early arrival and late departure) Constant fatigue, listlessness, or falling asleep in class Alcohol or drug abuse Delinquency (for example, thefts) States there is no caretaker
Sexual Abuse	Difficulty walking or sitting Torn, stained, or bloody underclothing Pain or itching in genital area Bruises or bleeding in external genitalia or vaginal or anal areas Sexually transmitted disease, especially in preteens Pregnancy	Unwillingness to change for gym or participate in physical education class Withdrawal, fantasizing, or infantile behavior Bizarre, sophisticated, or unusual sexual behavior or knowledge Poor peer relationships Delinquency or truancy Reports sexual assault by caretaker
Emotional Maltreatment	Speech disorders Lags in physical development Failure to thrive	Habit disorders (for example, sucking, biting, rocking) Conduct disorders (for example, antisocial, destructive) Neurotic traits (sleep disorders, inhibition of play) Psychoneurotic reactions (hysteria, obsession, compulsion, phobias, hypochondria) Behavior extremes: compliant, passive-aggressive, demanding Overly adaptive behavior: inappropriately adult or inappropriately infantile Developmental lags (mental, emotional) Attempted suicide

Source: National Center on Child Abuse and Neglect.

Figure 23-1A

Figure 23-1B

Figure 23-1C

A. The face is a common target for physical abuse. **B.** Stocking-glove burns of the hands and feet are almost always inflicted injuries. **C.** Rope or cord bruises are a commonly inflicted injury.

- Fearful behavior (nightmares, depression, unusual fears, attempts to run away)
- Abdominal pain, bedwetting, urinary tract infection, genital pain or bleeding, sexually transmitted disease
- Extreme sexual behavior that seems inappropriate for the child's age
- Emotional abuse:
  - Sudden change in self-confidence
  - Headaches or stomachaches with no medical cause
  - Abnormal fears, increased nightmares
  - Attempts to run away
- Emotional neglect:
  - Failure to gain weight (especially in infants)
  - Desperately affectionate behavior
  - Large appetite and stealing of food

Care for Child Abuse and Neglect

The care of the neglected infant or child is extremely important.

- Give appropriate first aid for injuries.
- Do not accuse parents or caregivers, especially at the scene.
- Report any suspected abuse to the local welfare and social service agency responsible for investigating the problem. Report what you saw and heard, not what you think.

▶ Domestic Violence

Domestic violence, also known as *partner abuse, spouse abuse,* or *battering,* occurs when one person inflicts injury—either emotional or physical—upon another person with whom they had or have a relationship.

It occurs between spouses and partners, parents and children, children and grandparents, and brothers and sisters. Domestic violence may be the single most common source of serious injury to women.

Recognizing Domestic Violence

Physical domestic violence includes slapping, punching, kicking, and choking. Women also have been shot, stabbed, and bludgeoned. Injuries tend to be on the head, neck, chest, breast, abdomen, and perineum rather than the extremities. The injuries listed here should raise suspicion about potential domestic violence:

- Bruises or injuries on the head, neck, or chest
- Type or extent of an injury that is inconsistent with the victim's explanation
- Substantial delay between when the injury occurred and when the victim sought help
- Injuries during pregnancy
- Evidence of alcohol or drug abuse
- Needs medical care as a result of a suicide attempt or rape

FYI

Are You Being Abused?

Just one "yes" answer means you're involved in an abusive relationship. If so, you're not alone and you have choices. No one deserves to be abused.

- Threatens to hurt you or your children
- Says it is your fault if he or she hits you; then promises it will not happen again (but it does)
- Puts you down in public or keeps you from contacting family or friends
- Throws you down, pushes, hits, chokes, kicks, or slaps you
- Forces you to have sex when you do not want to

Source: American College of Obstetricians and Gynecologists, www.acog.org.

Care for Domestic Violence

- Talking with the suspected abuser about the problem is not likely to help.
- If you are not aware of immediate danger, but you suspect abuse, check with welfare and social service agencies. Most cities and counties, according to state law, will investigate and protect vulnerable adults. The problem cannot be remedied until it is reported.

- Call the police if a person is in imminent danger.
- First aid includes calling 9-1-1 and treating any injuries.

▶ Elder Abuse

Elder abuse ranges from passive neglect to active assault and includes emotional abuse. Some physically abused elderly people report having had something thrown at them; some are pushed, grabbed, or shoved; others are slapped, bitten, or kicked. Elder abuse occurs most often in women older than 75 years. Signs of abuse may be quite obvious or subtle. Burns are a common form of elder abuse.

Recognizing Elder Abuse

When concerned about an older adult who might be abused, look for these signs:

- Physical injury: Examples of questionable injuries include bruises, cuts, burn or rope marks, and broken bones that cannot be explained. Other signs of potential problems include sudden changes in behavior, comments about being battered, or the refusal of the caregiver to allow you to visit the older person alone.
- Lack of physical care: Examples include dehydration, malnourishment, weight loss, and poor hygiene. Bed sores, soiled bedding, unmet medical needs, and comments about being mistreated also may indicate a problem. Lack of physical care can happen to older adults living in their homes, as well as those in institutional care, such as a long-term care facility.
- Unusual behaviors: Examples include agitation, withdrawal, fear or anxiety, apathy, or reports of being treated improperly.

Care for Elder Abuse

- Talking with the suspected abuser about the problem is not likely to help.
- If you are not aware of immediate danger, but you suspect abuse, check with welfare and social service agencies. Most cities and counties, according to state law, will investigate

and protect vulnerable adults. The problem cannot be remedied until it is reported.

- If you suspect elder abuse in an institutional setting, such as a nursing home, report your concerns to your state long-term care ombudsman. Each state has a long-term care ombudsman to investigate and address nursing home complaints.
- Call the police if a person is in imminent danger.
- First aid includes calling 9-1-1 when needed and treating any injuries.

prep kit

▶ Ready for Review

- Behavior that leads to violence or other inappropriate activities is known as a behavioral emergency.
- Depression is one of the most common and treatable of all mental illness.
- Suicide in the United States is increasingly a problem of adolescents, college-age students, and older people.
- First aid for an emotional injury means being supportive of people with emotional injuries, whether the injuries are a result of physical injury or excessive or unbearable strain on the victim's emotions.
- Because child abuse and neglect usually occur in the privacy of the home, no one knows exactly how many children are affected.
- Domestic violence may be the single most common source of serious injury to women.
- The types of physical abuse of elders vary from passive neglect to active assault.

▶ Vital Vocabulary

<u>behavioral emergency</u> Situations in which a person exhibits abnormal behavior that is unacceptable or cannot be tolerated by the victims themselves, or by family, friends, or the community.

▶ Assessment in Action

Your good friend has been married for about 3 years. He is normally a quiet, reserved person who cares deeply for others. Lately, you have seen him change; he has been argumentative, jokes inappropriately, and appears to have a hard time concentrating. He no longer engages in several of his hobbies and does little else when not at work. You then find out that he separated from his wife about 2 weeks ago.

Directions: Circle Yes if you agree with the statement; circle No if you disagree.

Yes No **1.** Your friend is exhibiting an overactive reaction to his situation.

Yes No **2.** You should avoid being too argumentative with your friend.

Yes No **3.** You should not give sedatives to calm him down.

Yes No **4.** Supervision and perhaps even some type of professional therapy may be helpful for your friend.

Yes No **5.** Letting him talk to you about his situation will make things worse.

▶ Check Your Knowledge

Directions: Circle Yes if you agree with the statement; circle No if you disagree.

Yes   No   **1.** Abnormal behavior may be due to a psychological condition or a physical condition.

Yes   No   **2.** Low blood glucose in a person with diabetes can affect behavior.

Yes   No   **3.** Depression cannot be treated.

Yes   No   **4.** The rate of suicide for men is higher than the rate for women.

Yes   No   **5.** Most people who talk about suicide are not serious.

Yes   No   **6.** The only way for you to react to an aggressive person is with anger.

Yes   No   **7.** A failure to gain weight may be a sign of emotional neglect in an infant.

Yes   No   **8.** Women are rarely subjected to domestic violence.

Yes   No   **9.** Burns are a common form of elder abuse.

Yes   No   **10.** Feeling shaky during an emergency is not normal.

24

Wilderness First Aid

chapter
at a glance

Wilderness First Aid

At some time, anyone living, working, traveling, or recreating in the wilderness will probably encounter dangers unfamiliar to most people. Regardless of precautions, injuries and illnesses happen.

Wilderness, as defined by the Wilderness Medical Society (WMS), is a remote geographic location more than 1 hour from definitive medical care. According to that definition, wilderness could describe a variety of situations, including the following:

- Recreation (for example, fishing, camping, hiking, hunting)
- Occupations in remote areas (such as farming, forestry, fishing)
- Urban areas with overwhelmed EMS after a natural or man-made disaster
- Residences in remote communities (such as farms, ranches, vacation homes)
- Developing countries

The millions of people in these wildernesses should be as medically prepared as possible to manage a problem for others and for themselves. First aid with a wilderness focus seems indispensable in the following situations:

- Occurrence of injuries and illnesses in the outdoors where adverse environmental conditions such as heat, cold, altitude, rain, or snow may be a major concern

- Delay of definitive medical care for hours or days because of location, bad weather, lack of transportation, or lack of communication
- Occurrence of injuries and illnesses not commonly seen in urban or suburban areas (for example, altitude illness, frostbite, wild animal attacks)
- The need for advanced medical care (for example, reduction of some dislocations, wound cleansing)
- Limited first aid supplies and equipment
- Need to make difficult decisions (CPR, evacuation) in a remote setting

Most first aid books and training courses describe situations in which the EMS response is expected within 10 to 20 minutes. In these cases, the first aider usually helps for only a few minutes before an ambulance arrives. When the victim is transported, the first aider's job is finished.

Wilderness first aid is similar to that needed in urban situations, except that extra or extended skills are needed. Consideration must be given to time, distance, and availability of medical care. A first aider in the wilderness may have to remain many hours or days with a sick or injured person.

▶ Cardiac Arrest

Because heart activity must be restored within a short time (which requires defibrillation and medications) for a cardiac arrest victim to survive, CPR has limited use in a wilderness or remote setting, especially if severe trauma such as massive head or chest injury, severe blood loss, or a severed spinal cord accompanies the cardiac arrest. In addition, CPR is difficult to continue during a wilderness evacuation.

The WMS recommends *stopping* CPR if:
- The victim revives.
- The rescuers are exhausted.
- The rescuers are in danger.
- The victim is turned over to higher level trained personnel.
- The victim does not respond to prolonged (about 30 minutes) resuscitation efforts.

The State of Alaska Cold Injuries Guidelines, the WMS, and the NAEMSP say that CPR should *not be started* if:
- The victim has been submerged in cold water for more than 1 hour.
- The victim has a core temperature of less than 50° F.

- The victim has obvious signs of death or fatal injuries (eg, rigor mortis, decapitation, decomposition).
- The victim is frozen (eg, ice formation in the airway).
- The victim has a chest wall that is so stiff that compressions are impossible.
- Rescuers are exhausted or in danger.
- Definitive care is not available within 3 hours.

CPR for Hypothermia Victims

The victim with severe hypothermia must be handled very gently. The cold heart is very prone to spontaneous ventricular fibrillation due to any movement. Even cautious movement of the victim may induce ventricular fibrillation.

The 2010 Guidelines for Cardiac Arrest in Special Situations say that if the victim is unresponsive and not breathing, you should begin CPR. Do not wait to check the victim's temperature, and do not wait until the victim is rewarmed, to start CPR. Prevent further heat loss by removing the victim's wet clothes; insulate and shield the victim from wind and additional cold exposure. Avoid rough handling and seek medical care as soon as possible. Continue CPR until the victim is evaluated by health care providers.

The temperature at which defibrillation should first be attempted in a severely hypothermic victim and the number of defibrillation attempts that should be made have not been established.

CPR for Avalanche Victims

Avalanche-related deaths are on the rise in North America due to winter recreational activities (eg, backcountry skiing and snowboarding, helicopter and snowcat skiing, snowmobiling, out-of-bounds skiing, ice climbing, mountaineering, and snowshoeing). The most common causes of avalanche-related death are suffocation (hypoxia), injury, hypothermia, or a combination of these three. If the victim is unresponsive and is not breathing, begin CPR. Use an automated external defibrillator (AED) as soon as it becomes available.

CPR for Drowning

The 2010 AHA Guidelines for CPR and emergency cardiovascular care (ECC) have CPR beginning with chest compressions in a C-A-B sequence. The guidelines make an exception for drowning, however, because victims with only respiratory arrest usually respond after a few rescue breaths.

The first and most important care for a drowning victim is immediate rescue breaths. Rescue breathing increases the victim's chance of survival. Rescue breathing can be started once the victim is in shallow water or out of the water. There is no need to attempt to clear the airway of water because only a small amount of water is aspirated by most drowning victims and is absorbed by the body. Do not try to remove water by performing abdominal thrusts.

As soon as possible, open the airway and check for breathing. If there is no breathing, give two rescue breaths that make the chest rise (if this was not done previously in the water). After the two breaths, immediately begin cycles of 30 chest compressions and two rescue breaths. An AED should be used as soon as it becomes available.

If vomiting occurs during CPR, turn the victim to the side and remove the vomitus using a finger or a cloth. If a spinal injury is suspected, the victim should be turned as a unit with no twisting. A suggestion is to keep the victim's nose and navel pointed in the same direction as they are turned.

CPR for Lightning-Strike Victims

The National Weather Service estimates an average of 70 deaths occur from lightning strikes in the United States each year. The main cause of death in these victims is cardiac arrest. When multiple victims are struck at the same time by lightning, rescuers should give the highest priority to victims who are unresponsive and not breathing by beginning CPR. An AED should be used as soon as it becomes available.

▶ Dislocations

In a wilderness situation, *reducing* (a technical term that means aligning) some dislocated joints is recommended. The WMS gives the following reasons for reducing a joint dislocation quickly after it happens:

- Reduction is easier immediately after the injury, before swelling develops.
- It is easier to transport a victim after reduction.
- Reduction dramatically relieves pain.
- The joint can be stabilized and better protected.

- Reduction lessens the possibility of jeopardizing circulation in the extremity. (If the blood supply is cut off, gangrene could develop, which could result in amputation.)
- Several simple dislocations can be reduced using simple and safe techniques.

A dislocation is considered simple if it involves the anterior (front) part of the shoulder, a finger, or the patella (the kneecap, not the knee itself). Do not attempt to reduce a dislocated elbow or hip. Elbow and hip dislocations resemble fractures; reduction techniques for those joints are painful and can cause further injury.

Shoulder Dislocation

Anterior (frontal) shoulder joint dislocations account for more than 90% of shoulder dislocations **Figure 24-1**.

Recognizing a Shoulder Dislocation

- The victim is in extreme pain.
- Because the problem often recurs, the victim can identify the dislocation if it has happened before.
- The upper arm is held away from the body in various positions and cannot be brought next to the body into a sling-type position.

Figure 24-1

The shoulder almost always dislocates anteriorly. Note the absence of the normal rounded appearance of the shoulder.

- The victim is unable to touch the uninjured shoulder with the hand of the injured extremity.
- Compare the injured shoulder with the uninjured one. The shoulder joint will appear squared off or flattened and a prominence may be seen or felt in the front of the shoulder.

Care for a Shoulder Dislocation

There are two methods for reducing a shoulder dislocation. With either method, stop if pain increases or resistance is met. Do not try pulling on the victim's arm with your foot in the victim's armpit. Check the circulation, sensation, and movement of the hand before and after reducing.

Traction and External Rotation

Traction and external rotation is the easiest and most effective method for reducing an anterior shoulder dislocation **Figure 24-2**.

1. Gently but steadily pull the arm out to the side while another rescuer provides countertraction against the chest wall, just below the armpit, using straps, a sleeping bag, clothing, or a flotation vest.

2. Tell the victim to relax. Massage may help.
3. As you pull, gently and steadily rotate the arm half to two-thirds of the way up to a baseball-throwing position (take 5 to 15 minutes). Keep the arm in that position; the muscles will fatigue within 15 minutes, allowing the joint to slip back into place.
4. After successful reduction, stabilize the arm with a sling and swathe (binder).

If there is only one rescuer, countertraction can be applied by the rescuer's padded or bare feet against the victim's chest (not armpits).

Simple Hanging Traction

Using the simple hanging traction method:

1. Lay the victim face down on a surface high enough so the injured arm can hang over the side. Place some cushioning (a folded towel or clothing) under the armpit, between the arm and the surface **Figure 24-3**.
2. Attach a 5- to 10-lb weight to the victim's lower arm, between the elbow and the wrist. Cushion and strap the weight, being careful not to impede circulation. Keep the victim's palm facing inward.

Figure 24-2

Applying traction (left) and external rotation (right) to anterior shoulder dislocation.

Figure 24-3

Simple hanging traction to reduce anterior shoulder dislocation.

Figure 24-4

Dislocation of the finger joint. Do not be tempted to try to "pop" the joint back into place.

3. It may take up to 60 minutes to stretch and tire the muscles, allowing the joint to pop back in.
4. After successful reduction, stabilize the arm with a sling and swathe.

If available, place a small pillow, folded towels, or some type of pad under the person's armpit. Secure a sling and swathe (binder) using the method shown in Chapter 16, *Splinting Extremities*.

Finger Dislocation

The fingers are injured easily, and even a minor injury may cause a dislocation **Figure 24-4**.

Recognizing a Finger Dislocation

- Deformity and inability to use or bend the finger
- Pain and swelling
- An abnormal position of the two adjoining bones; looks like a lump at the joint

Care for a Finger Dislocation

To reduce a finger dislocation, use one of two methods. Method 1 **Figure 24-5**:

Figure 24-5

Reducing a finger dislocation.

1. Hold the end of the finger with one hand and the rest of the finger in the other.
2. Gently hyperextend the dislocated joint (bend it backwards).
3. Pull gentle traction.
4. Push the dislocated bone into place.
5. Unbend the finger.
6. Buddy-tape it to the next finger.
7. Splint the finger in the position of function (fingers and hand in a cupping shape, as though holding a baseball).

Method 2:

1. Hold the end of the finger with one hand and the rest of the finger in the other.
2. Pull the end of the finger first in the direction it is pointing, then, while maintaining

traction, gently swing it back into the normal anatomic position.

3. Regardless of whether the reduction is successful, stabilize the joint in the position of function (fingers and hand in a cupping shape, as though holding a baseball).

Often, persons with this injury can reduce the finger dislocation themselves. In a remote location, you should try to reduce a finger dislocation only once. Stabilize and protect the finger by the *buddy-taping method*—using adhesive tape to secure the injured finger to an adjacent uninjured finger. Do not attempt to reduce a dislocation at the base of the index finger or at the base of the thumb—those areas may require surgery for reduction.

Kneecap Dislocation

For most dislocated kneecaps, you should only apply an ice pack and use a splint to stabilize the leg in place as you found it. For remote locations, however, always consider reducing a dislocated kneecap by using the following method. All dislocations, whether successfully reduced in the field or not, should be seen by a physician.

Recognizing a Kneecap Dislocation

Some victims have recurrent dislocations of the patella and can tell you what is wrong.

- The patella has moved to the outside of the knee joint (large bulge under the skin) with the leg bent **Figure 24-6**.
- The victim is in pain.
- Compare the injured portion with the patella on the other leg.

Care for a Kneecap Dislocation

1. Slowly straighten the knee as you gently push the kneecap back into its normal position. Straightening alone may replace the kneecap.
2. Stabilize the leg straight. The victim usually can walk on the injured leg.
3. With the knee extended (straight) and stabilized, the victim may be able to walk well enough for self-evacuation. Because of the heavy physical demands and usually higher altitudes in the backcountry, carrying a

Figure 24-6

A dislocated patella typically will appear with the patella displaced lateral to the knee and with the knee moderately flexed.

victim can take 8 to 16 rescuers rotating the task. In the wilderness, a ski pole or a tree branch makes a good walking aid. Helicopter evacuation usually is not justified for a kneecap dislocation.

▶ Spinal Injury

The necessity of stabilizing the spine after trauma is well known. An unconscious victim with a cervical spinal injury who is moved without stabilization may become quadriplegic or die. In urban settings, spine stabilization is almost always automatically applied for survivors of violent accidents, such as motor vehicle crashes or falls from a height.

In the wilderness, full-spine stabilization may not always be necessary—such a procedure can be difficult, impractical, impossible, or even dangerous during prolonged evacuation in severe environments. For example, an injured climber far above the timberline could wait for hours or days, depending on the distance someone has to go for help. The injured climber would have to wait in a hostile environment and risk death from avalanche, rockfall, or hypothermia. If the victim were cleared of a spinal injury, he or she could self-evacuate.

Spinal fractures can be difficult to determine, even by physicians reading radiographs. One study found that all of the spinal fracture cases reviewed had at least one of the following findings: midline neck tenderness, altered mental status, evidence of intoxication, or a separate painful injury away from the neck.

Recognizing a Possible Spinal Injury

Assessing a spinal injury can be done through a process of elimination. First, ask these questions:

- Is the victim alert and oriented? Has the victim been drinking alcohol or using drugs?
- Does the victim have any major painful injury? Distracting injuries include fractures, deep lacerations, severe contusions, and large burns.
- Is the victim reporting neck pain?
- Does the victim have tingling, numbness, or weakness in the extremities?

Next, perform these physical exams:

- Check for neck tenderness by pressing firmly on the bony part of the spine. This is a safe procedure, and there is little chance of injuring the spinal cord by feeling the bony spinal column as long as movement of the spine is prevented.
- Determine whether the victim has sensation in the hands and feet and whether he or she can move the fingers and toes.

Here is a simple protocol for clearing a spinal injury in the wilderness: The victim does not need to be stabilized in one position if he or she is completely alert, not intoxicated, has no distracting injuries, does not report neck pain, can feel normal touch, and can move the fingers and toes.

Follow these guidelines to assess a suspected spinal injury:

- The victim is responsive:
  - Determine whether the mechanism of injury was a violent impact force capable of damaging the bony spinal column. Examples include a fall from a height, a gunshot wound near the spine, and a high-velocity vehicle crash.
  - Ask questions: Does your neck or back hurt? What happened? Can you move your hands and feet? Can you feel me touching your fingers and toes?
  - Look and feel for DOTS (deformity, open wounds, tenderness, swelling) along the bony spinal column.
  - Assess the equality of strength of the extremities: Have the victim grip your hands; have the victim push his or her feet against your hand.
- The victim is unresponsive:
  - Determine the mechanism of injury.
  - Look for deformity, open wounds, and swelling along the spinal bones.
  - Feel for deformity and swelling along the spinal bones.
  - Obtain information from others at the scene to determine information relevant to mechanism of injury and victim's mental status before your arrival.

Care for a Spinal Injury

Providing effective spine stabilization in the wilderness often requires you to improvise methods. Initially, you can use your hands or knees to hold the victim's head in place. While kneeling at the victim's head, use your hands or knees to stabilize the victim's neck in relation to the long axis of the spine.

Improvised cervical collars such as a blanket or a SAM splint alone are inadequate. Improvise supports by placing dirt or sand in garbage bags, stuffing sacks, or rolling up extra articles of clothing. Place them on both sides of the victim's head and secure them in place.

Leave the victim on the ground and avoid moving him or her. If necessary to prevent heat loss, log roll the victim, keeping the spine straight, and place insulating materials underneath. For spinal injury procedures when EMS response time is less than 1 hour, see Chapter 12, *Head and Spinal Injuries*.

▶ Splinting Femur Fractures

Victims with a femur fracture can easily lose 2 quarts of blood in the thigh and develop massive swelling. Because EMS personnel have the training, experience, and equipment, it is best to let them apply traction splints, if possible. However, first aiders can use the

Q&A

Do improvised traction splints work?

Although the advantages of stabilizing a broken femur by applying a traction splint are cited in various manuals, there are dissenting opinions about the effectiveness of improvised traction splints. For example, the Outward Bound organization says, "Improvised traction splints for field use employing ski poles, canoe paddles, and other pieces of equipment are usually more architecturally interesting than medically useful. The simplest, safest, and most universal splint is firm immobilization on a long board or litter without traction." The WMS suggests stabilizing the fractured extremity to the uninjured leg with adequate padding and placing padding behind the knee to create a slight bend, which is more comfortable than being straight.

FYI

Avalanche Rescue

If you survive an avalanche, follow these steps to find other victims:

1. With a piece of equipment, clothing, or tree branch, mark the spot where a victim was last seen.
2. Search the area below the last-seen point for any clues of the victim. Make probes into likely burial spots with a ski, ski pole, or tree limb.
3. If beacons were being used, all survivors must immediately switch their units to the receive mode and listen for a beeping sound from buried beacons.
4. If a second avalanche is possible, place one person in a safe location to shout a warning so rescuers can flee to safety.
5. Send a person to notify the ski patrol immediately if you are near a ski area and there are several rescuers. If you are the only rescuer, do a fast surface search for clues before leaving to notify the ski patrol. In remote backcountry, all survivors should remain and search until they cannot or should not continue.

Rescue transceivers or beacons are an efficient way of locating victims. Organized probe lines have found more victims than any other method, but because of the time involved, most of the victims were dead. Trained search dogs can locate buried victims quickly, but they often are brought to the scene only after long periods of burial. One trained dog can search more effectively than 30 searchers.

methods in Chapter 16, *Splinting Extremities,* to stabilize a femur fracture.

▶ Avalanche Burial

Avalanches are falling masses of snow that may also contain rocks, soil, or ice. Since the early 1970s, the number of deaths caused by avalanches has increased rapidly as a result of the tremendous growth in backcountry winter mountain travel (eg, skiing, mountaineering, snowmobiling). Recent statistics show that the average annual number of deaths is about 20 per year in the United States and 10 in Canada.

Snow sets up solid after an avalanche. It is almost impossible for victims to dig themselves out, even if they are buried under less than a foot of snow. The pressure of several feet of snow sometimes is so great that victims are unable to expand their chests to breathe.

Most avalanche victims die of suffocation; therefore, in the absence of fatal injuries, speed of extrication from the avalanche and existence of an air pocket are the main factors that determine survival of a buried victim. There are no documented reports of anyone surviving a burial of 7 feet or more.

Recognizing an Avalanche Victim

Avalanches kill and injure in two ways. The first is from the serious injury the victim acquires while tumbling down an avalanche path. Trees, rocks, cliffs, and the wrenching action of snow are hazards. About one third of all deaths are related to trauma, especially trauma to the head and neck. The second way is snow burial, which causes suffocation in the other two thirds of avalanche deaths. Inhaled snow clogs the mouth and nose, and victims can suffocate quickly if they are buried with the airway already blocked.

Care for an Avalanche Victim

A completely buried victim has a poor chance of survival. During the first 15 minutes, more people are found alive than dead. Between 16 and 30 minutes after an avalanche, an equal number are found dead and alive (50% chance of survival). After 30 minutes, more are found dead than alive.

After you have first checked for further avalanche danger and then found a victim, follow these steps:

1. Quickly free the victim's head, chest, and stomach.
2. Send for help.
3. Clear the victim's airway and check breathing.
4. If not breathing, begin CPR.
5. Check for severe bleeding.
6. Examine for and stabilize a spinal injury.
7. Treat for hypothermia.

▶ Altitude Illness

If you live in or visit mountainous regions, you need to know about altitude illness. Altitude illness is not simply an exotic affliction of mountaineers but is a common environmental risk to which millions of people are exposed, often without adequate knowledge.

Altitude illnesses actually are a spectrum of a single problem, __hypoxia__. *Hypoxia* occurs when the body's tissues do not have enough oxygen. Altitude illnesses include *acute mountain sickness (AMS), high-altitude pulmonary edema (HAPE), and high-altitude cerebral edema (HACE)* `Table 24-1`.

The least serious altitude illness is acute mountain sickness and affects about one in four people from lower elevations who visit areas 6,000 to 12,000 feet above sea level. Such elevations are common at ski resorts and on mountain hiking trails.

The actual incidence of altitude illness varies with rate of ascent and altitude attained. About 67% of climbers on Mt Rainier in Washington have at least mild AMS because of rapid ascent to a moderately high altitude. The incidence of AMS in a study of Colorado skiers at lower altitudes (usually 1 day's ascent from Denver or lower) was only 15% to 40%.

Although anyone can get altitude illness, certain factors increase the risk. Under similar conditions, different people sometimes respond quite differently to altitude. For most people, at least four factors determine whether they will be sick or well at a higher altitude: (1) the speed of ascent (the slower the climb, the fewer the symptoms); (2) the altitude reached (the higher one goes, the more likely one will have problems); (3) health at the time (malnutrition, dehydration, fatigue, and any of several illnesses increase the risk); and (4) individual differences and genetic influences.

Table 24-1 Characteristics of Altitude Illnesses

	AMS	HAPE	HACE
Elevation	Above 8,000 ft	Usually above 10,000 ft	Above 12,000 ft
Time after ascent	1-2 days	3-4 days, possibly later	4-7 days, possibly later
Cause and symptoms	Symptoms of hypoxia: headache, sleep disturbance, fatigue, shortness of breath, dizziness, loss of appetite, vomiting	Symptoms of fluid in the lungs: shortness of breath, dry cough, mild chest pain, weakness, insomnia, rapid pulse, cyanosis, *rales* (crackles), or gurgling sounds	Symptoms of increased fluid and pressure on brain: severe headache (unrelieved), vomiting, Cheyne-Stokes breathing (irregular breathing pattern that includes periods of apnea [no breathing]), ataxia (irregular gait or lack of coordination), unconsciousness
First aid	Stop ascending or return to a lower altitude. Drink fluids. Rest. Take aspirin or ibuprofen. Take acetazolamide (see information on page 401).	Descend at least 2,000 ft. Seek medical attention *immediately.*	Descend 4,000 ft. Seek medical attention *immediately.*

HAPE and HACE occur when reduced oxygen causes capillary leakage and swelling of body tissues. Both conditions are life threatening.

Altitude illness occurs because oxygen levels decrease as elevation increases, and it takes a few days to adapt to the "thinner" air. At 11,500 feet, the amount of oxygen in the air is about 65% the amount at sea level, so the body struggles to maintain normal levels of oxygen. As the person breathes more deeply he or she "blows off" more carbon dioxide than normal, creating a more alkaline (less acidic) condition in the body, which in turn causes altitude illnesses.

Recognizing Altitude Illness

Altitude illness typically strikes during the first 12 hours, and a headache is the most common symptom. Other symptoms include loss of appetite, nausea, insomnia, fatigue, and shortness of breath with exertion. Three fourths of all people who travel from sea level to above 8,000 feet have at least one symptom (usually a headache), and the rest have two or more symptoms. Many people mistake the symptoms for a cold, the flu, or a hangover and wonder why it had to happen on their long-awaited mountain vacation.

Care for Altitude Illness

It is important to recognize the symptoms of altitude illness and take steps to treat it. In a small number of people, acute altitude illness can progress to HAPE, in which fluid builds up in the lungs, or HACE, in which fluid collects in the brain. Although they are uncommon, both conditions can be fatal in less than 12 hours. Seek medical help if any of the following, more serious symptoms appear: persistent cough, shortness of breath while resting, noisy breathing, loss of balance, confusion, or vomiting.

Most people who have altitude illness get better with rest as the body acclimatizes. However, anyone who has recently ascended to above 6,000 feet, is feeling ill, and whose condition does not improve in 1 to 2 days should see a physician. If that is not possible, the victim should descend 2,000 to 3,000 feet, rest, and drink plenty of fluids. Aspirin or a similar pain reliever can be taken for a mild headache. If rest and over-the-counter (OTC) medications do not provide relief, a physician should be consulted and might administer oxygen or prescribe medication.

FYI

Preventing Altitude Illness

You can take several measures to lower your risk of getting altitude sickness. Start slowly and avoid overexerting yourself. If possible, gain altitude slowly to allow your body to adjust. By going easy, you allow your body to acclimatize; that is, adjust to different conditions. Simply put, your body becomes more efficient at using oxygen. Unfortunately, the effects of acclimatization do not last after you return to your normal altitude. You must repeat the process whenever you return to higher elevations.

If you cannot or will not take the time, protective medications are available by prescription. Acetazolamide (Diamox) has been effectively used to prevent AMS for more than 30 years. Acetazolamide also seems to prevent HAPE and HACE, although that is almost impossible to prove because HAPE and HACE are rare.

Side effects of acetazolamide include increased urination and tingling or numbness in the fingers and toes. If you are allergic to sulfa drugs, you may be allergic to acetazolamide. Also, you should wear a sunscreen with a sun protection factor (also called SPF) of at least 15 while taking the drug, since it may increase the risk of sunburn.

Acetazolamide is effective for most lowlanders going to moderate altitudes and perhaps for high-altitude residents returning after a short stay at low altitude. It has been called an *artificial acclimatizer*. Just how much acetazolamide to take and when to take it are debated. Follow the prescribed dosage; for adults it is 125 mg twice a day starting as early as 2 days prior to ascent.

Because dehydration can be a factor at high altitudes, drink plenty of fluids such as water and juice. Mountain air is drier than air at lower elevations. You are drinking enough fluid when your urine is clear. Tea, coffee, and alcohol cause more frequent urination and may lead to dehydration. Eat lightly for a few days.

Avoid taking sleeping pills because they tend to cause shallow breathing while you sleep, which can make it difficult for your body to get enough oxygen. Likewise, do not smoke because it increases carbon monoxide levels in the blood, which diminishes the body's ability to use oxygen.

The condition of people with acute altitude illness usually improves, even at higher elevations, after a few days of rest, and they can continue with their plans. As long as the condition does not worsen and the victim can be carefully watched, a day or two of rest at a lower altitude may be sufficient.

All forms of altitude illness will improve when the victim simply descends a few thousand feet. If HACE or HAPE is suspected, early descent is wise, because these conditions are serious. The next best step after descent is to breathe additional oxygen so that the inspired oxygen pressure equals that at sea level. This will also relieve the headache and make breathing easier.

At 18,000 feet, humans reach their ceiling and cannot stay for more than a few weeks. Any sea-level person taken quickly to 20,000 feet will be almost incapacitated in less than half an hour, and death will occur soon thereafter.

Other Altitude-Related Illnesses

- *Pharyngitis* and *bronchitis*. Because of dry air, a sore throat and coughing may develop. Care involves drinking fluids, applying an OTC antibiotic ointment in the nostrils, and sucking on hard candy or throat lozenges.
- *Peripheral edema.* The hands, ankles, and/or face (around the eyes) may swell at high altitude. If possible, raise the affected arms and/

or legs. After descending or with acclimatization to higher altitudes, the swelling diminishes. Descend if signs of more serious altitude illness appear.

▶ Lightning

Lightning is awesome and frightening **Figure 24-7**. About 30% of lightning strikes to humans result in death. Lightning is one of the leading environmental causes of death in the United States.

In the past, farmers, sailors, and other outdoor workers in isolated areas tended to be the most frequently injured. Today, a larger proportion of victims are hikers, campers, golfers, and others who are outdoors for recreational purposes.

Figure 24-7

Lightning strike.

FYI

Altitude Increases Sunburn Risk

Skiers, hikers, and others who enjoy outdoor activities in the mountains have long believed that it took less time to sunburn in the mountains than at lower levels. Research confirms that the higher the altitude, the quicker a person will develop sunburn. UV (ultraviolet) light energy readings were taken at solar noon in direct sunlight on cloudless days at Vail, Colorado; Orlando, Florida; and New York, New York. The high-altitude regions in the United States include areas with some of the fastest population growth, and it is vital that people living or visiting these regions recognize the increase in UV exposure at higher altitudes and take precautions to prevent sunburn.

Source: Rigel DS, Rigel EG, Rigel AC. 1999. Effects of altitude and latitude on ambient UVB radiation. *J Am Acad Dermatol* 40:114-116.

FYI

Lightning's "Rule of 70s"

70% happen in June, July, and August.

70% happen between noon and 6:00 PM.

70% involve only one victim.

70% of the victims survive.

70% of the victims have a residual effect (hearing, vision, or neurologic impairment).

FYI

Myths About Lightning

- **Lightning strikes are always fatal.** Actually, studies report that lightning strikes kill only 20% to 30% of those struck. Generally, only people who sustain immediate cardiac arrest die.
- **A person who has been struck by lightning retains the charge—is "electrified"—and is dangerous to touch.** This false idea has led to a delay of resuscitation efforts and probably to some unnecessary deaths.
- **Lightning strike injuries allow a long resuscitation effort.** Although rescue breathing (when the person has a pulse) can effectively sustain life for long periods, CPR is usually ineffective after 30 minutes for cardiac arrest victims.
- **Lightning never strikes twice in the same place.** In fact, certain areas are prone to lightning due to height, location, or material. The Willis Tower and the Empire State Building are hit hundreds of times a year, as are mountaintops and radio and television antennas.
- **A person inside a building is safe from lightning injury.** Electrical current can travel along plumbing fixtures, telephone wires, and other appliances attached to the outside of the house by metal conductors.

Almost 70% of lightning deaths involve just one person; 15% involve groups of two; and groups of three or more account for another 15%. Lightning deaths occur more often during daytime hours when people are active and outdoors. Most occur during the months of June through September, when thunderstorms are most frequent. There are more thunderstorm days in the South than in any other region of the United States. Thunderstorms occur frequently over high mountains. People are better protected in urban areas where high buildings have metal frames and lightning devices.

How Lightning Injures

Lightning injures in five ways. A *direct strike* is actually being struck by lightning. Lightning is most likely to hit a person in the open who has been unable to find shelter. Any conductor of electricity that the victim carries, especially if it is metal and carried above the shoulder level (for example, an open umbrella or a bag of golf clubs slung over the shoulder) increases the chances of a direct hit.

A more frequent cause of injury is a *splash,* which occurs when lightning strikes a tree or a building and "splashes" onto a victim seeking shelter nearby. The electrical current seeks the path of least resistance and may jump to the person because bodies have less resistance than trees or other objects. Frequently, a splash can kill groups of animals as they stand near a fence or seek shelter under trees. *Contact injury* occurs when a person is holding an object that is directly hit or splashed by lightning.

Ground current is produced when lightning hits the ground or a nearby object. The current spreads like a wave in a pond. Although ground current is less likely to produce fatalities than direct hits or splashes, it often creates multiple victims and injuries. Large groups have been injured on baseball fields and hiking paths and during military maneuvers.

Finally, people can be injured by the explosive force of the *shock wave* produced as lightning strikes nearby. Victims actually can be thrown by this blast effect.

Differences Between Generated High-Voltage Electricity Injuries and Lightning Injuries

Lightning contact with the body is instantaneous, leading to flashover, where the current flashes over the body. The current flashes over the body as well as going through it. With flashover, the victim seldom has burns of any magnitude. Lightning injuries disrupt electrical activity in the heart and nervous system. Exposure to household electricity tends to be much more prolonged because the victim freezes to the circuit. The electrical energy surges through the tissues with little resistance to flow, causing thermal

FYI

Flash-to-Bang: How Close

Be aware of how close lightning is occurring. The flash-to-bang method is the easiest and most convenient way to estimate how far away lightning is occurring. Thunder always accompanies lightning even though its audible range can be diminished due to background noise in the immediate environment and its distance from you. To use the flash-to-bang method, count the seconds from the time the lightning is sighted to when the clap of the thunder is heard. Divide this number by five to obtain how far away (in miles) the lightning is occurring. For example, if you count 15 seconds between seeing the flash and hearing the bang, 15 divided by 5 equals 3. Therefore the lightning flash is about 3 miles away.

FYI

30/30 Rule: When to Find Shelter

The 30/30 rule states that people should seek shelter if the flash-to-bang delay (length of time in seconds between a lightning flash and its subsequent thunder) is 30 seconds or less, and that they remain under cover until 30 minutes after the final clap of thunder.

A 30-second lead time is necessary prior to a storm's arrival because of the possibility of distant strikes. A 30-minute wait after the last thunder clap is heard is necessary because the trailing storm clouds still carry a lingering charge. This charge can—and does—occasionally produce lightning on the back edge of a storm, several minutes after the rain has ended.

Studies have shown most people struck by lightning are struck not at the height of a thunderstorm, but before and after the storm has peaked. DO NOT wait for the rain to start before seeking shelter, and do not leave shelter just because the rain has ended. Half of all lightning deaths occur after a storm passes.

injury with severe tissue damage that can result in the loss of the damaged extremity. Electric current can also disrupt the body's electrical activity as does lightning.

Recognizing a Lightning Injury

- Breathing may be absent.
- Seizures, paralysis, and loss of responsiveness can result if the central nervous system is damaged.

FYI

Avoid Lightning Injury

- Be alert about weather conditions and predictions before going outdoors.
- Do not stand under a natural lightning rod such as a tall, isolated tree in an open area.
- Avoid projecting above the surrounding landscape, as you would do if you were standing on a hilltop, in an open field, on the beach, or fishing from a boat on the open water.
- Get out of and away from open water.
- Get away from tractors and other metal farm equipment.
- Get off and away from motorcycles, scooters, golf carts, and bicycles. Lay down golf clubs.
- Stay away from wire fences, clotheslines, metal pipes, rails, and other metallic paths that could carry lightning to you from some distance away.
- Avoid standing in small, isolated sheds or other small structures in open areas.
- In a forest, seek shelter in a low area under a thick growth of small trees.
- In open areas, go to a low place such as a ravine or valley.
- If you are hopelessly isolated in a level field or prairie and you feel tingling or your hair stand on end—indicating lightning is about to strike—drop to a baseball catcher's crouching position or stance and put your hands over both ears to help avoid an eardrum rupture. Do not lie flat on the ground. You want as small an area of your body as possible touching the ground to minimize the possibility of your body acting as a conductor.
- If you are indoors during a thunderstorm, avoid open doors and windows, fireplaces, and metal objects such as pipes, sinks, and plug-in electrical appliances. Avoid using the telephone.
- If you are in an automobile (without a cloth top), stay in it. The vehicle will diffuse the current around you to the ground. It is a myth that the rubber tires will provide insulation but it is true that the metal body affords protection.
- If a group of people is exposed, they should spread out and stay several yards apart. That way, should a strike hit, the smallest number will be seriously injured.

- Minor burns. Most people believe that a lightning strike victim will be severely burned. However, owing to the flashover effect, most victims have only minor burns. The entrance and exit burn points common with electrical current burns are rare with lightning. The types of burns seen with lightning strikes are *punctate burns* (small, circular injuries resembling cigarette burns), *feathering* or *ferning burns, linear burns,* and burns from ignited clothing and heated metal. On rare occasions, clothing is ignited by lightning. A victim wearing metal, such as a necklace or a belt buckle, or carrying coins in a pocket may be burned as the objects heat.

Care for a Lightning Injury

1. If more than one victim has been struck by lightning at the same time, go to the quiet and motionless victim first, check for breathing and, if absent, begin CPR.
2. If the victim is unresponsive but breathing, place the victim on his or her side.
3. Because spinal injuries can occur with lightning strikes, precautions should be taken to stabilize the spine.
4. Check for injuries.
5. Evacuate all victims to medical care.

▶ Wild Animal Attacks

Despite the fact that few large wild animals (bears, bison, cougars, and alligators) remain in the United States, attacks on humans still occur **Figure 24-8** . Wild animal attacks outside the United States are more common. Attacks, especially fatal attacks, are often reported and sensationalized in the media.

The incidence of injuries from wild animal attacks is not known. Reporting is not mandatory, and many attacks are not recorded. Perhaps one or two deaths occur each year in the United States. Outside the United States, animal attacks by hippopotami, crocodiles, elephants, cape buffalo, lions, and tigers are a much greater cause of injury and death.

Wild animal attacks occur most often in rural or wilderness settings, a long distance from medical care. Preventing wild animal attacks is largely common sense and awareness. An increasing number of parks and wilderness areas are posting warning signs. Recreationalists should be aware of and knowledgeable about the animal habitats through which they travel and take precautions in food handling so as not to attract animals.

Generally, if you encounter a large wild animal, try to remove yourself from the scene quietly and slowly. Running will elicit a predatory response. Never get between an adult animal and its offspring. In most cases, a general rule is to fight back if you are attacked. Vigorous physical resistance, including striking the attacking animal with fists, a weapon, or any other object, has been effective in repelling attacks by cougars, lions, tigers, brown and black bears, and even crocodiles. Exceptions to this recommendation are the grizzly bear and a mother black bear with cubs. In these cases, you should lie down and play dead.

Recognizing Wild Animal-Related Injuries

Not all injuries are bites. Severe injuries result from victims being thrown in the air, gored by an antler, butted, or trampled on the ground. Injuries include puncture wounds, bites, lacerations, bruises, fractures, rupture of internal organs, and evisceration.

Care for Wild Animal-Related Injuries

See Chapters 8, 9, and 10 for what to do for bleeding and wound care. Depending on the severity of the injury, either evacuate the victim to medical care or contact local authorities for evacuation.

▶ Wilderness Evacuation

Determining the best way to evacuate a victim (helicopter evacuation versus walking the victim out versus carrying the victim on a litter) must be based on several factors. The following list is adapted from the

Figure 24-8

Large animals do not always retreat from humans and may attack rescuers.

WMS Practice Guidelines and suggests factors for determining the level of evacuation:

- Severity of the illness or injury
- Rescue and medical skills of the rescuers
- Physical and psychological condition of the rescuers and the victims
- Availability of equipment and aid for the rescue
- The time it would take to evacuate the victim by other means as determined by distance, terrain, weather, and other conditions
- Cost

When requesting outside assistance, you must consider the safety of incoming rescuers, their time commitment, and the cost of the rescue.

As a general rule, you should delay travel plans or start evacuating a victim from the wilderness for any of the following reasons:

- The victim's condition is not improving.
- The victim is experiencing debilitating pain.
- The victim is unable to travel at a reasonable pace owing to a medical problem.
- The victim is passing blood via the mouth or rectum (not from an obviously minor source).
- The victim has signs and symptoms of serious altitude illness.
- Infections are not improving.
- Chest pain is not caused by a rib cage injury.
- Wounds are severe enough to require medical care.
- The victim's dysfunctional psychological status is impairing the safety of others.

When to Evacuate

Use these guidelines to decide whether a victim should be evacuated.

Immediate Evacuations

Rapidly evacuate the following injuries, where medical care is needed in 30 to 60 minutes or less:

- Open fractures
- Extremity injuries with deformity
- Extremity injuries in which circulation is absent
- Spinal injuries with no sensation in the fingers or toes or inability of the victim to move fingers or toes
- Severe altitude illness (signs of HACE or HAPE)
- Decreased level of consciousness

- Signs of shock
- Severe bleeding

In the wilderness, all bleeding should be controlled. Wounds should be cleaned and irrigated under pressure. The standard rule is not to remove blood-soaked dressings; locate the bleeding vessels and reapply pressure directly over the bleeding vessels. Never attempt to clamp or tie a vessel—more damage can result. Do not close a wound with adhesive strips, butterfly bandages, staples, or sutures.

Delayed Evacuations

Medical care should be obtained within 6 to 24 hours of injury:

- Limb injuries with deformity, severe pain, or inability to walk
- Severe frostbite
- Open wounds: Evacuate a wounded victim so that a physician can suture a wound within 6 hours for hand or foot injuries and within 24 hours for head or trunk injuries. (If necessary, closure can be done by a physician up to about the fourth day).
- Hypothermia: It is not necessary to evacuate a victim of mild hypothermia if the victim has normal mental status and is shivering. Evacuate victims who have severe hypothermia (shivering has stopped but the victim is still cold, altered mental status). It is impossible to rewarm a severely hypothermic victim in a wilderness or remote location. See Chapter 20, *Cold-Related Emergencies* for more information.

Guidelines for Ground Evacuation

If the victim is walking out, at least two people should accompany the victim. If the victim is being carried out, one or two people should be sent to notify authorities that assistance is needed and to give them specifics about the problem.

During a litter evacuation, there should be at least four, and preferably six, litter bearers at all times. Over rough terrain, eight carriers (six over smooth trail) should carry the litter 100 yards and then rest or rotate with eight other carriers. It is very demanding to carry a loaded litter for more than 15 minutes without a break.

Guidelines for Helicopter Evacuation

Helicopters can reduce the time the victim has to wait to receive medical care. Evacuate by helicopter only if

Figure 24-9

An EMS helicopter.

FYI

Hiking: How to Protect One's Health on the Trail

The popularity of backpacking and day hiking has greatly increased, but so have related injuries. A survey of 224 backpackers who hiked the entire 2,100-mile mountainous Appalachian Trail showed that 82% had injuries (mostly muscle sprains, strains, and stress fractures) and illnesses (mostly diarrhea, skin irritations, foot blisters, and colds). Medical help was needed in 25% of the incidents. Hikers lost an average of 5 days of hiking because of these problems. Because these problems are common, hikers should carry supplies such as water purification equipment, pain medicine, antibiotic ointment, and bandages.

Source: Crouse BJ, Josephs D. 1993. Health care needs of Appalachian Trail hikers. *J Fam Pract* 36:521–525.

CAUTION

DO NOT approach a helicopter until one of the aircraft personnel signals it is safe for you to approach.

DO NOT approach a helicopter from the rear, where the fast-spinning tail rotor is invisible and dangerous. Many people walk into spinning rotors each year.

DO NOT forget to protect against wind chill from the rotor blades in the winter or to protect the eyes against flying dirt and debris.

DO NOT approach from the uphill side. The rotor is closer to the ground on the uphill side **Figure 24-10**.

DO NOT stand up when approaching a helicopter. Keep as low as possible in a crouched position. Because the blade is flexible, it may dip as low as 4 feet off the ground.

Approach and leave downhill   Not this way

Sloping ground surface

Figure 24-10

Helicopter safety.

the following conditions apply **Figure 24-9**:

- The victim's life will be saved or the victim will have a significantly better chance for full recovery.
- The pilot believes conditions are safe enough for helicopter evacuation.

- Ground evacuation would be unusually dangerous or excessively prolonged or not enough rescuers are available for ground evacuation.

In general, helicopters are not beneficial if ground transport can get the victim to the hospital within 30 to 60 minutes.

▶ Signaling for Help

Many emergency conditions require a search for people in distress. Under such circumstances, it is always better if the people being sought know how to make their presence and their location conspicuous.

Signaling Aircraft

When creating a ground signal that people in an aircraft can see, remember that there are few straight lines or right angles in nature and that things are a lot smaller when viewed from the air. Bigger is almost always better. For ground signals, make a large "V" for immediate assistance or an "X" if medical assistance is needed. Make the lines of these signals as large as you can. Construct your signal so that each line is six times as long as it is wide, such as a "V" with each side 12 feet long and 2 feet wide. Contrast is another key to ground signals. Examples of materials to use include toilet paper, strips of plastic tarp, strips of tent material, tree branches, logs, and light-colored rocks. In snow and on open ground or sandy shores, signals may be tramped or dug into the surface using shadows to make the signals stand out.

Other Signals

A series of three of almost anything indicates "Help." Examples include three shouts, three shots, three blasts from a whistle, or three flashes from a light. Use smoke by day and bright flame by night if other signaling devices are not available. Add engine oil, rags soaked in oil, or pieces of rubber to your fire to make black smoke (best against a light background). Keep plenty of spare fuel on hand. If you are tending a fire as you wait for help, keep fuel handy and throw it on the fire when you hear an aircraft; do not wait, because it takes time for smoke to form and rise. Make sure to start the fire away from combustibles such as grass or trees.

A mirror is an effective means of sending a distress signal. On hazy days, aircraft pilots can see the flash of a mirror before survivors can see the aircraft, so it is wise to flash the mirror in the direction of a plane when you hear it, even when you cannot see it. Mirror flashes have been spotted by rescue aircraft more than 20 miles away.

To use a mirror, follow this procedure:

1. Hold the mirror up to the sun with one hand, and stretch your other hand out in front of you. Use your finger or thumb to block your view of your target.
2. Hit your extended finger or thumb with a reflection of the sun from the mirror.

Figure 24-11

Signaling.

3. Repeatedly flick the spot of light from the mirror across the finger or thumb and the target.
4. Try to hit the aircraft or rescuers with a flash as much as possible. Do not attempt to do series of three flashes—it is too difficult **Figure 24-11**.

FYI

Survival Kit: The Bare Essentials

Minimal items	Purpose
One or two large plastic trash bags or an emergency blanket ("space blanket") made of Mylar	Protects against weather (wind, rain, snow). Wear one trash bag by cutting a hole in the bottom of the bag for your head; use the second bag to cover your legs.
Whistle (Mini Fox 40 or Windstorm)	Signal for help.
Signal mirror	Signal for help.
Metal match with striker (magnesium)	Start a fire.
Waterproof match case containing windproof and waterproof matches	Start a fire.
Waterproof match case or empty film canister containing several cotton balls smeared with petroleum jelly (such as Vaseline) or commercial tinder tabs	Petroleum jelly is flammable. Make tinder using cotton balls smeared with petroleum jelly. When using, open a cotton ball up to catch sparks from metal match.
Knife (multitool) and/or wire blade survival saw	Cutting
Food (such as energy bars and MREs [US military surplus meals-ready-to-eat])	Provides calories and a psychological boost

▶ Ready for Review

- Be as medically prepared as possible to manage a problem for others and for yourself.
- Because heart activity must be restored within a short time for a cardiac arrest victim to survive, CPR has limited use in a wilderness or remote setting.
- In a wilderness situation, reducing some dislocated joints is recommended.
- Always stabilize an unresponsive victim.
- Victims with a femur fracture can lose 2 quarts of blood in the thigh and develop massive swelling. These injuries should be splinted.
- Since the early 1970s, the number of deaths caused by avalanches has increased rapidly.
- Altitude illnesses actually are a spectrum of a single problem: hypoxia.
- Determining the best way to evacuate a victim must be based on several factors.
- Many emergency conditions require a search for people in distress.

▶ Vital Vocabulary

hypoxia A low oxygen content in the blood; lack of oxygen in inspired air.

prep kit

▶ Assessment in Action

You have been enjoying a 5-day backpack trip in the high mountains of Colorado. Being from sea level, you knew the high altitude would take some getting used to but your group is doing very well. On day 4, you must ascend a 1,000-foot pass to get to your final campsite. After an hour of never-ending switchbacks, you arrive at the highest point of the trip—13,500 feet above sea level. At this elevation, several members in your group report a severe headache and fatigue. Two members cannot seem to "catch their breath."

Directions: Circle Yes if you agree with the statement; circle No if you disagree.

Yes No **1.** Because you are above 12,000 feet, you suspect they are suffering from HAPE or HACE.

Yes No **2.** Plenty of fluids should be given to the victims.

Yes No **3.** You should stay at this elevation until they feel well enough to hike down the other side of the pass.

Yes No **4.** After descent to your final campsite (3,000 feet below the pass), if the victims' conditions do not improve, you should seek medical care.

▶ Check Your Knowledge

Directions: Circle Yes if you agree with the statement; circle No if you disagree.

Yes   No   **1.** Injuries in the wilderness rarely happen.

Yes   No   **2.** CPR in the wilderness should be stopped if the victim does not respond after 30 minutes.

Yes   No   **3.** Reduction of a dislocation dramatically relieves pain.

Yes   No   **4.** When it comes to spinal stabilization, never improvise!

Yes   No   **5.** After an avalanche, it is easy for victims to dig themselves out.

Yes   No   **6.** Speed of ascent can affect altitude illness.

Yes   No   **7.** Headache is a common symptom of altitude illness.

Yes   No   **8.** A victim of altitude illness should keep moving.

Yes   No   **9.** Most lightning deaths occur during the night.

Yes   No   **10.** Most lightning victims will have only minor burns.

Rescuing and Moving Victims

Victim Rescue

▶ Water Rescue

Reach-throw-row-go identifies the sequence for attempting a water rescue. The first and simplest rescue technique is to reach for the victim. Reaching requires a lightweight pole, ladder, long stick, or any object that can be extended to the victim. Once you have your "reacher," secure your footing and have a bystander grab your belt or pants for stability. Secure yourself before reaching for the victim.

You can throw anything that floats—an empty picnic jug, an empty fuel or paint can, a life jacket, a floating cushion, a piece of wood, or an inflated spare tire—whatever is available Table 25-1 . If there is a rope handy, tie it to the object to be thrown so you can pull the victim in, or, if you miss, you can retrieve the object and throw it again. The average untrained rescuer has a throwing range of about 50 feet.

If the victim is out of throwing range and there is a rowboat, canoe, motor boat, or boogie board nearby, you can try to row to the victim. Maneuvering these craft requires skill learned through practice. Wear a personal flotation device for your own safety. To avoid capsizing, never pull the victim in over the side of a boat; instead, pull the victim in over the stern (rear end) or tow the victim to safety.

If reach, throw, and row are impossible and you are a capable swimmer trained in water lifesaving procedures, you can go to the drowning victim by swimming. Entering even calm water makes a swimming

Table 25-1 Effect of Flotation Devices on Survival Times	
Situation (50° F water)	Predicted Survival Time (hours)
No Flotation Device	
Drownproofing	1.5
Treading water	2.0
With Flotation Device	
Swimming	2.0
Holding still	2.7
HELP (heat escape lessening position)	4.0
Huddle position	4.0

rescue difficult and hazardous. All too often a would-be rescuer becomes a victim as well.

Near-Drowning

In the United States, there are about 4,000 deaths each year due to drowning. In addition to the drownings, there are many cases of extreme, permanent disability that result from near-drowning.

Drowning means suffocation by immersion in water or other liquid. *Near-drowning* occurs when a victim survives an immersion incident. About two thirds of drowning victims are younger than 30 years. Most are males.

Usually, the initial reaction to drowning is panic. Then violent struggling occurs. Frequently, as victims become short of breath, they swallow water during attempts to breathe, and the water is often vomited. Further attempts to breathe may then result in aspiration of water, vomitus, or foreign bodies into the lungs. Sometimes the vocal cords (larynx) close and will not allow any water to enter the lungs. A seizure may occur, followed by death.

Drownings are classified into three basic types. In *dry drownings* (10% to 15%), no water passes the vocal cords. Presumably, in these cases, the cords shut tightly (*laryngospasm*) when water touches them. Other things being equal, a near-drowning without aspiration is easier to resuscitate because water has not entered the airway.

In *wet drownings* (85% of near-drownings), water, vomitus, or foreign bodies are aspirated into the lungs. Fresh water in the lungs enters the bloodstream and

has a profoundly destructive effect on blood cells (which swell and burst) and leads to cardiac arrest (ventricular fibrillation). In saltwater drownings, water is taken from the bloodstream and enters the lungs. As much as 25% of the total blood volume can be lost as fluids move into the lungs. The victims drown in their own fluids as much as in the saltwater itself.

A *secondary drowning* is one in which a victim who was resuscitated dies within 96 hours. Aspiration pneumonia (due to inhalation of vomitus) is a late complication of near-drowning and occurs 48 to 72 hours after the episode. Near-drowning victims should be hospitalized or closely monitored.

CAUTION

DO NOT swim to and grasp a drowning person unless you are trained in lifesaving.

FYI

Typical Drowning Situations

Immediate-Disappearance Syndrome
- Victim enters water but does not return to the surface
- Little chance of rescue
- Caused by:
  1. Diving from height and striking the head
  2. Hyperventilation before underwater swimming
  3. Cold-induced heart attack

Distressed Nonswimmer
- Struggles 20 to 60 seconds before sinking
- Signs of distress: flailing arms, head tilted back, no vocalizing, appears to be playing

Sudden-Disappearance Syndrome
- Victim fully clothed
- Victim apparently able to swim but is fatigued, a poor swimmer, and/or cold
- Victim disappears after 5 to 10 minutes on surface (after clothing loses entrapped air)

Hypothermia-Induced Drowning
- Victim seriously affected after about 15 minutes of exposure to cold water
- Rule of 50s: Average unaware, unpracticed, and unprotected 50-year-old man would approach the 50-50 life-or-death point after 50 minutes of exposure to 50° F water.

Source: Adapted from David S. Smith.

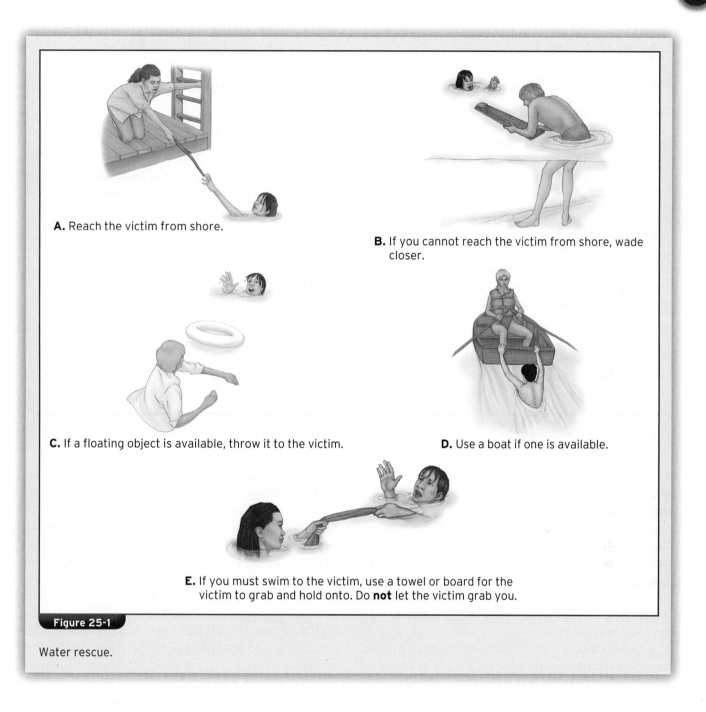

A. Reach the victim from shore.

B. If you cannot reach the victim from shore, wade closer.

C. If a floating object is available, throw it to the victim.

D. Use a boat if one is available.

E. If you must swim to the victim, use a towel or board for the victim to grab and hold onto. Do **not** let the victim grab you.

Figure 25-1

Water rescue.

Care for Drowning

1. Survey the scene (see Chapter 2, *Action at an Emergency*), then carry out a water rescue **Figure 25-1**.

2. If the victim was diving (or it is unknown whether he or she was diving), suspect a possible spine injury. Keep the victim in-line floating on the water surface until properly trained rescuers arrive with a backboard.

3. Check breathing and treat accordingly. Any nonbreathing victim who has been submerged in cold water should be resuscitated unless submerged for more than 60 minutes.

4. If no spinal injury is suspected, after the victim has been resuscitated, place the victim on his or her side to allow fluids to drain from the airway.

Cold-Water Immersion

Immersion in cold water is a potential hazard for anyone who participates in activities in the oceans, lakes, and streams of all but the tropical regions of the world.

FYI

American Academy of Pediatrics Recommendations for Preventing Childhood Drowning (by Age Group)

4 years and younger

- Never leave children alone in bathtubs, spas, or wading pools or near nearly filled buckets, toilets, irrigation ditches, or other standing water.
- Recognize that swimming lessons do not "drownproof" children.
- Fence the entire pool so that it is separated from the house. Pool covers are not a substitute for fences.
- Learn CPR and keep a telephone and emergency equipment—such as life preservers and a shepherd's crook—poolside.

5 to 12 years

- Provide with swimming lessons that include safety rules.
- Never let the children swim alone or without adult supervision.
- Make sure the children wear approved flotation devices when playing in or near a body of water.
- Teach the children the dangers of jumping or diving into water and of being on thin ice.

13 to 19 years

- In addition to relaying the preceding safety tips, counsel about the dangers of substance abuse combined with swimming, diving, or boating.
- Teach adolescents how to perform CPR.

Source: Pediatrics 112(2):437-439. 2003.

The US Coast Guard defines *cold water* as water with a temperature of less than 70° F. However, water does not need to be that cold for a person to become hypothermic. A person can become hypothermic in water that is 77° F. Most North American lakes, rivers, and coasts are colder than that year-round. The risk of immersion hypothermia in North America is nearly universal most of the year. A person immersed in cold water loses heat about 25 times faster than someone exposed to cold air.

The US Coast Guard and other rescue organizations recommend that survivors get as much of their bodies out of the water as possible to minimize cooling rate and maximize survival time. A widespread misunderstanding of the concept of wind chill often causes people to conclude that survivors have higher heat losses if they are exposed to wind, especially if they are wet, than if they are immersed in water. During recreational activities at beaches, lakes, and swimming pools, most people have experienced feeling colder after leaving the water than they do while swimming. That reinforces the misunderstanding, which has sometimes led accident victims to abandon a safe position atop a capsized vessel and reenter the water, usually with tragic results.

Cold-water immersion is associated with two potential medical emergencies: drowning and hypothermia. Numerous case histories and statistical evidence document the prominence of cold-water immersion as a cause of drowning and hypothermia. Perhaps the most famous occurrence of cold-water immersion was the sinking of the ocean liner *Titanic* on April 14, 1912. After striking an iceberg, the ship sank in calm seas. Of the 2,201 people on board, only 712 were rescued, all from the ship's lifeboats. The remaining 1,489 people died in the water, despite the arrival of a rescue vehicle within 2 hours. Nearly all of those victims were wearing life preservers, yet the cause of death was officially listed as drowning. More likely, the cause of death was immersion hypothermia.

The speed at which a person cools depends on several factors:

- *Body fat.* The more body fat a person has, the slower cooling occurs. More fat increases survival chances.
- *Body type.* Bigger people cool more slowly than smaller people. Children cool faster than adults. Women have more fat but are usually smaller, so they cool at the same rate as men.
- *Physical fitness.* Cardiovascular fitness can help meet the stress of cold-water immersion,

but physically fit people usually have less subcutaneous fat for insulation.

- *Water temperature.* The colder the water, the faster a person cools.
- *Clothing.* Clothing can insulate, and some types of fabric, such as wool, are better than others.
- *Alcohol.* People who have been drinking alcohol are more likely to get into dangerous situations. Alcohol impairs judgment and coordination. Research studies have implicated alcohol in 10% to 50% of all drownings. Alcohol dilates the skin's blood vessels, which allows more body heat to escape.
- *Behavior.* Swimming and treading water increase the flow of warm blood from the body's core to the muscles, increasing the cooling rate. Thus, swimmers often die first because they are more likely to try to tread water or swim rather than float. Likewise, so-called *drownproofing,* a technique of bobbing in the water (like a jellyfish), markedly increases heat loss as water circulates around the head.

A *heat escape lessening position (HELP)* has been devised, in which the victim draws the knees up close to the chest, presses the arms to the sides, and remains as quiet as possible **Figure 25-2**. For two or more people, huddling quietly and closely together (huddle position) will decrease heat loss from the groin and the front of the body. Both of these positions require personal flotation devices (life jackets).

Surviving long periods of submersion has been explained by the diving reflex found in mammals. Some say that the diving reflex slows the heart rate, shunts blood to the brain, and closes the airway. Recent research, however, suggests that the diving reflex is present in marine mammals such as seals, porpoises, whales, and walruses but not in humans. If the diving reflex is discounted, the most likely explanation for prolonged submersion survival is that cold water produces hypothermia, which reduces the body's demand for oxygen and protects the brain.

▶ Ice Rescue

If a person has fallen through the ice near the shore, extend a pole or throw a line with a floatable object attached to it. When the person has hold of the object, pull him or her toward the shore or the edge of the ice.

Figure 25-2

HELP or huddle. **A.** A person wearing a flotation device can minimize heat loss and increase chances of survival by assuming the heat escape lessening position (HELP) in which the knees are pulled up to the chest and the arms crossed. **B.** Groups of three or more can conserve heat by wrapping their arms around one another and pulling into a tight circle or huddle.

Figure 25-3

Ice rescue: Lie flat to distribute the weight over a larger surface area.

If the person has fallen through the ice away from the shore and you cannot reach him or her with a pole or a throwing line, lie flat and push a ladder, plank, or similar object ahead of you **Figure 25-3**. You can also tie a rope to a spare tire and the other end to an anchor point on the shore, lie flat, and push the tire ahead of you. Pull the person ashore or to the edge of the ice.

CAUTION

DO NOT go near broken ice without support.

▶ Electrical Emergency Rescue

Electrical injuries can be devastating. Just a mild shock can cause serious internal injuries. A current of 1,000 V or more is considered high voltage, but even the 110 V of household current can be deadly.

When a person receives an electrical shock, electricity enters the body at the point of contact and travels along the path of least resistance (nerves and blood vessels). The current travels rapidly, generating heat and causing destruction.

Most indoor electrocutions are caused by faulty electrical equipment or the careless use of electrical appliances. Before you touch the victim, turn off the electricity at the circuit breaker, fuse box, or outside switch box or unplug the appliance if the plug is undamaged.

If the electrocution involves high-voltage power lines, the power must be turned off before anyone

approaches the victim. If you approach a victim and feel a tingling sensation in your legs and lower body, stop. You are on energized ground, and an electric current is entering one foot, passing through your lower body, and leaving through the other foot. You should raise one foot off the ground, turn around, and hop to a safe place. Wait for trained personnel with the proper equipment to cut the wires or disconnect them. If a power line falls over a car, tell the driver and passengers to stay in the car. A victim should try to jump out of the car only if an explosion or fire threatens and then without making contact with the car or the wire.

CAUTION

DO NOT touch an appliance or the victim until the current is off.
DO NOT try to move downed wires.
DO NOT use any object, even dry wood (broomstick, tools, chair, stool) to separate the victim from the electrical source.

▶ Hazardous Materials Incidents

Almost any highway crash scene involves the potential danger of hazardous chemicals. Clues that indicate the presence of hazardous materials include the following:

- Look for warning signs on the vehicle (for example, "explosive," "flammable," "corrosive"). If you are unable to read the placard or labels, do not move closer and risk exposure. If you are able to read the placard with the naked eye, you may be too close and should consider moving farther away. **Figure 25-4** shows a chart illustrating the hazardous materials warning placards, and **Figure 25-5** shows a chart illustrating the warning labels.
- Watch for a leak or spill from a tank, container, truck, or railroad car with or without hazardous material placards or labels.
- A strong, noxious odor can denote a hazardous material.
- A cloud or strange-looking smoke from the escaping substance "says" stay away.

Stay well away and upwind from the area. Only people who are specially trained in handling hazard-

Figure 25-4

Hazardous materials warning placards.

Figure 25-5

Hazardous materials warning labels.

ous materials and who have the proper equipment should be in the area.

▶ Motor Vehicle Crashes

In most states, you are legally obligated to stop and give help when you are involved in a motor vehicle crash. If you arrive at a crash shortly after it happens, the law does not require you to stop, although it might be argued that you have a moral responsibility to provide any aid that you can.

1. Stop and park your vehicle well off the highway or road and out of active traffic lanes. Park at least five car lengths from the crash. If the police have taken charge, do not stop unless you are asked to do so. If the police or other emergency vehicles have not arrived, call or send someone to call 9-1-1 or the local emergency number as soon as possible. Ways to call include the following:
   - Finding a pay phone or roadside emergency phone
   - Using a cellular phone or CB (citizen's band) radio
   - Using a phone at a nearby house or business
2. Turn on your vehicle's emergency hazard flashers. Raise the hood of your vehicle to draw more attention to the scene.
3. Make sure everyone on the scene is safe.
   - Ask the driver to turn off the ignition or turn it off yourself.
   - Ask bystanders to stand well off the roadway.
   - Place flares or reflectors 250 to 500 feet behind the crash scene to warn oncoming drivers of the crash. Do not ignite flares around leaking gasoline or diesel fuel.
4. If the driver or passenger is unresponsive or might have spinal injuries, use your hands to stabilize the person's head and neck.
5. Check and keep monitoring the victim's breathing. Treat any life-threatening injuries.
6. Whenever possible, wait for EMS personnel to extricate the victims from vehicles because

they have training and the proper equipment. In most cases, keep the victims' conditions stabilized inside the vehicle.

7. Allow the EMS ambulance to take victims to the hospital.

CAUTION

DO NOT rush to get the victims out of a car that has been in a crash. Contrary to opinion, most vehicle crashes do not involve fire, and most vehicles stay in an upright position.

DO NOT move or allow victims to move unless there is an immediate danger such as fire or oncoming traffic.

DO NOT transport victims in your car or any other bystander's vehicle.

▶ Fires

Should you encounter a fire, you should:

1. Get all the people out of the vehicles and area quickly.
2. Call the emergency telephone number (usually 9-1-1).

Then—and *only* then—if the fire is small and if your own escape route is clear, should you fight the fire yourself with a fire extinguisher. You may be able to put out the fire or at least hold damage to a minimum. Because a fire can spread quickly, efforts to contain it within the first 5 minutes of a blaze can make a substantial difference in the eventual outcome.

To use a fire extinguisher, aim directly at whatever is burning and sweep across it at the base of the flames. Extinguishers expel their contents quickly; it takes just 8 to 25 seconds for most home models containing dry chemicals to empty.

If clothing catches fire, tear the article off, in a motion away from the face. Keep the victim from running, because running fans the flames. Wrap a rug or a woolen blanket around the victim's neck to keep the fire from the face or throw a blanket on the victim. In some cases, you may be able to smother the flames by throwing the victim to the floor and rolling him or her in a rug.

CAUTION

DO NOT let victims run if their clothing is on fire.

DO NOT become trapped while fighting a fire. Always keep a door behind you so you can exit if the fire gets too big.

▶ Threatening Dogs

When you enter any emergency scene, look for signs of a dog and proceed with caution if the animal is not threatening. Ask the owner to control a threatening dog. If you cannot be delayed, consider using a fire extinguisher, water hose, or pepper spray. For a vicious dog, call the police for assistance.

▶ Farm Animals

Emergencies involving farm animals can be dangerous to rescuers. Horses kick and bite. Cattle kick, bite, gore, or squeeze people against a pen or barn. Pigs can deliver severe bites.

- Approach a situation involving animals with caution.
- Do not frighten an animal. Speak quietly to reassure it.
- If food is available, use it to lure the animal away from the victim.

▶ Confined Spaces

A *confined space* is any area not intended for human occupancy that may have or develop a dangerous atmosphere. They have limited openings for entrance and exit. There are three types of confined spaces: below ground, ground level, and above ground. Below-ground confined spaces include manholes, below-ground utility vaults and storage tanks, old mines, cisterns, and wells. Ground-level confined spaces include industrial tanks and farm storage silos. Above-ground confined spaces include water towers and legged storage tanks.

An accident in a confined space demands immediate action. If someone enters a confined space and signals for help or becomes unresponsive, follow these steps:

1. Call 9-1-1 for immediate assistance.
2. Do not rush in to help.
3. When help arrives, try to rescue the victim without entering the space.
4. If rescue from the outside cannot be done, only trained and properly equipped (respiratory protection plus safety harnesses or lifelines) rescuers should enter the space and remove the victim.

5. Once the victim is removed, provide care. Additional training is required if first aiders may be on-call in helping rescue confined space victims.

Triage: What to Do With Multiple Victims

You may encounter emergency situations in which there are two or more victims. This often occurs in multiple vehicle accidents or disasters. After making a quick scene survey, decide who must be cared for and transported first. This process of prioritizing or classifying injured victims is called *triage*. **Triage** comes from the French word *trier*, to sort. The goal is to do the greatest good for the greatest number of victims. Triage may require unpleasant decisions to withhold care from victims who are unlikely to survive so that lifesaving care can be given to those more likely to survive.

▶ Finding Life-Threatened Victims

A variety of systems are used to identify care and transportation priorities. To find the people needing immediate care for life-threatening conditions, first tell all victims who can get up and walk to move to a specific area. Victims who can get up and walk rarely have life-threatening injuries. These victims (*walking wounded*) are classified as needing delayed care (see the following definitions). Do not force a victim to move if he or she reports pain.

Find the life-threatened victims by performing only a primary check on all remaining victims. Assess motionless victims first. You must move rapidly (spend less than 60 seconds with each victim) from one victim to the next until all have been assessed. Classify victims according to the following care and transportation priorities:

1. Immediate care: Victim needs immediate care and transport to medical care as soon as possible.
   - Breathing difficulties
   - Severe bleeding
   - Severe burns
   - Signs of shock
   - Open chest or abdominal injuries

2. Delayed care: Care and transport can be delayed up to 1 hour.
   - Burns without airway problems
   - Major or multiple bone or joint injuries
   - Back injuries with or without suspected spinal cord damage
3. Walking wounded: Care and transportation can be delayed up to 3 hours.
   - Minor fractures
   - Minor wounds
4. Dead: Victim is obviously dead or unlikely to survive because of the type and extent of the injuries. This includes most cases of cardiac arrest due to injury.

Do not become involved in treating the victims at this point, but ask knowledgeable bystanders to provide care for immediate life-threatening problems (eg, bleeding).

Reassess victims regularly for changes in their condition. Only after victims with immediate life-threatening conditions receive care should people with less serious conditions be given care.

You may have to care for multiple victims without adequate help until more highly trained emergency personnel arrive. You will usually be relieved when more highly trained emergency personnel arrive on the scene. You may then be asked to provide first aid, to help move victims, or to help with ambulance or helicopter transportation.

Moving Victims

A victim should not be moved until he or she is ready for transportation to a hospital, if required. All necessary first aid should be provided before moving a victim. A victim should be moved only if there is an immediate danger, such as the following:
- There is a fire or danger of a fire.
- Explosives or other hazardous materials are involved.
- It is impossible to protect the scene from hazards.
- It is impossible to gain access to other victims in the situation who need lifesaving care (such as in a vehicle crash).

A cardiac arrest victim is usually moved unless he or she is already on the ground or floor because CPR must be performed on a firm, level surface.

FYI

Principles of Lifting

- Know your capabilities. Do not try to handle a load that is too heavy or awkward; seek help.
- Use a safe grip. Use as much of your palms as possible.
- Keep your back straight. Tighten the muscles of your buttocks and abdomen.
- Bend your knees to use the strong muscles of the thighs and buttocks.
- Keep your arms close to your body and your elbows flexed.
- Position your feet shoulder width apart for balance, one in front of the other.
- When lifting, keep and lift the victim close to your body.
- While lifting, do not twist your back; pivot with your feet.
- Lift and carry slowly, smoothly, and in unison with the other lifters.
- Before you move a victim, explain to him or her what you are doing.

CAUTION

DO NOT move a victim unless absolutely necessary, such as if the victim is in immediate danger or must be moved to shelter while waiting for EMS personnel to arrive.

DO NOT make the injury worse by moving the victim.

DO NOT move a victim who could have a spinal injury unless absolutely necessary due to other threats to life such as fire.

DO NOT move a victim without stabilizing the injured part.

DO NOT move a victim unless you know where you are going.

DO NOT leave an unconscious victim alone except for taking a short time to call 9-1-1.

DO NOT move a victim when you can send someone for help. Wait with the victim.

DO NOT try to move a victim by yourself if other people are available to help.

▶ Emergency Moves

The major danger in moving a victim quickly is the possibility of aggravating a spinal injury. In an emergency, every effort should be made to pull the victim in the direction of the long axis of the body to provide as much protection to the spinal cord as possible. If the victims are on the floor or ground, you can drag them away from the scene by using the various techniques shown in **Figure 25-6** to **Figure 25-19**.

▶ Nonemergency Moves

All injured parts should be stabilized before and during moving. If rapid transportation is not needed, it is helpful to practice on another person about the same size as the injured victim.

Stretcher or Litter

The safest way to carry an injured victim is on some type of stretcher or litter, which can be improvised. Before using it, test an improvised stretcher by lifting a rescuer about the same size as the victim.

Figure 25-6

Shoulder drag. Use for short distances over a rough surface; stabilize the victim's head with your forearms.

Figure 25-7

Ankle drag. This is the fastest method for a short distance on a smooth surface.

Figure 25-8

Blanket pull. Roll the victim onto a blanket, and pull from behind the victim's head.

- *Blanket-and-pole improvised stretcher.* If the blanket is properly wrapped, the victim's weight will keep it from unwinding **Figure 25-20**.
- *Blanket with no poles.* The blanket is rolled inward toward the victim and grasped for carrying by four or more rescuers.
- *Board-improvised stretcher.* These are sturdier than a blanket-and-pole stretcher but heavier and less comfortable. Tie the victim on to prevent him or her from rolling off **Figure 25-21**.
- *Commercial stretchers and litters.* These usually are not available except through EMS.

Figure 25-9

Human crutch (one person helps victim to walk). If one leg is injured, help the victim to walk on the good leg while you support the injured side.

Figure 25-10

Cradle carry. Use this method for children and lightweight adults who cannot walk.

Figure 25-11

Fire fighter's carry. If the victim's injuries permit, you can travel longer distances if you carry the victim over your shoulder.

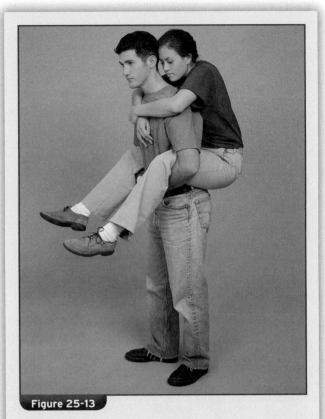

Figure 25-13

Piggyback carry. Use this method when the victim cannot walk but can use the arms to hang onto the rescuer.

Figure 25-12

Pack-strap carry. When injuries make the fire fighter's carry unsafe, this method is better for longer distances.

Figure 25-14

Two-person assist. This method is similar to the human crutch.

Figure 25-15

Two-handed seat carry.

Figure 25-16

Four-handed seat carry. This is the easiest two-person carry when no equipment is available and the victim cannot walk but can use the arms to hang onto the two rescuers.

Figure 25-17

Extremity carry.

Figure 25-18

Chair carry. This method is useful for a narrow passage or up or down stairs. Use a sturdy chair that can take the victim's weight.

Figure 25-20

Blanket-and-pole improvised stretcher.

Figure 25-21

Board-improvised stretcher.

Figure 25-19

Hammock carry. Three to six people stand on alternate sides of the injured person and link hands beneath the victim.

▶ Ready for Review

- Reach-throw-row-go identifies the sequence for attempting a water rescue.
- If a person has fallen through the ice near the shore, extend a pole or throw a line with a floatable object attached to it.
- Electrical injuries can be devastating.
- Almost any highway crash scene involves the potential danger of hazardous chemicals.
- In most states, you are legally obligated to stop and give help when you are involved in a motor vehicle crash.
- Should you encounter a fire, you should:
  - Get all people out fast.
  - Call 9-1-1.
- When you enter any emergency scene, look for signs of an animal and proceed with caution if the animal is not threatening.
- Emergencies involving farm animals can be dangerous to rescuers.
- A confined space is any area not intended for human occupancy that may have or develop a dangerous atmosphere.

- The goal of triage is to do the greatest good for the greatest number of victims.
- A variety of systems are used to identify care and transportation priorities.
- A victim should not be moved until he or she is ready for transportation to a hospital, if required.
- The major danger in moving a victim quickly is the possibility of aggravating a spinal injury.
- All injured parts should be stabilized before and during moving.

prep kit

▶ Vital Vocabulary

<u>triage</u> A system used for sorting victims to determine the order in which they will receive medical attention.

▶ Assessment in Action

You are fishing at the nearby lake. Several swimmers and others in canoes are also enjoying the lake. One swimmer decides to swim to the other side but begins to struggle about 30 feet off shore.

Directions: Circle Yes if you agree with the statement; circle No if you disagree.

Yes No **1.** This type of drowning situation is called distressed nonswimmer.

Yes No **2.** You are a very strong swimmer so you should immediately jump in the lake to rescue the victim.

Yes No **3.** You could try throwing a floating object to the victim.

Yes No **4.** The best option in this situation would be to use a canoe to rescue the victim.

▶ Check Your Knowledge

Directions: Circle Yes if you agree with the statement; circle No if you disagree.

Yes No **1.** You should attempt to move downed power lines away from a victim by using a broom or other wooden object.

Yes No **2.** Strong, unusual odors or clouds of vapor are possible indications of the presence of hazardous materials.

Yes No **3.** To keep from becoming trapped while attempting to extinguish a fire, you should always keep a door behind you for rapid exit.

Yes No **4.** In a situation involving several victims, those with breathing difficulties need immediate attention.

Yes No **5.** A major concern in moving a victim quickly is the possibility of aggravating a spinal injury.

Yes No **6.** "Row-throw-reach-go" represents the safe order for executing a water rescue.

Yes No **7.** In most states, you are legally obligated to stop and give help when you are involved in a motor vehicle crash.

Yes No **8.** The first thing to do in case of a fire is to use a fire extinguisher and try to put out the fire.

Yes No **9.** When using a fire extinguisher, aim it at the base of the flames.

Yes No **10.** When several people are injured, those crying or screaming should receive your attention first.

26 Disaster Preparedness

▶ Disaster Preparedness

Disasters are a fact of life. Each year thousands of disasters, large and small, natural and caused by humans, strike somewhere in the world. Many people have survived disasters, thanks to good luck and will-power, but that is not enough. Training about disasters needs to be modified from "nice to know" to "must know."

Valuable information about disasters is discussed in this chapter. This information is adapted from US government documents provided by the Federal Emergency Management Agency (FEMA), the US Department of Homeland Security, the National Weather Service, and the US Geological Survey.

▶ Natural Disasters

Natural disasters such as earthquakes, floods, hurricanes, and tornados claim many lives each year. Becoming informed about the dangers of natural disasters and the steps you can take to protect yourself and others can help minimize injuries and deaths.

Earthquake

An earthquake is a sudden, rapid shaking of the earth caused by the breaking and shifting of rock deep beneath the earth's surface. This

Figure 26-1

Devastation resulting from the California earthquake that crippled San Francisco in 1989.

shaking can cause buildings and bridges to collapse; disrupt gas, electric, and phone service; and sometimes trigger landslides, avalanches, flash floods, fires, and huge, destructive ocean waves known as *tsunamis*. Earthquakes can occur at any time of the year **Figure 26-1**.

What to Do During an Earthquake

Follow these safety guidelines if you experience an earthquake:

- If you are indoors, take cover under a sturdy desk, table, or bench or against an inside wall. If the earthquake is severe, crouch next to a large, sturdy object such as a refrigerator or file cabinet. Should the ceiling collapse, a triangle of space next to the object will provide a safe place. Stay away from glass, windows, outside doors, walls, and anything that could fall. If there is not a table or desk nearby, cover your face and head with your arms and crouch down, a door frame may offer some protection. Stay inside until the shaking has stopped and you are sure exiting is safe. It is dangerous to try to leave a building during an earthquake because objects can fall on you. Beware of aftershocks, and follow the same precautions as for an earthquake.
- If you are in bed, stay there, and protect your head with a pillow, unless you are under a heavy light or fan fixture that could fall. If the earthquake is severe, move to the floor next to but not under the bed. This will also provide a safe space if the ceiling collapses.

- If you are in a high-rise building, expect the fire alarms and sprinklers to go off during an earthquake. Do not use the elevators; use the stairs.
- If you are outdoors, find a clear spot away from buildings, trees, streetlights, and power lines. Drop to the ground and stay there until the shaking stops.
- If you are in a vehicle, pull over and stay there with your seatbelt fastened until the shaking has stopped. If the earthquake is severe and you are under a highway overpass, exit your car and lie next to, but not underneath your vehicle. The falling debris may crush the roof of the car, but beside the car will be a safe place for you to stay until help arrives.
- If you are trapped in debris, do not panic. Move carefully.
  - Do not use a flame for light due to gas leaks.
  - Do not move about or kick up dust.
  - Cover your mouth with a handkerchief or clothing.
  - Tap on a pipe or wall so rescuers can locate you.
- Learn how to turn off your gas supply where it enters the house. Turn off the gas if you smell gas or have to evacuate.
  - If you smell gas, do not use light switches or any other devices that can spark.

Flood

With the exception of fire, floods are the most common and widespread of all natural disasters. Most communities have experienced some type of flooding after heavy storms or winter snow thaws **Figure 26-2**. Pay attention to flash flood warnings even if skies are clear in your location because run-off can occur from storms miles away. Be especially aware of storms in hills above you. Flash floods occur when heavy rain causes run-off into channels and low-lying areas. The flood can be very fast and can occur miles from the rain, often catching people off-guard.

What to Do During a Flood

Follow these safety guidelines if conditions exist that could cause a flood:

- Be aware of the likelihood of flooding in your area. If there is any possibility of a flood or

Figure 26-2

Hurricane Katrina caused massive floods in New Orleans.

flash flood, move immediately to higher ground. Be aware of streams, drainage channels, canyons, and other areas prone to flooding quickly and suddenly.

- Listen to the radio or television stations for local information.
- If local authorities issue a flood watch, prepare to evacuate.
    - Secure your home, if you have time. Move essential items to upper floors.
    - If instructed, turn off utilities at the main switches or valves. Disconnect electrical appliances. Do not touch electrical equipment if you are wet or standing in water.
    - If you are not evacuating, you still need to prepare for the worst. If you do not have access to adequate bottled water, you can fill the bathtub with water in case water becomes contaminated or services are cut off. Before filling the tub, sterilize it with a diluted bleach solution (1 part bleach to 10 parts water).
- Do not walk through moving water. Six inches of moving water can knock you off your feet. Use a stick or pole to check the firmness of the ground and water depth in front of you.
- Do not drive into flooded areas. A foot of water can float a vehicle. Two feet of water can carry away most vehicles, including sport utility vehicles and pickups.
- If flood water rises around your car and you cannot drive out, abandon the car and move to higher ground, but only if you can do so safely.

Heat Wave

In extreme heat and high humidity, cooling of the body by evaporation is slowed and it is difficult for the body to maintain normal temperature **Figure 26-3**. People living in urban areas may be at greater risk from the effects of a prolonged heat wave than those living in rural areas. Asphalt and concrete store heat longer and gradually release heat at night. A devastating heat wave struck Europe in 2003, resulting in thousands of injuries and deaths.

What to Do During a Heat Wave

Follow these safety guidelines if you experience a heat wave emergency:

- Stay in the coolest available location. Stay indoors as much as possible. If air-conditioning is not available, stay on the lowest floor out of the sunshine. Circulate the air with a fan, and use cool, wet cloths to help keep your body temperature down.
- Drink plenty of water regularly, even if you do not feel thirsty.
- Avoid drinking alcoholic beverages because they cause further dehydration.
- Never leave children or pets alone in vehicles.
- Dress in loose-fitting clothes. Lightweight, light-colored clothing reflects heat and sunlight and helps maintain normal body temperature.
- Protect your face and head outdoors by wearing a wide-brimmed hat.
- Avoid too much sunshine. Sunburn slows the skin's ability to cool itself.
- Avoid strenuous work during the warmest part of the day (usually 10 AM to 3 PM).
- Spend at least 2 hours of the day in an air-conditioned place. If your home is not air-conditioned, consider spending the warmest part of the day in public buildings (for example, libraries, movie theaters, and shopping malls).
- Check on family, friends, and neighbors who do not have air-conditioning and who spend much of their time alone. Refer to Chapter 19 for first aid procedures for heat-related emergencies (for example, heat stroke, heat exhaustion, and heat cramps).

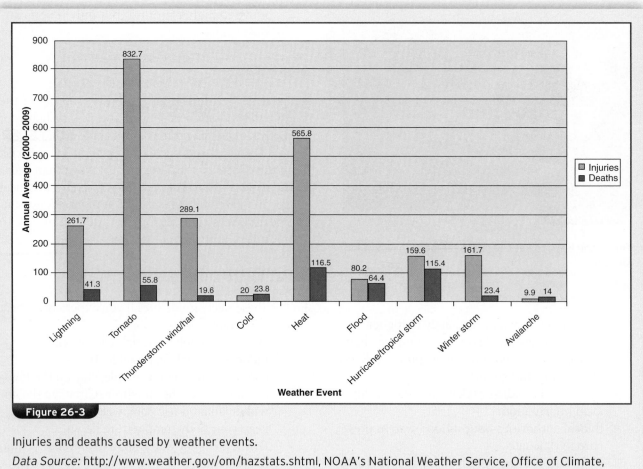

Figure 26-3

Injuries and deaths caused by weather events.

Data Source: http://www.weather.gov/om/hazstats.shtml, NOAA's National Weather Service, Office of Climate, Water, and Weather Services.

Hurricane

A hurricane is a tropical storm with winds that have reached a constant speed of at least 74 miles per hour. As a hurricane nears land, it can bring torrential rains, high winds, and flooding from the ocean, called storm surges. All Atlantic and Gulf of Mexico coastal areas are subject to hurricanes or tropical storms. August and September are the peak months of hurricane activity during the storm season, which lasts from June to November **Figure 26-4**. In the Pacific Ocean these storms are called typhoons.

Figure 26-4

Hurricanes are among the most costly and dangerous disasters.

What to Do During a Hurricane

Follow these safety guidelines if you experience the threat of a hurricane:

- Listen to the radio or television stations for local information. If a hurricane *watch* is issued, you usually have 24 to 36 hours before the hurricane hits land.

- Secure your home. Close any storm shutters. Secure outdoor objects or bring them indoors. Attach boards to window frames or tape windows to prevent or reduce the risk of broken glass. Park cars remaining at home along the side of the house. Make sure that all vehicles have a full tank of gas.

- If you are not evacuating, you need to prepare for the worst. Gather several days' supply of water and food for each household member. If you do not have access to adequate bottled water, fill the bathtub with water in case water becomes contaminated or services are cut off. Before filling the tub, sterilize it with a diluted bleach solution (1 part bleach to 10 parts water).
- If you are evacuating, prepare backpacks to take your disaster supplies with you to the shelter.
- When preparing to evacuate, fuel your vehicle and review evacuation routes. If instructed, turn off utilities at the main valves or switches before departing your residence.
- Evacuate to an inland location early if:
  - Local authorities announce an evacuation and you live in an evacuation zone.
  - You live in a mobile home near the path of the hurricane.
  - You live in a high-rise building near the path of the hurricane.
  - You live on the coast, on a flood plain near a river, or near an inland waterway.
  - You think you are in danger.
- Leave immediately if local authorities order an evacuation. Follow evacuation routes; stay away from coastal areas, riverbanks, and streams; and tell others where you are going.
- If you are not required to evacuate or are unable to evacuate, stay indoors and away from windows and glass doors during the hurricane.
- To protect yourself against the strong wind:
  - Take refuge in a small interior room, closet, or hallway.
  - Close all interior doors; secure and brace exterior doors.
  - In a multiple-story building, go to the first or second floor and stay in interior rooms away from the windows.
  - Lie on the floor under a table or other sturdy object if a hurricane or any associated tornado approaches.
- Phone lines are likely to be busy with emergency traffic. Avoid using the phone except for serious emergencies.

Q&A

What part does first aid play in disasters?

The value of first aid training for laypersons has increased during natural and man-made disasters. When a sudden disaster strikes, survivors often constitute the only source of initial help because medical help takes time to mobilize or is insufficient.

Reports from bombings in New York and London state that first aid by bystanders saved lives. In the Madrid bombings, 67 percent of the injured victims arrived at the hospital in nonambulance vehicles. Victim transport by bystanders occurs in many mass casualty disasters if ambulance transport is lacking. Officials interviewed after disasters strongly agree that first aid training for laypersons decreases death.

Source: Van de Velde, S, et al. 2009. Effectiveness of nonresuscitative first aid training in laypersons: a systematic review. *Ann Emerg Med.* 54(3):447-457.

Landslides

Landslides occur in almost every US state when masses of rock, earth, or debris move down a slope. They may be small or large and can move at slow or high speeds. They are usually associated with periods of heavy rainfall or rapid snowmelt.

What to Do During a Landslide

Follow these safety guidelines if conditions exist that could cause a landslide:

- Stay alert. Many landslides occur when people are sleeping.
- If you are in an area susceptible to landslides, consider evacuating if it is safe to do so.
- Listen for unusual sounds that might indicate moving debris, such as trees cracking, boulders knocking together, or rumbling.
- If you are near a stream or channel, be alert for any sudden increase or decrease in water flow and for a change from clear to muddy water. Such changes may indicate landslide activity upstream, so be prepared to move quickly.
- Be alert when driving. Embankments along roadsides are susceptible to landslides. Watch the road for collapsed pavement, mud, fallen rocks, and other indications of possible debris flow.

• If you remain at home, move to a second level if possible to distance yourself from the direct path of landslide debris.

Tornado

A tornado is a violent windstorm characterized by a twisting, funnel-shaped cloud. It is spawned by a thunderstorm (or sometimes as a result of a hurricane). Tornado season is generally March through August, although tornadoes can occur at any time of the year. Every state is at some risk from this hazard, but tornados are most frequently reported east of the Rocky Mountains **Figure 26-5** .

What to Do During a Tornado

Follow these safety guidelines if you experience a tornado. If you are at home:

• Go immediately to a windowless interior room, storm cellar, basement, or the lowest

Figure 26-5A

Figure 26-5B

A. Tornados are most frequently reported east of the Rocky Mountains. **B.** The tornado in Wichita Falls, Texas, in 1979 was one of the worst tornadoes in US history.

level of the building. If there is no basement, go to an inner hallway or a smaller inner room without windows, such as a bathroom or closet.

• Get under a piece of sturdy furniture (such as a heavy table or desk) and hold on to it.

If you are outdoors:

• If possible, get inside a building.

• If shelter is not available or there is no time to get indoors, lie in a ditch or low-lying area or crouch near a strong building.

If you are at work or school:

• Avoid places with wide-span roofs such as auditoriums, cafeterias, large hallways, and shopping malls.

• Go to a predetermined shelter area (signs are usually posted).

• Get under a piece of sturdy furniture (such as a heavy table, desk, or workbench).

If you are in a vehicle:

• Do not try to outrun a tornado.

• Get out of the vehicle immediately and take shelter in a nearby building. If there is no time to get indoors, get out of the car and lie in a ditch or low-lying area away from the vehicle.

Tsunami

A **tsunami** (pronounced soo-nahm′ee) is a series of waves generated by an undersea disturbance (for example, an earthquake). From the area of disturbance, the waves travel outward in all directions, much like the ripples caused by throwing a rock into a pond. Tsunamis reaching heights of more than 100 feet have been recorded near coastlines, although most waves are less than 18 feet high. Areas of greatest risk are less than 50 feet above sea level and within 1 mile of the shoreline. Drowning is the most common cause of death due to a tsunami.

What to Do During a Tsunami

Follow these safety guidelines if conditions exist that could cause a tsunami:

• Listen to the radio or television stations for the latest local emergency information. If you are advised to evacuate, do so immediately.

• Stay away from the area until local authorities say it is safe to return.

- Do not go to the shoreline to watch for a tsunami. If you can see the wave, you are too close to escape it. Because a tsunami is a series of waves, do not assume that one wave means the danger is over.

Volcano Eruption

A volcano is a mountain that opens downward to a reservoir of molten rock below the earth's surface. When the pressure from gases and molten rock becomes strong enough to cause an explosion, eruptions occur. Gases and rock shoot up through the opening and spill over the mountainsides and/or spew into the air. Most injuries and deaths are due to ash, falling rocks, landslides, and floods, rather than hot flowing lava.

What to Do During a Volcano Eruption

Follow these safety guidelines if a volcano erupts:
- Follow the evacuation order issued by local authorities. Avoid areas downwind from the volcano.

If caught indoors:
- Close all windows, doors, and chimney and stove dampers.

If caught outdoors:
- Seek shelter indoors.
- Avoid low-lying areas where poisonous gases can collect and flash floods and lava- and mudflows can be dangerous.
- Put all machinery inside a garage or barn.

Protect yourself:
- Wear long-sleeved shirts and pants.
- Use goggles to protect your eyes.
- Use a dust mask or hold a damp cloth over your face to keep from breathing in the hot ash or gases.

Storm Watch vs Storm Warning

Government agencies such as the National Weather Service issue alerts when threats arise. A watch, such as a tornado watch, is issued when conditions are ripe for the development of that threat. A warning is issued if the threat is actually occurring or has been detected.

- Stay out of the area around the erupting volcano. Trying to watch an erupting volcano can be deadly.

Wildfire

Forest, brush, and grass fires can occur at any time of the year, but mostly during long, dry hot spells. The majority of these fires are caused by human carelessness or ignorance **Figure 26-6** .

What to Do During a Wildfire

Follow these safety guidelines if a wildfire occurs:
- Listen to local radio or television stations for the latest emergency information.
- If advised to evacuate, do so immediately. Choose a route away from the fire hazard. Watch for changes in the speed and direction of fire and smoke. Do not block firefighting entrance routes.

Winter Storm

Heavy snowfall and extreme cold can immobilize an entire region. Even areas that usually experience mild winters can be hit with a major snowstorm or extreme cold **Figure 26-7** .

What to Do During a Winter Storm

Follow these safety guidelines if a winter storm occurs. If indoors:

Figure 26-6

Wildfires can move quickly, threatening lives and homes.

Figure 26-7

Major winter snowstorms can tie up a city.

- Listen to the local radio or television stations or NOAA (National Oceanic and Atmospheric Administration) weather radio for weather reports and emergency information.
- Conserve fuel by lowering the thermostat to 65° F during the day and 55° F at night. Close off unused rooms.
- Eat regularly and drink ample fluids, but avoid caffeine and alcohol.
- If using kerosene heaters, maintain ventilation, refuel the heater outside, and keep heaters at least 3 feet from flammable objects.
- Never use heat sources designed for outside use in a closed space.

If outdoors:

- Dress warmly (that is, several layers of loose fitting clothing, a hat, and a scarf to cover your mouth and protect your lungs).
- Avoid overexertion (for example, shoveling snow or pushing a car), which can bring on a heart attack.
- Be aware of signs of frostbite and hypothermia.
- Keep dry by changing wet clothing, which does not insulate well.

If trapped in a vehicle during a winter storm:

- Pull off the highway. Turn on the vehicle's hazard lights. Hang a distress flag from the window or radio antenna.
- Stay inside the vehicle. Rescuers are more likely to find you. Do not set out on foot unless you can see a building close by where you know you can take shelter.

- Run the engine and heater about 10 minutes each hour to keep warm. When the engine is running, open a window slightly for ventilation, and clear snow from the exhaust pipe to prevent carbon monoxide poisoning.
- Exercise (for example, clap your hands and move your arms and legs occasionally) to maintain body heat, but avoid overexertion.
- In extreme cold, use floor mats, seat covers, road maps, newspapers, and other available resources for insulation. Huddle with other passengers.
- Take turns sleeping. One person should be awake at all times to look for rescue crews.
- Drink fluids to avoid dehydration.
- Watch for signs of frostbite and hypothermia.
- Be careful not to waste battery power.
- At night, turn on the inside light so work crews or rescuers can see you.
- Once the winter storm passes, you may need to leave the car and proceed on foot.

FYI

Winter Travel Supplies

When traveling during the winter, carry disaster supplies in the vehicle. The kit should include the following:

- Shovel
- Windshield scraper
- Flashlight
- Extra batteries
- Battery-powered radio
- Water
- Snack food
- Gloves and mittens
- Hat
- Blanket
- Tow chain or rope
- Tire chains
- Bag of road salt and sand
- Fluorescent distress flag
- Jumper or booster cables
- Road maps
- Emergency flares
- Cellular telephone
- Emergency heating candles and container

▶ Technological Hazards

Hazardous Materials Incidents

Chemicals are found everywhere. They can become hazardous during their production, storage, transportation, and disposal. It is not always possible to identify a situation as one involving hazardous materials, but clues such as a leaking cargo trailer, color-coded placards (signs) on abandoned drums, and unusual odors can be good indicators **Figure 26-8**.

What to Do During a Hazardous Materials Incident

Follow these safety guidelines if a hazardous materials incident occurs:

- If you witness an incident that you believe to be a hazardous materials incident, call 9-1-1 or your local emergency telephone number.
- Stay away from the incident site.
- If caught outside, remember that gases and mists are usually heavier than air. Try to stay upstream, uphill, and upwind. Try to go at least one-half mile from the danger area.
- If in a vehicle, stop and seek shelter in a permanent building if possible. If you must remain in the vehicle, keep the windows and vents closed and shut off the air-conditioner and heater.
- If asked to evacuate your home, do so immediately.

Figure 26-8

Fumes leaking from a cargo truck could be an indication of a hazardous materials incident.

- If requested to stay indoors rather than evacuate:
  - Follow all instructions and close all exterior doors, windows, vents, and fireplace dampers.
  - Turn off air-conditioners and ventilation systems.
  - Go into an above-ground room with the fewest openings to the outside; close the doors and windows; tape around the sides, bottom, and top of the door; and cover each window and vent in the room with a single piece of plastic sheeting.
  - Listen to local emergency broadcasts.
  - When advised that it is safe to leave your shelter, open all doors and windows and turn on air-conditioning and ventilation systems to flush out any chemicals that infiltrated the building.

Nuclear Power Plants

Nuclear power plants operate in most states and produce about 20% of the nation's power. Nearly 3 million Americans live within 10 miles of an operating nuclear power plant. Although these plants are closely monitored and regulated, unintentional radiation exposures are possible. Local and state governments, federal agencies, and electric utility companies have emergency response plans for nuclear power plant incidents.

What to Do During a Nuclear Power Plant Emergency

Follow these safety guidelines in a nuclear power plant emergency:

- Stay tuned to local radio and television stations. Local authorities will provide specific information and instructions.
- Evacuate if you are advised to do so.
- If told not to evacuate, remain indoors. Close the doors and windows and turn off the air-conditioner, ventilation fans, furnace, and other air intakes. Go to a basement or other underground area if possible. Keep a battery-powered radio with you at all times.
- Do not use the telephone unless absolutely necessary. Lines will be needed for emergency calls.

FYI

Disaster Myths

Myth: Disasters are truly exceptional events.

Reality: They are a normal part of daily life and in many cases are repetitive events.

Myth: Disasters kill people without respect for social class or economic status.

Reality: The poor and marginalized are more at risk of death than are rich people or the middle classes.

Myth: People can survive for many days when trapped under the rubble of a collapsed building.

Reality: The vast majority of people brought out alive from the rubble are saved within 24 or perhaps even 12 hours of impact.

Myth: When disaster strikes, panic is a common reaction.

Reality: Most people behave rationally in a disaster. While panic is not to be ruled out entirely, it is of such limited importance that some leading disaster sociologists regard it as insignificant or unlikely.

Myth: After disaster has struck, survivors tend to be dazed and apathetic.

Reality: Survivors rapidly start reconstruction. Activism is much more common than fatalism (this is the so-called "therapeutic community"). Even in the worst scenarios, only 15–30 percent of victims show passive or dazed reactions.

Myth: Looting is a common and serious problem after disasters.

Reality: Looting is rare and limited in scope. It mainly occurs when there are strong preconditions, as when a community is already deeply divided.

Myth: Disease epidemics are an almost inevitable result of the disruption and poor health caused by major disasters.

Reality: Generally, the level of epidemiological surveillance and health care in the disaster area is sufficient to stop any possible disease epidemic from occurring. However, the rate of diagnosis of diseases may increase as a result of improved health care.

Myth: In order to manage a disaster well, it is necessary to accept all forms of aid that are offered.

Reality: It is better to limit acceptance of donations to goods and services that are actually needed in the disaster area.

Myth: Unburied dead bodies constitute a health hazard.

Reality: Not even advanced decomposition causes a significant health hazard. Hasty burial demoralizes survivors and upsets arrangements for death certification, funeral rites, and, where needed, autopsy.

Myth: One should donate used clothes to victims of disasters.

Reality: This often leads to accumulations of huge quantities of useless garments that victims cannot or will not wear.

Myth: Companies, corporations, associations, and governments are always very generous when invited to send aid and relief to disaster areas.

Reality: They may be, but in the past disaster areas have been used as dumping grounds for outdated medicines, obsolete equipment, and unusable goods, all under the cloak of apparent generosity.

Myth: There is usually a shortage of resources when disaster occurs and this prevents them from being managed effectively.

Reality: The shortage, if it occurs, is almost always very temporary. There is more of a problem in deploying resources well and using them efficiently than in acquiring them. Often, there is also a problem of coping with a superabundance of certain types of resources.

Source: Alexander D E. Misconception as a barrier to teaching about disasters. *Prehosp Disaster Med.* March–April 2007, page 97.

- If you suspect exposure, take a thorough shower. Change clothes and shoes. Put all exposed clothing in a plastic bag. Seal the bag and place it out of the way.
- Seek medical care for any symptoms, such as nausea, that may be related to radiation exposure.

▶ National Security Emergencies

Terrorism

<u>Terrorism</u> is the use of force or violence against persons or property in violation of the criminal laws of the United States for purposes of intimidation, coercion, or ransom. Acts of terrorism range from threats of terrorism, assassinations, kidnappings, hijackings, bomb scares and bombings, and cyber attacks (computer based) to the use of chemical, biologic, and nuclear weapons **Figure 26-9** .

The Homeland Security Advisory System is designed to provide quick, comprehensive information about the potential threat of terrorist attacks or threat levels. Threat conditions can apply nationally, regionally, by industry, or by specific target. You should be aware of the current Homeland Security threat level at all times **Table 26-1** .

Chemical and Biologic Agents

<u>Chemical warfare agents</u> are poisonous vapors, aerosols, liquids, or solids that have toxic effects on people, animals, or plants. They can be released by bombs; sprayed from aircraft, boats, or vehicles; or used in liquid form to create a hazard to people and the environment. Some chemical agents may be odorless and tasteless. They can have an immediate effect (a few seconds to a few minutes) or a delayed effect (several hours to several days). Although potentially lethal, chemical agents are difficult to deliver in lethal concentrations. Outdoors, the agents often dissipate rapidly.

<u>Biologic agents</u> are organisms or toxins that can kill or incapacitate people, livestock, and crops. The three basic groups of biologic agents likely to be used as weapons are bacteria, viruses, and toxins.

What to Do During a Chemical or Biologic Attack

If a chemical or biologic weapon attack occurs near you, authorities will instruct you on the best course of action, which may be to evacuate the area immediately,

Table 26-1 Homeland Security Advisory System	
Threat Level	**Protective Measures You Should Take**
Severe	Avoid high-risk areas such as public gatherings.
	Listen attentively to news for advisories and instructions.
	Contact employers to determine work status.
High	Review evacuation and sheltering measures for different types of attacks (chemical, biologic, or radiologic).
Elevated	Watch and report any suspicious activity. Contact school(s) to determine their emergency procedures.
Guarded	Review home disaster plan and update supplies.
	Meet with your family to discuss what to do, where to go, and how to communicate if an attack occurs.
Low	Develop a home disaster plan and disaster supply kit.

Figure 26-9

The September 11, 2001, terrorist attacks on the World Trade Center in New York City.

seek shelter at a designated location, or take immediate shelter where you are and seal the premises. The best way to protect yourself is to take emergency preparedness measures ahead of time and get medical attention as soon as possible, if needed.

Follow these additional safety guidelines if a chemical or biologic attack occurs:

- Listen to the local radio or television stations for instructions from authorities, such as whether to remain inside or to evacuate.
- If instructed to remain in your home, office building, or other shelter during a chemical or biologic attack:
  - Turn off all ventilation, including furnaces, air-conditioners, vents, and fans.
  - Seek shelter in an internal room, preferably one without windows. Seal the room with duct tape and plastic sheeting.
  - Avoid the furnace or utility room.
  - Do not use any major appliances (for example, the furnace, oven or range, clothes dryer, or washing machine).
- Remain in protected areas where toxic vapors are reduced or eliminated, and take a battery-operated radio with you.
- If caught in an unprotected area, try to get upwind of the contaminated area, try to find shelter inside a building as quickly as possible, and listen to the radio for official instructions.

Nuclear and Radiologic Weapons

Nuclear explosions can cause deadly effects such as blinding light, intense heat (thermal radiation), initial nuclear radiation, blast fires started by the heat pulse, and secondary fires caused by the destruction. Surface level explosions also produce radioactive particles called *fallout* that can be carried by wind for hundreds of miles.

Terrorist use of a radiologic dispersion device—often called a dirty bomb—is considered far more likely than use of a nuclear device. These radiologic weapons are a combination of conventional explosives and radioactive material designed to scatter dangerous and sublethal amounts of radioactive material over a general area. There is no way of knowing how much warning time there would be before an attack by a terrorist using a nuclear or radiologic weapon.

What to Do During a Nuclear or Radiologic Attack

Follow these safety guidelines if a nuclear or radiologic attack occurs:

- Avoid looking at the flash or fireball; it can blind you.

FYI

Disaster Preparedness

The US Department of Homeland Security offers these general guidelines for food and water needs for survival during emergency situations.

Water

- One gallon of water per person per day, for drinking and sanitation.
- Keep at least a 3-day supply of water per person.
- Children, nursing mothers, and people who are ill may need more water.
- If you live in a warm weather climate, more water may be necessary.

Food

- Store at least a 3-day supply of nonperishable food.
- Select foods that require no refrigeration, preparation, or cooking and little or no water.
- Pack a manual can opener and eating utensils.
- Choose foods your family will eat:
  - Ready-to-eat canned meats, fruits, and vegetables
  - Protein or fruit bars
  - Dry cereal or granola
  - Peanut butter
  - Dried fruit
  - Nuts
  - Crackers
  - Canned juices
  - Nonperishable pasteurized milk
  - High-energy foods
  - Vitamins
  - Food for infants
  - Comfort foods

First Aid Kit

- See Appendix A for suggestions for your first aid kit.

- If you hear an attack warning:
  - Take cover as quickly as you can, below ground if possible, and stay there until instructed to do otherwise.
  - If caught outside and unable to get inside immediately, take cover behind anything that might offer protection. Lie flat on the ground and cover your head.
  - If the explosion is some distance away, it could take 30 seconds or more for the blast wave to hit. Be aware of a second, returning blast wave.
  - Protect yourself from radioactive fallout by taking shelter, even if you are many miles from the source of the explosion.
  - Keep a battery-powered radio with you, and listen for official information. Follow the instructions given. Local instructions should always take precedence; officials in your area know the local situation best.

▶ Summary

"The farther you are from the last disaster, the closer you are to the next one" is an often-quoted statement made by emergency preparedness specialists. This is an age of catastrophe. Every American will likely be an unfortunate victim or witness to at least one disaster during his or her lifetime. The tragedy is that each citizen can be better prepared than he or she is now for that disaster. When a disaster strikes, you must be ready to act.

prep kit

▶ Ready for Review

- Disasters are a fact of life and you need to be prepared.
- Natural disasters such as earthquakes, floods, hurricanes, and tornados claim many lives each year.
- Chemicals are found everywhere; they can be hazardous during their production, storage, transportation, and disposal.
- Terrorism is the use of force or violence against persons or property in violation of the criminal laws of the United States for purposes of intimidation, coercion, or ransom.
- When disaster strikes, you must be ready to act.

▶ Vital Vocabulary

<u>biologic agents</u> Organisms or toxins that can kill or incapacitate people, livestock, and crops.

<u>chemical warfare agents</u> Poisonous vapors, aerosols, liquids, or solids that have toxic effects.

<u>terrorism</u> Use of force or violence against persons or property in violation of criminal laws for purposes of intimidation, coercion, or ransom.

<u>tsunami</u> A series of waves generated by an undersea disturbance.

▶ Assessment in Action

Seismologists have been predicting a large earthquake for your region of the country within the next 10 years. While at work on the top floor of your three-story office building, the predictions come true. Sudden shaking begins and you feel the building move. Wall hangings and items on shelves begin to fall to the ground.

Directions: Circle Yes if you agree with the statement; circle No if you disagree.

Yes　No　**1.** This is most likely not the "big one," so you can continue your work as normal.

Yes　No　**2.** You should take cover under your desk.

Yes　No　**3.** You should call 9-1-1 to report the emergency.

Yes　No　**4.** You should know all the exit routes from your building.

Yes　No　**5.** If you smell gas, you should not delay your evacuation from the building.

▶ Check Your Knowledge

Directions: Circle Yes if you agree with the statement; circle No if you disagree.

Yes　No　**1.** Earthquakes most often occur in the winter.

Yes　No　**2.** Never walk through moving water.

Yes　No　**3.** People in urban areas may be at greater risk from the effects of a prolonged heat wave than those in rural areas.

Yes　No　**4.** Hurricane season is from April until August.

Yes　No　**5.** Hide in a room with open windows if you are in the path of a tornado.

Yes　No　**6.** Never go near the shoreline to watch for a tsunami.

Yes　No　**7.** If you are trapped inside your car during a winter storm, run the engine and heater 10 minutes each hour to keep warm.

Yes　No　**8.** If you witness a hazardous materials incident, get up close to find out the name of the hazardous material before calling 9-1-1.

Yes　No　**9.** You should be aware of the Homeland Security threat level at all times.

Yes　No　**10.** All chemical agents have a smell or taste.

appendix
A

First Aid Supplies

▶ First Aid Supplies

Many injuries and sudden illnesses can be cared for without medical attention. For these situations and for situations requiring medical attention later, it is a good idea to have useful supplies on hand for emergencies.

Supplies in a first aid kit should be customized to include those items likely to be used on a regular basis. For example, a kit for the home may be different from one at a workplace or one found on a boat.

The list here includes nonprescription (over-the-counter) medications. Some drug products lose their potency over time, especially after they have been opened. Therefore, buying a large, family size of a product that you use infrequently may not be economical. Note the expiration date on every medication.

Keep all medicines out of the reach of children. Read and follow all directions for properly using medications. Consider keeping your first aid supplies in either a fishing tackle box or a tool box.

First Aid Kits

The following recommended items should be stocked inside a first aid kit in the workplace, at home, and for travel. First aid kits should be:

- Impact resistant and made of durable material to protect against moisture, dust, and contamination
- Portable and easily carried by a handle
- Of sufficient size to store the equipment listed
- Clearly marked as being a first aid kit by words and/or symbols
- Regularly inspected and updated for completeness and content condition

Workplace First Aid Kit

Equipment	Minimum Quantity
1. Adhesive strip bandages (1″ × 3″)	20
2. Triangular bandages (muslin, 36″–40″, 52″–56″)	4

Gauze pads

Nonstick pads

Figure A-1

Gauze pads and nonstick pads.

3. Sterile eye pads (2⅛″ × 2⅝″)	2
4. Sterile gauze pads (4″ × 4″) **Figure A-1**	6
5. Sterile nonstick pads (3″ × 4″) Figure A-1	6
6. Sterile trauma pads (5″ × 9″) **Figure A-2**	2
7. Sterile trauma pads (8″ × 10″) Figure A-2	1
8. Sterile conforming roller gauze (2″ width) **Figure A-3**	3 rolls
9. Sterile conforming roller gauze (4½″ width) Figure A-3	3 rolls
10. Waterproof tape (1″ × 5 yards)	1 roll
11. Porous adhesive tape (2″ × 5 yards)	1 roll
12. Elastic roller bandages (4″ and 6″) **Figure A-4**	1 each
13. Antiseptic skin wipes, individually wrapped **Figure A-5**	10

Figure A-2

Trauma dressings.

Figure A-4

Elastic roller bandages.

Figure A-3

Gauze rolls and conforming, self-adhering roller bandages.

Figure A-5

Antiseptic towelettes and alcohol prep pads.

14. Medical-grade exam gloves (medium, large, extra large), conforming to FDA requirements   2 pairs per size

     Figure A-6

15. Mouth-to-barrier device, either a face mask with a one-way valve or a disposable face shield Figure A-6   1

Figure A-6

Exam gloves and face mask.

Figure A-7

EMT shears, bandage scissors, regular scissors, tweezers, and knife.

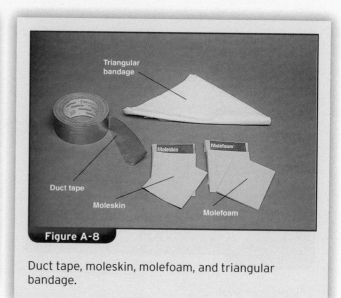

Figure A-8

Duct tape, moleskin, molefoam, and triangular bandage.

16. Disposable instant-activating cold packs ... 2
17. Resealable plastic bags (quart size) ... 2
18. Padded malleable splint (4″ × 36″) ... 1
19. Emergency blanket, Mylar ... 1
20. EMT shears (with one serrated edge) **Figure A-7** ... 1
21. Splinter tweezers (about 3″ long) ... 1
22. Biohazard waste bag (3½ gallon capacity) ... 2
23. First aid and CPR manual and list of local emergency telephone numbers ... 1

Home First Aid Kit

The American College of Emergency Physicians recommends that a home first aid kit include the following:

1. Acetaminophen, ibuprofen, and aspirin tablets: for headaches, pain, fever, and simple sprains or strains of the body. (Aspirin should not be used for relief of flu symptoms or given to children.)
2. Antihistamine: to relieve allergies and inflammation. Use appropriate dosages and make sure the medicine is age appropriate.
3. Cough suppressant: to relieve coughing. Use appropriate dosages and make sure the medicine is age appropriate.
4. Decongestant tablets: to relieve nasal congestion from colds or allergies. Use appropriate dosages and make sure the medicine is age appropriate.
5. Antiseptic wipes: to disinfect wounds or clean hands.
6. Thermometer: to take temperature. For infants younger than 1 year, use a rectal thermometer.
7. Calamine lotion: to relieve itching and irritation from insect bites and stings and poison ivy.
8. Hydrocortisone ointment: to relieve irritation from rashes.
9. Elastic wraps: for wrapping wrist, ankle, knee, and elbow injuries.
10. Triangular bandage: for wrapping injuries and making arm slings **Figure A-8** .
11. Scissors with rounded tips.
12. Adhesive tape **Figure A-9** and 2″ gauze: for dressing wounds.
13. Disposable, instant-activating ice bags: for icing injuries and treating high fevers.
14. Bandages of assorted sizes **Figure A-10** : for covering minor cuts and scrapes.
15. Antibiotic ointment: for burns, cuts, and scrapes.
16. Gauze in rolls and in 2″ and 4″ pads: for dressing wounds.

Figure A-9

Eye patches, knuckle and fingertip bandages, and tape.

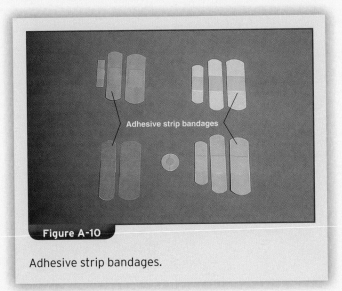

Figure A-10

Adhesive strip bandages.

17. Bandage closures, ¼″ and 1″: for taping cut edges together.
18. Tweezers: to remove small splinters and ticks.
19. Safety pins: to fasten splints and bandages.
20. Medical-grade exam gloves to protect your hands and reduce the risk of infection when treating open wounds.

21. First aid manual.
22. List of emergency phone numbers.

Travel First Aid Kit

The American College of Emergency Physicians recommends that a travel first aid kit include the following:

1. Aspirin, acetaminophen, or ibuprofen: for headaches, pain, fever, and simple sprains or strains of the body. (Aspirin should not be used for relief of flu symptoms or given to children.)
2. Antiseptic wipes: to disinfect wounds or clean hands, tweezers, scissors, and thermometer.
3. Calamine lotion: to relieve itching and irritation from insect bites and stings and poison ivy.
4. Gauze in rolls and 2″ and 4″ pads: to dress larger cuts and scrapes.
5. Antihistamine/decongestant cough medicine.
6. Antinausea/motion sickness medication.
7. Bandages of assorted sizes, including adhesive bandages.
8. Adhesive tape and 2″ gauze: for dressing wounds.
9. Elastic wraps: for wrapping wrist, ankle, knee, and elbow injuries.
10. Triangular bandage: for wrapping injuries and making arm slings.
11. Scissors with rounded tips.
12. Medical-grade exam gloves: to reduce the risk of infection.
13. Disposable, instant-activating ice bags: for icing injuries and treating high fevers.
14. Antifungal cream (tolnaftate 1% or clotrimazole 1%): good for athlete's foot or ringworm.
15. Antibiotic ointment: for burns, cuts, and scrapes.
16. Thermometer with case.
17. Sunscreen: SPF 30 or higher **Figure A-11**.
18. Insect repellent: those that contain 35%–55% DEET with stabilizer.
19. Antidiarrheal medications, tablets or liquid; follow directions carefully.
20. Antimalaria medications (if indicated).
21. Water-purifying pills or liquid or mechanical filtration devices.

Figure A-11

Insect repellent, aloe vera gel, sunscreen, instant ice pack, commercially available burn dressing, and lip balm.

Figure A-12

Emergency blanket, cotton-tipped swabs, safety pins, and SAM splint.

22. Corticosteroid cream, such as hydrocortisone cream.
23. Tweezers: to remove small splinters and ticks.
24. Safety pins: to fasten splints and bandages **Figure A-12**.

Medication Information

As a first aider, you might be in a situation that requires you to give a victim certain medications (or to assist a victim in taking his or her own medication). A knowledgeable first aider should be familiar with the following medications:

Over-the-counter pain relievers:
- Acetaminophen
- Aspirin
- Ibuprofen
- Naproxen

Physician-prescribed medications:
- Metered-dose inhaler
- Nitroglycerin
- Epinephrine

Over-the-counter medications carried in a first aid kit or available from the victim:
- Oral glucose

▶ Pros and Cons of Popular Pain Relievers

Acetaminophen

Brand names: Tylenol
Advantages: Relieves pain and fever, does not irritate stomach
Disadvantages: Heavy or prolonged use can damage liver

Aspirin

Brand names: Bufferin, Anacin, Bayer
Advantages: Relieves pain, fever, inflammation; useful for heart attacks and their prevention
Disadvantages: Interferes with blood clotting; might trigger stomach bleeding; can cause Reye's syndrome in children with viral infections

Ibuprofen

Brand names: Advil, Nuprin, Motrin
Advantages: Relieves pain, fever, and inflammation

Disadvantages: Interferes with clotting; can cause stomach bleeding, ulcers, irritation; heavy or prolonged use can damage liver and kidneys

Naproxen

Brand name: Aleve
Advantages: Relieves pain, fever, and inflammation; one dose lasts 8 to 12 hours
Disadvantages: Can cause stomach bleeding, ulcers, irritation; prolonged use can harm kidneys

▶ Nitroglycerin

Give a victim nitroglycerin (trade name Nitrostat) if the following conditions exist:
- The victim is an adult.
- The victim has chest pain.
- The victim has physician-prescribed sublingual tablets or spray.

Do *not* give a victim nitroglycerin if any of the following conditions applies:
- The victim has a head injury.
- The victim is an infant or a child.
- The victim has already taken three doses.

Medication forms: tablet (about one tenth the size of an aspirin), sublingual spray, and patch.
Dosage: One dose.

Procedure

Once you have decided to administer nitroglycerin, follow these steps:

1. Check the expiration date of nitroglycerin.
2. Ask the victim about the last dose taken.
3. Ask the victim to lift his or her tongue. Place the tablet or spray dose under the tongue or have the victim do so. Do not touch the tablet—wear gloves because your skin can absorb nitroglycerin and your blood pressure may be affected.

4. Have the victim keep his or her mouth closed (if doing so will not interfere with easy breathing) with the tablet under the tongue (without swallowing) until the tablet dissolves and is absorbed.

Actions

Nitroglycerin takes the following actions:
- Relaxes (dilates) blood vessels
- Reduces the workload of the heart

Side Effects

Side effects of nitroglycerin include the following:
- Lower blood pressure (victim should sit or lie down)
- Headache
- Heart rate changes

▶ Epinephrine Auto-Injector

Give a victim epinephrine (trade name Adrenaline, Epi-pen) if both of the following conditions exist:
- The victim exhibits signs of a severe allergic reaction (includes breathing distress or shock).
- The victim has physician-prescribed medication.

Medication form: liquid from automatic needle-and-syringe injection system.

Dosage

- Adult: One adult auto-injector (0.3 mg)
  Figure B-1
- Child/infant: One infant/child auto-injector (0.15 mg)

Figure B-1

Auto-injectors.

Procedure

Use these steps when administering epinephrine:
1. Obtain the victim's physician-prescribed auto-injector.
2. Remove the safety cap.
3. Place the tip of the auto-injector against the victim's thigh.
4. Push the injector firmly against the thigh to inject medication.
5. Hold the injector in place for 10 seconds.
6. Call 9-1-1.

Actions

Epinephrine takes the following actions:
- Dilates the bronchioles (small tubes in lungs)
- Constricts blood vessels

Side Effects

Epinephrine has the following side effects:
- Increased heart rate
- Dizziness
- Headache
- Chest pain
- Nausea
- Vomiting
- Anxiety

▶ Metered-Dose Inhaler

Give a victim a metered-dose inhaler (trade names Albuterol, Proventil, Ventolin) if the victim is experiencing asthma, difficulty breathing with wheezing.

Dosage

- Adult/child: 1 to 2 inhalations

Procedure

Use these steps when administering a metered-dose inhaler:
1. Obtain the victim's physician-prescribed inhaler.
2. Coach the victim to take one to two inhalations while pressing the inhaler. The victim must inhale all medication in one breath.

3. Coach the victim to hold breath for 5 seconds after inhalation.

4. Wait 5 minutes before repeating dose.

Actions

A metered-dose inhaler takes the following actions:

- Stimulates the nervous system
- Causes bronchodilation

Side Effects

A metered-dose inhaler has the following side effects:

- Hypertension
- Increased heart rate
- Anxiety
- Restlessness

▶ Oral Glucose

Give a victim oral glucose if all of the following conditions exist:

- The victim has low blood glucose (hypoglycemia, insulin reaction).
- The victim is able to swallow.
- The victim is alert and able to follow instructions.

Dosage

Adult: 1 tube of gel or three tablets

Procedure

Use these steps when administering oral glucose:

1. Coach the victim to squeeze oral glucose between a cheek and the gum, then let it dissolve.

2. If the victim experiences a decline in responsiveness or there is no improvement in the low glucose after 15 minutes, call 9-1-1. If the patient remains alert, repeat the dose while awaiting EMS arrival.

Actions

When oral glucose is absorbed by the body, it provides glucose for cell use.

Side Effects

Oral glucose has the following side effects:

- Nausea
- Vomiting

appendix C

Health Care Provider Basic Life Support

A health care provider is a person who provides health care as part of his or her job responsibilities. Examples include physicians, nurses, paramedics, and athletic trainers. Health care providers work in a variety of settings such as emergency medical services, hospitals, medical clinics, and athletic facilities. These professionals perform basic life support techniques differently than lay persons. Lifeguards are often taught two-rescuer CPR procedures.

▶ One-Rescuer Adult CPR

If you see a motionless person, do the following:

1. *Check for responsiveness* **Figure C-1**.
   - Check the scene for hazards.
   - Tap the victim's shoulder.
   - Shout, "Are you OK?"
2. *If no response, call 9-1-1 and get an AED.*
   - If you are alone with the victim, shout for help.
   - If someone responds, send him or her to call 9-1-1 and get an AED.
   - If no one responds, call 9-1-1 and get an AED, if available.
3. *Check pulse* **Figure C-2**.
   - Keep the victim's head tilted with your hand that is nearest the head.
   - Using your hand nearest the victim's feet, locate the Adam's apple (larynx) with two or three fingers.
   - Slide your fingers down into the groove of the neck on the side closest to you (do not use your thumb because you might feel your own pulse).
   - Feel for the carotid pulse for 5 to 10 seconds.
   - If there is a pulse:
     - Give a normal breath every 5 to 6 seconds.
     - Each breath lasts 1 second.
     - Use the head tilt–chin lift method.

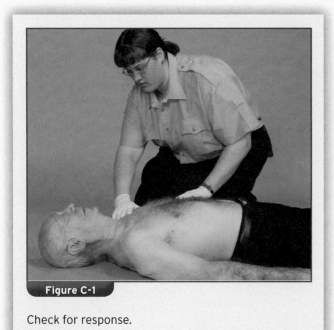

Figure C-1

Check for response.

Figure C-2

Check circulation by checking pulse.

4. *Begin cycles of 30 compressions and two breaths.*
- The victim should be on a firm, flat surface facing upward (supine).
- Find the hand position by placing the heel of one hand on the center (middle) of the chest (lower half of the sternum) and the heel of the other hand on top of the first hand. Interlace the fingers and either hold or extend your fingers up off the chest **Figure C-3**.
- Give chest compressions by:
  - Placing your shoulders directly over your hands on the chest
  - Keeping your arms straight and your elbows locked
  - Pushing straight down at least 2″
  - Giving 30 compressions at a rate of at least 100 per minute. Push hard; push fast
  - Allowing chest to recoil completely after each compression
- Open the airway (head tilt–chin lift), and give two normal breaths (1 second each) to make the chest rise **Figure C-4**. If a cervical (neck) spine injury is suspected, open the airway using a jaw thrust without head extension **Figure C-5**. If the jaw thrust method does not adequately open the airway, use the head tilt–chin lift maneuver.
- Give five cycles (2 minutes) of CPR.
- Continue CPR until one of these happens:
  - The victim recovers.
  - An AED becomes available.
  - You are relieved by trained rescuers.
  - You are completely exhausted.

5. *When an AED is available:*
- Turn on the AED.

Figure C-4

Give two breaths.

Figure C-3

Give chest compressions.

Figure C-5

Jaw-thrust method.

- Attach adhesive pads to bare skin on the victim's chest and then attach the cable to the AED (use child pads for children, if available).
- The AED analyzes the victim's heart rhythm (no one should be touching victim).
- If shock is indicated by the AED (no one should be touching the victim), press the shock button.
- Start CPR with chest compressions.
- After five cycles of CPR, analyze the rhythm with the AED.
- If shock is not indicated by the AED:
  - Start CPR with chest compressions.
  - After five cycles of CPR, analyze the rhythm with the AED.

Figure C-6

Bag-mask.

▶ Two-Rescuer CPR for Adults and Children

Having two or more rescuers has two advantages:
- One rescuer can call 9-1-1 and obtain an AED, if available.
- It is less exhausting for the rescuers because one can give chest compressions while the other performs rescue breathing, and they are switching after every five cycles of CPR Table C-1.

- There is less interruption between the compressions and breaths.

If a mask is available, a mouth-to-mask or bag-to-mask method should be used Figure C-6. The rescuer providing breaths should be at the victim's head while the other rescuer, who is giving chest compressions, should be at the victim's side. Ideally, the rescuers should be on opposite sides of the victim to enable a quicker switch.

Table C-1 Two-Health Care Provider Basic Life Support

1. Check for responsiveness.	• Check the scene for hazards. • Tap the victim's shoulder. • Shout, "Are you OK?"
2. If no response, call 9-1-1 and get an AED.	• If you are alone with the victim, shout for help. • If someone responds, send him or her to call 9-1-1 and get an AED. • If no one responds, call 9-1-1 and get an AED, if available.
3. Position the victim facing up on a firm, flat surface.	

4. Check carotid pulse.	• Keep the victim's head tilted with your hand that is nearest the head.
	• Using your hand nearest the victim's feet, locate the Adam's apple (larynx) with two or three fingers.
	• Slide your fingers down into the groove of the neck on the side closest to you (do not use your thumb because you might feel your own pulse).
	• Feel for carotid pulse for 5 to 10 seconds.
	• If there is a pulse:
	  • Give normal breath every 5 to 6 seconds
	  • Each breath lasts 1 second
	  • Use the head tilt–chin lift method
	  • If there is no pulse, begin CPR.

Rescuer 1	Rescuer 2
• Gives 30 chest compressions (15 compressions for a child age 1 to puberty [about 12 to 14 years of age]) while counting out loud.	• Keeps airway open with head tilt–chin lift during compressions.
• Pauses after 30 compressions for two breaths to be given by Rescuer 2.	• Gives two normal breaths (last 1 second each during pause).
• After five cycles of 30 chest compressions/two breaths, reassesses the victim, and if pulse is absent, quickly switches with Rescuer 2.	• Quickly switches with Rescuer 1 after five cycles of 30 compressions.
• Rescuer 1 performs what Rescuer 2 previously did.	• Rescuer 2 performs what Rescuer 1 previously did.
Use AED when it arrives.	

appendix D

FEMA Disaster Supplies Checklists

Table D-1 First Aid Supplies

Supplies	Home	Vehicle	Work
Adhesive bandages, various sizes			
5″ × 9″ sterile dressing			
Conforming roller gauze bandage			
Triangular bandages			
3″ × 3″ sterile gauze pads			
4″ × 4″ sterile gauze pads			
Roll 3″ cohesive bandage			
Germicidal hand wipes or waterless, alcohol-based hand sanitizer			
Antiseptic wipes			
Pairs large, medical grade, non-latex gloves			
Tongue depressor blades			
Adhesive tape, 2″ width			
Antibacterial ointment			
Cold pack			
Scissors (small, personal)			
Tweezers			
Assorted sizes of safety pins			
Cotton balls			
Thermometer			
Tube of petroleum jelly or other lubricant			
Sunscreen			
CPR breathing barrier, such as a face shield			
First aid manual			

Table D-2 Nonprescription and Prescription Medicine Kit Supplies

Supplies	Home	Vehicle	Work
Aspirin and non-aspirin pain reliever			
Antidiarrhea medication			
Antacid (for stomach upset)			
Laxative			
Vitamins			
Prescriptions			
Extra eyeglasses/contact lenses			

Table D-3 Sanitation and Hygiene Supplies

Item		Item	
Washcloth and towel		Heavy-duty plastic garbage bags and ties for personal sanitation uses and toilet paper	
Towelettes, soap, hand sanitizer		Medium-sized plastic bucket with tight lid	
Toothpaste, toothbrushes		Disinfectant and household chlorine bleach	
Shampoo, comb, and brush		A small shovel for digging a latrine	
Deodorants, sunscreen		Toilet paper	
Razor, shaving cream		Contact lens solution	
Lip balm, insect repellent		Mirror	
Feminine supplies			

Table D-4 Equipment and Tools

Tools		Kitchen Items	
Portable, battery-powered radio or television and extra batteries		Manual can opener	
NOAA Weather Radio, if appropriate for your area		Mess kits or paper cups, plates, and plastic utensils	
Flashlight and extra batteries		All-purpose knife	
Signal flare		Household liquid bleach to treat drinking water	
Matches in a waterproof container (or waterproof matches)		Sugar, salt, pepper	
Shut-off wrench, pliers, shovel, and other tools		Aluminum foil and plastic wrap	
Duct tape and scissors		Resealable plastic bags	
Plastic sheeting		Small cooking stove and a can of cooking fuel (if food must be cooked)	
Whistle			
Small canister, ABC-type fire extinguisher		**Comfort Items**	
Tube tent		Games	
Compass		Cards	
Work gloves		Books	
Paper, pens, and pencils		Toys for kids	
Needles and thread		Food	
Battery-operated travel alarm clock			

Table D-5 Food and Water

Supplies	Home	Vehicle	Work
Water			
Ready-to-eat meats, fruits, and vegetables			
Canned or boxed juices, milk, and soup			
High-energy foods such as peanut butter, jelly, low-sodium crackers, granola bars, and trail mix			
Vitamins			
Special foods for infants or persons on special diets			
Cookies, hard candy			
Instant coffee			
Cereals			
Powdered milk			

Table D-6 Clothes and Bedding Supplies

Item	
Complete change of clothes	
Sturdy shoes or boots	
Rain gear	
Hat and gloves	
Extra socks	
Extra underwear	
Thermal underwear	
Sunglasses	
Blankets/sleeping bags and pillows	

Table D-7 Documents and Keys

Item	Stored
Personal identification	
Cash and coins	
Credit cards	
Extra set of house keys and car keys	
Copies of the following:	
Birth certificate	
Marriage certificate	
Driver's license	
Social Security cards	
Passports	
Wills	
Deeds	
Inventory of household goods	
Insurance papers	
Immunization records	
Bank and credit card account numbers	
Stocks and bonds	
Emergency contact list and phone numbers	
Map of the area and phone numbers of places you could go	

answer key

Chapter 7
1. No; 2. Yes; 3. No; 4. No; 5. Yes; 6. Yes; 7. Yes; 8. Yes; 9. Yes; 10. No

Chapter 8
1. No; 2. No; 3. Yes; 4. Yes; 5. Yes; 6. No; 7. Yes; 8. Yes; 9. Yes; 10. No

Chapter 9
1. Yes; 2. No; 3. Yes; 4. Yes; 5. Yes; 6. No; 7. Yes; 8. No; 9. No; 10. Yes

Chapter 10
1. No; 2. Yes; 3. Yes; 4. No; 5. No; 6. Yes; 7. No; 8. No; 9. Yes; 10. Yes

Chapter 11
1. No; 2. No; 3. Yes; 4. No; 5. Yes; 6. Yes; 7. Yes; 8. No; 9. Yes; 10. No

Chapter 12
1. No; 2. No; 3. No; 4. Yes; 5. No; 6. Yes; 7. No; 8. Yes; 9. Yes; 10. No

Chapter 13
1. Yes; 2. Yes; 3. No; 4. No; 5. Yes; 6. Yes; 7. No; 8. Yes; 9. No; 10. Yes

Chapter 14
1. Yes; 2. Yes; 3. Yes; 4. Yes; 5. No; 6. No; 7. No; 8. Yes; 9. No; 10. Yes

Chapter 15
1. Yes; 2. No; 3. Yes; 4. No; 5. No; 6. Yes; 7. Yes; 8. No; 9. No; 10. Yes

Chapter 16
1. Yes; 2. No; 3. Yes; 4. Yes; 5. No; 6. Yes; 7. No; 8. No; 9. Yes; 10. Yes

Chapter 17
1. Yes; 2. Yes; 3. Yes; 4. Yes; 5. Yes; 6. No; 7. Yes; 8. No; 9. Yes; 10. Yes

Chapter 18
1. Yes; 2. No; 3. No; 4. No; 5. No; 6. No; 7. Yes; 8. Yes; 9. Yes; 10. Yes

Chapter 19
1. Yes; 2. No; 3. No; 4. Yes; 5. Yes; 6. Yes; 7. Yes; 8. No; 9. No; 10. Yes

Chapter 20
1. Yes; 2. No; 3. Yes; 4. Yes; 5. Yes; 6. No; 7. No; 8. Yes; 9. Yes; 10. No

Chapter 21
1. Yes; 2. Yes; 3. Yes; 4. Yes; 5. Yes; 6. No; 7. Yes; 8. No; 9. Yes; 10. Yes

Chapter 22
1. Yes; 2. No; 3. No; 4. Yes; 5. No; 6. Yes; 7. Yes; 8. No; 9. Yes; 10. Yes

Chapter 23
1. Yes; 2. Yes; 3. No; 4. Yes; 5. No; 6. No; 7. Yes; 8. No; 9. Yes; 10. No

Chapter 24
1. No; 2. Yes; 3. Yes; 4. No; 5. No; 6. Yes; 7. Yes; 8. No; 9. No; 10. Yes

Chapter 25
1. No; 2. Yes; 3. Yes; 4. Yes; 5. Yes; 6. No; 7. Yes; 8. No; 9. Yes; 10. No

Chapter 26
1. No; 2. No; 3. Yes; 4. No; 5. No; 6. Yes; 7. Yes; 8. No; 9. Yes; 10. No

index

photo credits

Chapter 1
Opener © MANCEAU/age fotostock

Chapter 2
2-1 © AbleStock; **page 18** Courtesy of Lara Shane/FEMA

Chapter 3
Opener © Robert J. Beyers II/ShutterStock, Inc.

Chapter 4
4-1B © Jonathan Noden-Wilkinson/ShutterStock, Inc.; **4-5A-B** Courtesy of the MedicAlert Foundation®. © 2006, All Rights Reserved. MedicAlert® is a federally registered trademark and service mark.

Chapter 5
Opener © Berta A. Daniels, 2010 ; 5-2 © Berta A. Daniels, 2010

Chapter 6
Opener © Berta A. Daniels, 2010; 6-3, 6-4 From *Arrhythmia Recognition: The Art of Interpretation*, courtesy of Tomas B. Garcia, MD.; 6-8 LIFEPAK® 1000 Defibrillator (AED) courtesy of Physio-Control. Used with Permission of Physio-Control, Inc., and according to the Material Release Form provided by Physio-Control.

Chapter 8
Opener © E. M. Singletary, M.D. Used with permission.

Chapter 9
Opener Courtesy of Rhonda Beck; 9-2 © SHOUT/Alamy Images; 9-7 © Dr. P. Marazzi/Photo Researchers, Inc.; 9-8 © Chuck Stewart, MD.; 9-10 © Maximillian Weinzierl/Alamy Images

Chapter 11
Opener © E. M. Singletary, M.D. Used with permission.; 11-1 © Suzanne Tucker/ShutterStock, Inc.; 11-7 © E. M. Singletary, M.D. Used with permission.; 11-10A © Chuck Stewart, MD.

Chapter 12
12-3 © Scott Camazine/Photo Researchers, Inc.; 12-4 Courtesy of Rhonda Beck

Chapter 13
Opener © Piotr Marcinski/ShutterStock, Inc.

Chapter 14
Opener © Medical-on-Line/Alamy Images

Chapter 15
Opener © Corbis/age fotostock

Chapter 17
Opener © Don Hammond/age fotostock

Chapter 18
18-2 Courtesy of the American Association of Poison Control Centers; 18-4 © Doug Menuez/Photodisc/Getty Images; 18-5 Courtesy of DEA; 18-6 © Ben Smith/ShutterStock, Inc.; 18-8 © Thomas Photography LLC/Alamy Images; 18-9 © Thomas J. Peterson/Alamy Images; 18-10 Courtesy of US Fish & Wildlife Service; 18-11 © pinkannjoh/age fotostock

Chapter 19
Opener © Amee Cross/ShutterStock, Inc.; 19-1 © Chuck Stewart, MD.; 19-5 © AbleStock; 19-6 Courtesy of Ray Rauch/U.S. Fish and Wildlife Services; 19-7 Courtesy of South Florida Water Management District; 19-8 © Rolf Nussbaumer/age fotostock; 19-11A © Borut Gorenjak/ShutterStock, Inc.; 19-11B © Dwight Lyman/ShutterStock, Inc.; 19-11C © pixelman/ShutterStock, Inc.; 19-11D © Heintje Joseph T. Lee/ShutterStock, Inc.; 19-12 Courtesy of Scott Bauer/USDA; 19-13 Courtesy of Daniel Wojcik/USDA; 19-15 © photobar/ShutterStock, Inc.; 19-16 Courtesy of Kenneth Cramer, Monmouth College; 19-17 © Nick Simon/ShutterStock, Inc.; 19-18 © David Desoer/ShutterStock, Inc.; 19-20 Courtesy of James Gathany/CDC; 19-22 © AbleStock; 19-23 Courtesy of NOAA; 19-24 © Nir Levy/ShutterStock, Inc.; 19-25 © Roger Dale Calger/ShutterStock, Inc.; 19-26 © AbleStock

Chapter 20
Opener © Sascha Burkard/ShutterStock, Inc.; 20-2 © Simon Price/Alamy Images; 20-3 Courtesy of Neil Malcom Winkelmann

Chapter 21
Opener © Ashley Cooper/Alamy Images

Chapter 23
23-1A, 23-1B, 23-1C Courtesy of Ron Dieckmann, M.D.

Chapter 24
Opener © StockShot/Alamy Images; 24-7 © Riccardo Bastianello/ShutterStock, Inc.; 24-8 © AbleStock; 24-9 Courtesy of Mark Woolcock

Chapter 25
Opener Courtesy of Jocelyn Augustino/FEMA; 25-4, 25-5 Source: U.S. Department of Transportation

Chapter 26
Opener Courtesy of Goddard Space Flight Center/NASA; 26-1 Courtesy of D. Perkins/USGS; 26-2 Courtesy of Jocelyn Augustino/FEMA; 26-4 © Photos.com; 26-5B Courtesy of the National Weather Service Forecast/NOAA; 26-6 Courtesy of John Hutmacher/USFS; 26-7 © Igumnova Irina/ShutterStock, Inc.; 26-9 Courtesy of Andrea Booher/FEMA

Appendix B
Page 448 Courtesy of Dey, L.P.